Digestive System Physiology

Second edition

PAUL A. SANFORD

Associate Professor of Physiology, College of Medicine, King Saud University,
Riyadh, Saudi Arabia. Formerly Senior Lecturer in Physiology,
The Middlesex Hospital Medical School, London

Edward Arnold

A division of Hodder & Stoughton

LONDON   MELBOURNE   AUCKLAND

© 1992 Edward Arnold

First published in Great Britain 1981
First edition 1981
Second edition 1992

For Wooly and 2X

British Library Cataloguing in Publication Data

Sanford, Paul A.
  Digestive System Physiology. – 2Rev. ed. –
  (Physiological Principles in Medicine
  Series)
  I. Title   II. Series
  612.3

  ISBN 0–340–56020–7

Typeset in Caledonia by   Anneset, Weston-super-Mare, Avon.
Printed and bound in Great Britain for Edward Arnold, a division
of Hodder & Stoughton Limited, Mill Road, Dunton Green,
Sevenoaks, Kent TN13 2YA by St. Edmundsbury Press, Bury St.
Edmunds, Suffolk and Hartnolls Ltd., Bodmin, Cornwall

General preface to series

Student textbooks of medicine seek to present the subject of human diseases and their treatment in a manner that is not only informative, but interesting and readily assimilable. It is important, in a field where knowledge advances rapidly, that principles are emphasized rather than details, so that what is contained in the book remains valid for as long as possible.

These considerations favour an approach which concentrates on each disease as a disturbance of normal structure and function. Rational therapy follows logically from a knowledge of the disturbance, and it is in this field where some of the most rapid advances in Medicine have occurred.

A disturbance of normal structure without any disturbance of function may not be important to the patient except for cosmetic or phsychological reasons. Therefore, it is disturbances in function that should be stressed. Preclinical students should aim at a comprehensive understanding of physiological principles so that when they arrive on the wards they will be able to appreciate the significance of disordered function in disease. Clinical students must be presented with descriptions of disease which stress the disturbances in normal physiological functions that are responsible for the symptoms and signs which they find in their patients. All students must be made aware of the growing points in physiology which, even though not immediately applicable to the practice of Medicine, will almost certainly become so during the course of their professional lives.

In this Series, the major physiological systems are each covered by a pair of books, one preclinical and the other clinical, in which the authors have attempted to meet the requirements discussed above. A particular feature is the provision of numerous cross-references between the two members of a pair of books to facilitate the blending of a basic science and clinical expertise that is the goal of this Series. This coordination, which is initiated at the planning stage and continues throughout the writing of each pair of books, is achieved by frequent discussions between the preclinical and clinical authors concerned and between them and the editors of the Series.

MH
KBS
JTF

Preface to the first edition

Sunday is the one day on which I can relax and read newspapers. During the week reviews are not read, crosswords are unfinished and the headlines only glanced at to provide confirmation for the stories heard on radio and television.

On the sports pages of the *Sunday Times* I find the stories of Michael Parkinson. I remember his hatred of golf. With passion he would recall epics of football and cricket, but he looked upon golf as nothing more than an elaborate means of spoiling a Sunday morning walk. This reminded me of a famous physiologist who regarded the gastrointestinal tract as a sophisticated way of producing manure. I hope to force the reader to the conclusion that, even though the gastriontestinal tract produces that material which is so valuable to plant growth, it is something more.

I was apprehensive when invited to write a prelinical text on gastroenterology. However, the concept of pairs of books was appealing. I was being given the opportunity to provide students with an essential scientific background. This chance I accepted. In addition, without diluting the physiological content, I have tried to whet the preclinical students' appetites by frequently referring to clinical situations. Furthermore, by working closely with Michael Hobsley I have been able to guide interested readers to relevant chapters in his clinical text. I hope that clinical students also find the book useful. Thus, when a particular malfunction is being considered, they can rediscover the basis of the functions of normal tissue. With such a knowledge many diseases are understandable alterations of normal function and therapy becomes an easier problem.

Having written this book I hope that students will *enjoy* it. Not only those in medical schools but also the many who are studying for scientific qualifications. Some, no doubt, will find it an irritating text. I do myself in some sections. I use the word 'may' on perhaps too many occasions because I have tried not to present a clear-cut but false picture. Others will criticize my allotment of space to different subjects. I make no apology. Rather I would ask that those stimulated to make the criticism should use the bibliographies to extend their coverage. If I have caused students to make use of other texts because they find my subject interesting, then I shall have been at least partially successful.

A comment on bibliographies

I hope that readers will not be discouraged either when they see the bibliographies at the end of the chapters, or when, from time to time, they come across the names of prominent workers in the text. I must emphasize that it is *not* essential to read the bibliographies. I am fully aware that most students have little time for extra reading. Nevertheless, if the subject is stimulating, an odd hour or two can be found. The lists provide a guide to some of the papers I have found useful in increasing my understanding of the subject.

I anticipate that only a few of the workers mentioned in the text will be remembered. Several are included because they were the pioneers in gastro-enterology and it would be a pity if I did not make the students aware of some of the contributions of those such as Pavlov, Cannon and Bayliss and Starling. Many of the others mentioned remain extremely active. If readers are interested in discovering the current concepts in this still rapidly expanding subject, one approach would be to search the literature for the views of these active researchers. However, I have to admit that some of those involved in recent studies in gastroenterology are not to be found in this text. These include a number for whom I have the greatest respect. I hope they will not be offended by the omission.

PAS

London 1981

Preface to the second edition

I wonder how many authors have introduced new editions of their books with the statement, 'Considerable advances have been made in recent years . . .' or words to that effect? Certainly, I was tempted to do so. A decade has passed since the original publication during which new concepts have appeared and old ones considerably altered. It is easier now to envisage at least some of the many transport processes in secretion and absorption that exist along the gastrointestinal tract. More is known of the mechanisms by which they are controlled. Even motility is becoming clearer, emerging from the morass those working in the field feared had been created. Nevertheless, many questions remain unanswered.

One subject which has evolved at an alarming rate is that of the peptides regulating gastrointestinal functions. The number of such substances discovered in the gastrointestinal tract continues to grow. Some peptides are released from endocrine-like cells and exert their effects either locally (paracrine) and/or in the classical way, at more distant sites. Others are detected in nerve endings. These are regarded as neurotransmitters or factors modulating neurotransmitter release. The situation is complicated not least by the finding that many nerves are capable of releasing several potentially active agents. Interestingly, some peptides can be detected in both nerve fibres and in endocrine-like cells. Their functions may not be identical when released from different sites.

Furthermore, many of the peptides present in the gut are also found in the brain. This serves as a useful reminder that many of the gastrointestinal processes are controlled by local mechanisms and are relatively independent of the central nervous system. (Indeed some have asked whether the gastrointestinal tract should be regarded as a 'brain' or 'higher centre'.)

Those who would like to establish how far 'behind the times' the author is when they read this book should, perhaps, be directed to a number of publications which provide excellent 'up-to-date' coverage of gastrointestinal functions. They will find 'Current Opinion in Gastroenterology' (Current Science, Philadelphia, USA) a valuable journal in which recent advances are reviewed and evaluated. A survey of the world literature is also provided. An eye might be kept on the 'Annual Review of Physiology' (Annual Reviews, Palo Alto, USA) in which a section is devoted to gastrointestinal physiology. Three research journals also frequently publish well-written and informative reviews. These are 'Gut' (British Medical Association, London), 'Gastroenterology' (Elsevier Science, New York) and the 'American Journal of Physiology' (American Physiological Society, Bethesda, MD, USA).

Riyadh 1992   PAS

Contents

1

Food intake and its control

Before studying the many and complex processes occurring along the gastrointestinal (GI) tract it is worth considering which substances are part of our diet. To what is the GI tract exposed? How much food is ingested and what controls food intake? Furthermore, it is important to recognize that it is not only ingested substances that must be handled by the GI tract. At least 8 litres of fluid are secreted each day as saliva, bile and gastric, pancreatic and intestinal juices. These fluids contain a variety of organic and inorganic constituents which must be absorbed and further utilized.

Approximately forty substances, some of which are seen in Table 1.1, are

Table 1.1 Suggested daily intakes of energy and some nutrients for sedentary young adult males

Energy 10–11 MJ	Thiamin 1.0 mg
Protein 60–65 g	Vitamin A 750 μg
Calcium 500 mg	Riboflavin 1.6 mg
Iron 10 mg	Ascorbic acid 30 mg
Vitamin D 0 μg	

Notes
1. There are huge differences in the recommended intakes of these dietary components. Thus it is suggested that man eats grams of protein, milligrams of iron and ascorbic acid but only micrograms of vitamin A (retinol equivalents) and vitamin D. As vitamin D results from the action of ultraviolet light on the skin dietary sources may not be essential for adults exposed adequately to sunlight. However, housebound individuals may need a 10 μg supplement daily.
2. Even with a particular group of the population the suggested intakes vary depending on the activities of the individuals. For example 33 per cent more energy and protein are suggested in the diet of the very active as compared with the sedentary adult male.
3. Large differences can be seen in the recommended intakes of dietary factors for different groups of the population. Thus a 20 per cent greater intake of iron than above may be insufficient for women with large menstrual losses. Also 140 per cent more calcium in the diet is regarded as necessary during lactation.

The Department of Health and Social Security published their Report on Health and Social Subjects 15 (1979), 2nd impression (1981), in which the requirements of various groups of people in the United Kingdom were considered.

considered essential for proper development and resistance to disease. The water and energy needs of the body are the first priority. If these are not met breakdown in function will occur. The total energy needs of the body are known. However, these are not constant and depend, for example, on the occupation of the individual. The proportion of the energy requirement supplied by carbohydrate, fat and protein, the major energy sources, also varies. In some countries energy intake is governed by personal choice. In others less fortunate the availability of energy rich foods is the controlling factor. Many subjects appear in good health on diets of very different composition.

Carbohydrates

Carbohydrates provide most energy in nearly all human diets, varying from as little as 40 per cent of the total in many rich countries to 90 per cent in some poor regions.

Monosaccharides

The simplest carbohydrates are the monosaccharides with 3–6 carbon atoms per molecule (Table 1.2). Several hexoses (6 carbons) and pentoses (5 carbons) are present in the diet either free or in combined forms.

Hexoses and their derivatives

Glucose is the only sugar detected in a free state in fasting man. Traces are found in some fruits, e.g. grapes. However, it is widely distributed in the combined form as starch, glycogen and several disaccharides, e.g. lactose and sucrose.

Fructose occurs in honey and some fruits but is ingested more regularly combined with glucose as the disaccharide sucrose. Galactose and mannose do not appear in the free form. They are found, however, in combined forms, e.g. glucose combined with galactose produces the disaccharide lactose.

Sorbitol is an interesting hexose derivative. It is found in the rowan berry and produced commercially from glucose by converting its aldehyde ($-CHO$) group of alcohol ($-CH_2OH$). It is absorbed slowly but almost completely (90 per cent) from the GI tract. The sugar alcohol is useful in 'diabetic foods' because it is 60 per cent as sweet as sucrose, has little effect on blood glucose levels and can be metabolized to provide energy.

Pentoses

Pentoses are not important energy sources. Nevertheless, derivatives of ribose and 2–deoxyribose are present in all cells as essential components of nucleic acids and high energy phosphate compounds, e.g. ATP. These pentoses are not essential in the diet. They can be synthesized.

Di- and trisaccharides

Several di– and trisaccharides pass down the GI tract. These include sucrose, maltose, lactose and raffinose. The first is commonly found on the dining

Table 1.2 Some monosaccharides found in free or combined form, and disaccharides of diet

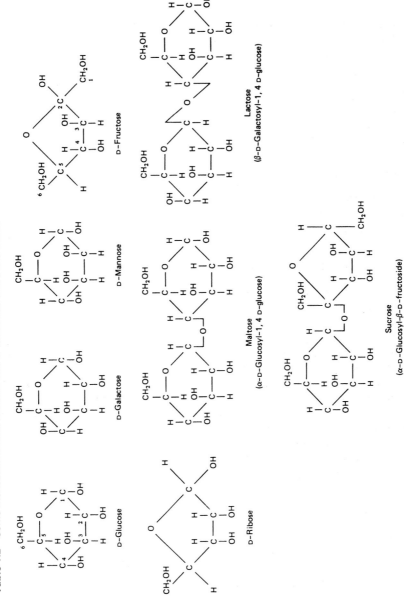

table. It is the product of one molecule of glucose combining with one of the fructose and can be manufactured from cane sugar and sugar beet. Maltose is composed of two glucose units and is formed in the breakdown of starch in the malting of barley. The third disaccharide, lactose, is a sugar unique to mammals and present as the principal sugar of milk. An example of the trisaccharides is to be found in molasses. This is raffinose, resulting from the combination of glucose, fructose and galactose.

Polysaccharides

Starch

This utilizable carbohydrate is stored in granules in seeds and roots of many plants. It consists of two polymers, amylose and amylopectin. The former constitutes 15–20 per cent of the total and consists of long unbranched chains of several hundred glucose units. The major component is amylopectin, a glucose polymer with branching chains. Starch grains are completely insoluble in water. However, moist heat causes them to swell and become more soluble.

Glycogen

This polymer is the animal equivalent to starch. It is made up of 3000 to 60 000 glucose units with branching chains of 12–18 units. The richest sources are animal livers and shellfish.

Cellulose

The fibre supporting plants is mainly cellulose. This carbohydrate is made up of 3000 or more glucose units linked in a different way from those of starch. The result is that cellulose is resistant to hydrolysis by enzymes secreted into the GI tract. Thus glucose is not available to provide energy. Cellulose and other complex carbohydrates present in plant cell walls are, however, far from useless. They provide bulk for intestinal peristalsis. Some suggest that a high roughage diet may decrease the incidence of large bowel malignancies (*see* Chapter 6).

Fats

Fats are not necessary dietary components in man except for relatively small amounts of essential polyunsaturated fatty acids. Nevertheless, they perform several valuable functions. They:

1. Have a high energy content and therefore reduce the dietary bulk.
2. Slow gastric emptying, and as a result they have a high satiety value.
3. Improve the palatability of food and aid swallowing by providing lubrication.
4. Make available a wider range of cooking methods, and thus provide variety.
5. Provide essential fatty acids and fat soluble vitamins, A, D, E and K.

Fats are also incorporated into many essential structures. Their separation by the distinguished French physiologist, Térroine, into 'l'element constant' (structural) and 'l'element variable' (fuel) illustrates this point. Most accept that fats should form 20–25 per cent of the dietary energy intake. In the UK, fats constitute 42 per cent of this intake. Approximately 30 per cent is derived from visible fat, e.g. butter and cooking fats. The remainder is obtained from foods.

Triglycerides

Quantitatively the most important fats are the tryglycerides (Table 1.3). These are esters of the trihydric alcohol glycerol and fatty acids. Over forty fatty acids are found in nature, and each glycerol unit normally carries three different acids. The acids present in the triglycerides vary with their source. Thus, freshwater plants and animals contain predominantly unsaturated C16, 18, 20 and 22 fatty acids, palmitic acid being the only saturated acid and constituting 10–18 per cent of the total fatty acids. Unsaturated C20 and C22 fatty acids are found in the marine world, while on land oleic acid (unsaturated) and palmitic acid (saturated) predominate.

Phospholipids

The phospholipids cover a variety of substances derived from α-glycerophosphate and combined with fatty acids and nitrogen containing alcohols, e.g. choline, serine or ethanolamine. They include the structurally important lecithins incorporated into all membranes.

Sterols

These are important and widely distributed. They have the same basic ring structure. This group includes (a) cholesterol found in all foods of animal origin, particularly in eggs; and (b) bile salts, which play an essential role in the digestion of fat.

The vital requirement of fat in the diet was established in 1929 when Burr and Burr maintained rats on fat-free diets. Such animals failed to grow and developed eczematous skin conditions. The essential components, the polyunsaturated fatty acids, play a major role in the synthesis of protaglandins regarded as vital in the control of many cellular processes. Probably, arachidonic acid is the physiologically active component in the diet. However, man needs only perhaps 1 g per day, an amount supplied by the poorest of diets.

Proteins

Proteins are dietary sources of energy but as such are less important than fats and carbohydrate. Approximately 30 g body protein are broken down daily and used to provide energy. This must be replaced. Dietary proteins provide the cells with the 'building materials' for doing this.

Under the heading of proteins are many large molecules with different

Table 1.3   Constituents of fat

Triglycerides

$$
\begin{array}{ccccccc}
CH_2OH & & R^1COOH & & CH_2. & O. & CO. & R^1 \\
|\ & & & & |\ & & & \\
CHOH & + & R^2COOH & \longrightarrow & CH. & O. & CO. & R^2 \\
|\ & & & & |\ & & & \\
CH_2OH & & R^3COOH & & CH_2. & O. & CO. & R^3
\end{array}
$$

Glycerol   Fatty acids   Triglyceride

Saturated fatty acids — general formula is $CH_3.(CH_2)_n.COOH$ where n = even no. from 2-24.

Commonest are	lauric (n = 10)
	myristic (n = 12)
Widely distributed	palmitic (n = 14)
	stearic (n = 16)

Unsaturated fatty acids — with one or more double bonds.

One double bond, e.g. oleic acid (18 C atoms) — forms 30% or more total fatty acids
                                                                  of most fats.
Two double bonds, e.g. linoleic acid (18 C atoms)
Three double bonds, e.g. linolenic acid (18 C atoms)
                         eicosatrienic acid (20 C atoms)
Four double bonds, e.g. arachidonic acid (20 C atoms)

Phospholipid components (in addition to fatty acids)

$$
\begin{array}{l}
CH_2OH \\
|\ \\
CHOH \quad OH \\
|\ \quad\ \ / \\
CH_2{-}O{-}P{=}O \\
\qquad\quad \backslash \\
\qquad\qquad OH
\end{array}
$$

Glycerophosphate

$H_2N{-}CH_2{-}CH_2{-}OH$

Ethanolamine

$$
\begin{array}{l}
CH_2{-}OH \\
|\ \\
CH_2 \\
|\ \quad CH_3 \\
|\ \ / \\
N{-}CH_3 \\
|\ \ \backslash \\
|\ \quad CH_3 \\
OH
\end{array}
$$

Choline

$$
\begin{array}{l}
CH_2{-}OH \\
|\ \\
H{-}C{-}NH_2 \\
|\ \\
COOH
\end{array}
$$

Serine

e.g. egg yolk lecithin

$$
\begin{array}{l}
CH_2{-}O{-}(\text{stearic acid}) \\
|\ \\
CH{-}O{-}(\text{oleic acid}) \\
|\ \\
CH_2{-}O{-}(\text{phosphate}){-}(\text{choline})
\end{array}
$$

Table 1.3   cont.

Sterol cholesterol

permutations of the same amino acids (Table 1.4). There are two types of amino acid, those that can by synthesized (non-essential) and those that cannot be produced at a rate commensurate with the needs of the body (essential).

In man, eight amino acids are essential – with arginine and histidine also required by children. Dietary proteins may differ from human tissue proteins in their composition. The quality of dietary protein must be considered, therefore, before a daily requirement can be suggested, as the body will be unable to synthesize tissue protein or to retain amino acids from protein with an essential amino acid missing. The term 'biological value' of protein has been introduced to describe the quality of protein with gradings from 100 (e.g. egg), where all amino acids can be completely utilized, to zero, where one essential amino acid is absent. The system, though useful, provides no information as regards the value of mixed dietary proteins. Thus two dietary proteins, each with a different essential amino acid missing may form a useful dietary source, e.g. maize and milk. In maize the lysine content is limited, although plentiful in milk. However, the methionine content of milk protein is low but can be supplemented by maize, which is relatively rich in methionine. The improvement of the biological value of protein is called complementation. The dietary sources of protein may at first sight be surprising. The obvious sources such as cheese, fish and eggs, contribute only 5 per cent of the intake. Much greater proportions are derived from foods commonly considered to be carbohydrate energy sources, e.g. bread, flour and cereals (28 per cent). These values reflect the relative amounts of the different foodstuffs eaten.

Water and mineral salts

Water

Water is the most important dietary constituent. While many can tolerate 30 days' starvation without apparent ill effects, the survival time is considerably

Table 1.4   Principal amino acids

Amino acid	Abbreviation	R

α-amino acid structure

$$R-\underset{\underset{NH_2}{|}}{\overset{\overset{H}{|}}{C}}-COOH$$

where −COOH = carboxyl group → acidic properties

−NH$_2$ = amine group → basic properties

R = variable

Amino acid	Abbreviation	R
Glycine	Gly	H−
Alanine	Ala	CH_3-
Valine*	Val	$(CH_3)_2.CH-$
Leucine*	Leu	$(CH_3)_2.CH.CH_2-$
Isoleucine*	Ile	$C_2H_5CH(CH_3)-$
Serine	Ser	CH_2OH-
Threonine*	Thr	$CH_3.CH(OH)-$
Aspartic acid	Asp	$HOOC.CH_2-$
Glutamic acid	Glu	$HOOC.CH_2.CH_2-$
Lysine*	Lys	$H_2N.(CH_2)_4-$
Ornithine	Orn	$H_2N.(CH_2)_3-$
Arginine[+]	Arg	

Arginine R group:

$$\underset{HN}{\overset{H_2N}{>}}C-NH-(CH_2)_3-$$

Histidine[+]   His

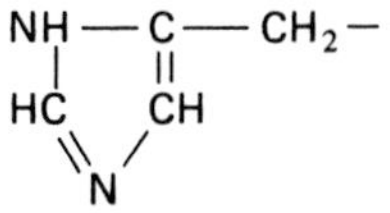

$$NH-\underset{HC}{\overset{|}{C}}\underset{\underset{N}{\diagdown\diagup}}{\overset{\|}{\underset{CH}{C}}}-CH_2-$$

Phenylalanine*   Phe

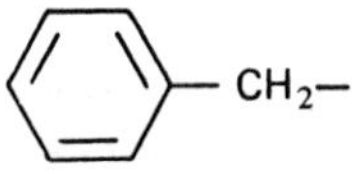

Tyrosine   Tyr

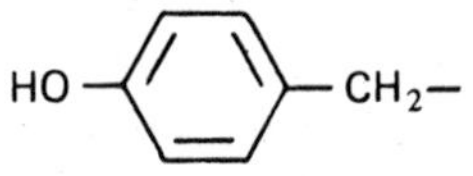

Tryptophan*   Trp

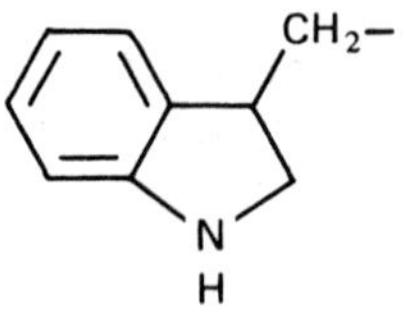

Table 1.4 cont.

Amino acid	Abbreviation	R
Cysteine	Cys	$HS-CH_2-$
Methionine*	Met	$CH_3-S-(CH_2)_2-$
Proline	Pro	Formula not simply R
Hydroxyproline	Hyp	

*Essential amino acids; [+]essential amino acids additionally required by children.

shorter if water is unavailable. Death may occur within 2–3 days under extremes of climate, although survival for 18 days has been recorded where temperature and humidity were moderate. Approximately 70 per cent of body weight is water and this proportion remains constant, losses and gains being balanced. Water is obtained from three sources. Approximately 500 ml per day is derived from cellular oxidation processes. This component is small in relation to man's needs, although some species can subsist indefinitely on it, e.g. the desert Kangaroo rat. The greater proportion of man's water intake is derived from fluids and the water content of food eaten. All food contains some water, fruits such as the orange and peach having a moisture content of 75–90 per cent. However usually man's intake is a function of his social habits and greater than his body's requirements.

Sodium

The major cation of extracellular fluid is sodium and its depletion is associated with dehydration in which the blood volume is reduced and the haematocrit increased. The characteristic symptom of sodium depletion is muscular cramp, well known to miners who replace salt-containing sweat with water or other low salt, but socially more acceptable, beverages. The normal dietary sodium intake is in the range of 70 – 350 mmol. This is greatly in excess of the minimal requirement (20 mmol), unless sweating occurs. In general, foods are low in sodium content, but in processing and preserving many are salted, e.g. butter and bacon.

Potassium

Potassium is the major intracellular cation and is present normally in low concentrations in extracellular fluid (5 mmol/l). Potassium deficiencies are difficult to detect, particularly as plasma potassium may be elevated if tissues are breaking down. The chief features of potasssium deficiency are muscular weakness (e.g. cardiac) and mental confusion. The potassium content of food is very variable (moderate sources are nuts, fruit and beef) and the dietary intake is about 65 mmol/day. However, deficiency is rarely a result primarily of dietary problems but may result from (a) adrenal tumours which lead to large urinary potassium losses, and (b) the diarrhoea of protein malnutrition (kwashiorkor).

Iron

Iron is a component of haemoglobin, myoglobin, cytochromes and several enzymes, e.g. cytochrome oxidase. The iron content of the adult is 3–4 g of which 1 g can be stored as ferritin in the liver, spleen and bone marrow. Daily losses amount to 0.5–1 mg, mainly in faeces. This component is derived from bile and cells lining the intestine. A further variable loss occurs in sweat, urine and hair. An additional 0.5–1 mg per day is lost during menstruation. A good diet contains 10–15 mg iron per day. This, obviously, is very much greater than the normal loss, indicating that absorption is by no means complete (see page 177). In the UK, cereals supply the largest proportion of the iron intake (35 per cent), mainly because flour is enriched to contain 1.65 mg/100 g. Meat (28 per cent) and vegetables (18 per cent) are also useful sources, the richest of the latter being the potato. In addition to providing iron, this extremely useful tuber is a major course of ascorbic acid, and contributes 15 per cent and 8 per cent of thiamine and niacin intake respectively.

Calcium and phosphate

These components form the greater part of bone structure and teeth. The serum contains 9–11 mg/100 ml calcium, of which about half is ionized, and most of the remainder is bound to albumin. A fall of $[Ca^{++}]$ leads to tetany because of an increased sensitivity of motor nerves. As with iron, only a fraction of the dietary intake is available. Absorption is reduced by soluble oxalates (rich sources are spinach and rhubarb) which precipitate the cation. Phytic acid, found in bran of cereals, can combine with six molecules of calcium to produce an insoluble complex. However, this is not as serious a problem as was once thought. Wheat contains phytase which releases the calcium. Less of this enzyme is available in oats (e.g. porridge), which led some to suggest that those in the northern parts of the UK might be calcium deficient and likely to suffer from deformations of their lower limbs. It now seems that the GI tract can adapt, at least partially, to provide an enzyme so that calcium is released and can be absorbed.

Vitamins

The vitamins are organic substances which are not synthesized adequately by the body, yet are essential in small catalytic amounts for the proper functioning of cells. The quantities required vary from 1 μg/day for vitamin B_{12} to 30 mg/day for vitamin C. Many of the compounds listed in Table 1.5 have

Table 1.5 The physiological actions of vitamins, their dietary sources and the symptoms and diseases associated with their deficiency

Vitamin	Physiological actions	Dietary sources	Symptoms of deficiency and diseases
A or retinol (β-carotene, widely distributed in plants, can form retinol)	1. Essential for vision in dim light. A retinol metabolite is a vital component of visual purple (rhodopsin) 2. Involved in maintenance of epithelial surfaces 3. Development of skeleton including skull and vertebral column	Fish liver oils (richest natural sources); green vegetables (cabbage and lettuce), red fruits and vegetables (carrots); also butter, cheese and eggs	Night blindness; squamous metaplasia of epithelia; cells become flattened and heaped; damage to brain and spinal cord
D D$_3$ (cholecalciferol) D$_2$ (ergocalciferol) (formed by exposing ergosterol, a fungal sterol, to UV light)	1. Essential for bone formation 2. Promotes the absorption of calcium and phosphate by the small intestine 3. Promotes phosphate absorption by the kidney	Fish liver oils (many obtain vitamin by action of UV light on 7-dehydrocholesterol in stratum granulosum of skin)	Rickets Softened and deformed bones
K	1. Formation of prothrombin in liver 2. Regulation of synthesis of clotting factors VII, IX and X	Fresh green leafy vegetables (broccoli, cabbage, spinach) NB Many diets are K deficient, **but** large bowel bacteria (e.g. *Esch. coli*) can synthesize the vitamin	Deficiency due to malabsorption leads to spontaneous or excessive bleeding Deficient blood coagulation in newborn with sterile intestine
E (the tocopherols)	It may prevent cell damage, e.g. the destructive oxidation of polyunsaturated fatty acids in cell membranes	Vegetable oils, e.g. wheat germ and sunflower seed	Dietary deficiency thought unlikely: in animal studies (rats) muscles weaken, fetuses die *in utero*, and males become sterile

C or ascorbic acid	Necessary for the formation of intercellular ground substance that binds cell in bone, teeth and connective tissue C contributes to hydroxyproline formation; this amino acid forms 13% of collagen, a component of ground substance	Citrus fruits, currants. NB A regular ration of citrus fruits on RN boats to prevent scurvy earned the British sailor the nickname 'limey'	Scurvy
B_1 or thiamin	The pyrophosphate (thiamin) is the carboxylase coenzyme. The enzyme is involved in the decarboxylation of pyruvic acid (i.e. in carbohydrate breakdown). Those cells having a specific requirement for glucose will be susceptible to B_1 lack, e.g. brain	Seeds of plants, e.g. the germ of cereals, nuts, peas and beans; also yeast	Mental changes resembling anxiety states
Nicotinic acid (niacin) and its amine nicotinamide	This is a component of the coenzymes NAD and NADP; these are concerned with tissue oxidation	Meat, fish and wholemeal cereals. NB Man can synthesize nicotinic acid from tryptophan	Pellagra
Riboflavin	Necessary for normal growth. Riboflavin is a component of active flavoproteins capable of reversible oxidation—reduction reactions	Liver, milk, eggs and green vegetables	A great variety of lesions, e.g. dermatitis, hair loss and conjunctivitis
B_{12} (the cobalamins)	1. Necessary for DNA formation (the nucleotide of thymine). Hence those cells dividing rapidly are the ones most affected, e.g. bone marrow and GI tract 2. Maintenance of myelin in the nervous system	Liver	Megaloblastic anaemia (pernicious)

Folic acid and related substances	Important for the transfer of one-carbon units. It receives one-carbon radicals from glycine, tryptophan etc. and can donate them in the synthesis of purines and pyrimidines	Liver (ox), oysters, spinach and orange juice	Megaloblastic anaemia
B_6 — pyridoxine and related compounds	1. Important as part of the enzyme system involved in porphyrin synthesis (including haemoglobin) 2. Valuable in nicotinic acid formation from tryptophan	Widely distributed. Rich sources are liver, meat and bran	No distinctive features of deficiency. However, rare cases of hypochromic anaemia not responding to iron therapy may reflect a deficiency of haemoglobin synthesis due to B_6 lack
Pantothenic acid	A constituent of coenzyme A and present in all living matter	Widely distributed, e.g. liver, kidney, egg yolk and yeast	Deficiency unlikely in man. In rats growth failure and greying of hair recorded. In chicks dermatitis is typical
Biotin	Forms part of several enzyme systems, e.g. (a) incorporation of CO_2 from HCO_3^- into pathway of fatty acid synthesis, (b) formation of oxaloacetate from pyruvate (important in glucose formation from pyruvate)	Liver, kidney and yeast. Large bowel bacteria can synthesize biotin	Dermatitis in individuals feeding on raw eggs. Eggs contain avidin, a protein which renders the vitamin unavailable

few similarities and their previous classification into water- and lipid-soluble vitamins is useful only to indicate those that would be lost if fat digestion was abnormal.

Preparation and preservation of food

An analysis of uncooked or 'natural' food can be misleading. During preparation and in many processes used in preserving, several components are modified. This results in both losses and gains of valuable substances. Thus heat inactivates enzymes which would otherwise break down useful nutrients and also releases substances which would have been unavailable, e.g. niacin in cereals, is released from complexes by heat under alkaline conditions. In contrast, however, heat destroys some protein and vitamins, e.g. B_1 and C. Nevertheless, most nutrients are extremely stable.

The major losses in processing are caused by the leaching out of water-soluble vitamins and minerals during washing and blanching. Proteins may be modified in two ways: (1) by amino acid destruction, and (2) by formation of linkages between – NH_2 groups of amino acids and reducing groups of other foodstuffs (the Maillard reaction). The latter changes are often desirable, e.g. in providing flavouring and colouring to biscuits and meat extracts.

Control of food intake

In many areas of physiology the mechanisms by which processes are controlled are incompletely defined. This could certainly be said for the control of food intake. By asking the following questions students should find it easier to understand what is known about a particular mechanism and appreciate in which areas progress remains to be made.

1. What factors stimulate or inhibit it?
2. What and where are the receptors which recognize the various stimulatory and inhibitory factors?
3. How is information dispatched from these receptors to the 'centres' controlling the physiological event?
4. Where are these 'centres'? Remember that they are not always found in (a) the brain and spinal cord or (b) discrete, well-defined areas.
5. Is anything known as regards the functioning of these 'centres' or must they be described as 'black boxes'?
6. How are instructions delivered from these 'centres' to modify individual processes?
7. How do the 'centres' modify specific physiological processes?

Centres concerned with food intake.

An important role for the hypothalamus is well established. Almost 40 years ago Anand and Brobeck reported that the destruction of a small well localized area of the lateral hypothalamus (LH) in rats was followed by the complete absence of spontaneous eating. This area was tentatively called the feeding centre (Fig. 1.1). None of the animals ate any food during the entire period of

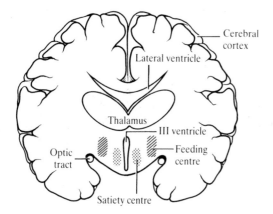

Cerebral cortex

Lateral ventricle

Thalamus

III ventricle

Optic tract

Feeding centre

Satiety centre

Fig. 1.1 Diagrammatic representation of the brain showing the hypothalamic feeding and satiety centres

their postoperative survival even when food was placed near them or inside their mouths. In contrast bilateral lesions involving the ventromedial hypothalamus (VMH), or the regions between it and the LH, induced hyperphagia and obesity.

The ventromedial nuclei were described as satiety centres and thought to exhibit an inhibitory control over the 'feeding centres'. This concept of two centres controlling food intake became well accepted. Indeed some of those who assimilate the world's literary classics and analyse the characters found there suggest that Joe, the obese boy introduced by Charles Dickens in *Pickwick Papers*, may have had a small benign tumour pressing on and slowly destroying his satiety centre.

More recently it has been recommended that the LH and VMH should no longer be regarded as the sites of feeding and satiety centres. It is suggested that the hypothalamus is a part of a more complex system involving many other cerebral structures, especially the limbic system, for the control of food intake.

The concept of areas being involved in either hunger or satiety is, however, extremely useful. The question remains as to when hunger is experienced and when is there no urgency to take food. Hunger is associated with the postabsorptive state when the body energy stores are being mobilized. In contrast satiety is linked with the postprandial state when excess energy sources are stored and metabolism is satisfied by energy derived from the nutrients recently absorbed. In some way the body recognizes the change from energy storage to energy mobilization. The question is how? One possibility is that hunger is the result of a decrease in cellular metabolism. Nicolaidis and Even (1985) have reported that the onset of eating is preceded by a reduction in the 'metabolisme de fond' (MF or basal metabolism). This was measured in animals as the total metabolism less the metabolic costs of locomotion. As the animals took food the MF increased. When it reached a peak value the feeding process was terminated. These observations led to the ischymetric hypothesis (from the Greek ischys = power) in which hunger and satiety are said to be dependent on the intensity of cell power production.

Factors stimulating or inhibiting hunger and satiety.

Some believe that there may not be specific hunger stimuli and that hunger may be the result of the removal of satiety signals. If this is so what are the satiety signals? Many of them occur before absorption has taken place as the result of food present in the gastrointestinal tract. The most potent signal is thought to be gastric distension which results in the activation of mechanoreceptors and an increased activity of vagal afferent fibres from the stomach to the CNS. Indeed the fact that nutrients in the small intestine can induce early satiety may be explained by the slowing of gastric emptying and the maintenance of a degree of gastric distension.

How could the luminal contents of the small intestine achieve this? One suggestion is that nutrients may act by releasing cholecystokinin (CCK) from the intestinal wall. This hormone has an important role to play in the control of gall-bladder contractions and the secretion of pancreatic enzymes. However, recently another function of CCK has emerged. CCK has been found to be:

1. Exclusively localized at sites in the circular smooth muscle.
2. Capable of contracting the pyloric sphincter.
3. Capable of increasing the pressure of the pyloric canal.

Thus CCK may slow gastric emptying and contribute to satiety (Fig. 1.2).

Such mechanisms may partly explain the observations of N.W. Read and his colleagues (1988). They administered lipid (a 50 per cent corn oil emulsion) either intrajejunally or intraileally to human volunteers. Subsequently these subjects were offered a previously selected and enjoyable meal. It was found that the lipid infusions resulted in less food being eaten than when lipid was not introduced into the small intestine. Furthermore the meal was taken by choice for a shorter time. However, not only a reduction in gastric emptying and therefore greater gastric distension was induced by intrajejunal lipid infusions. Sensations of hunger and rates of food ingestion were also reduced. This suggests a more direct effect of intrajejunal lipid on satiety.

The knowledge that gastric distension is an important satiety signal has been used in attempts to reduce, temporarily at least, the weight of obese

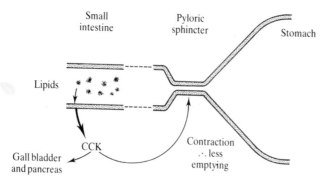

Fig. 1.2 By reducing gastric emptying CCK may maintain gastric distension and contribute to satiety

subjects. Thus Ramhamadany, Fowler and Baird (1989) recently reported their observations with 24 obese women. Acid resistant thermoplastic balloons were introduced into the stomachs of half of these and subsequently inflated with 400 ml. of air. The remaining women were given a sham procedure. None of the subjects were told whether an inflated balloon was inserted. All of them were advised to take 800 Calories (3.34 MJ) per day. A significantly greater weight loss was recorded in those receiving the balloons. It was concluded that balloons offered a safe and effective method of losing weight in well motivated obese subjects.

Clearly as food is released from the stomach the distension stimulus will be lost. The rate at which gastric emptying proceeds depends on the chemical composition of the chyme which enters the duodenum and the physical nature of the gastric contents. As nutrients are absorbed from the intestines and insulin is released from the pancreas hepatic metabolism is shifted from mobilization and the provision of energy to storage. This change results in an important second satiety signal (Fig. 1.3) which can be maintained until the intestines have been emptied. At this time the major satiety signals will have disappeared, calories must again be mobilized and hunger is experienced. Several questions should be asked:

1. How might satiety be produced when liver metabolism is altered?
2. Can nutrients act at sites other than the liver and contribute to satiety?
3. Is insulin a satiety hormone?

How might satiety be produced when liver metabolism is altered?

It appears that there is a reduced discharge in afferent fibres in the vagus when glucose is readily available from the small intestine. In this situation innervated hepatocytes alter their activity. Thus the CNS receives less input

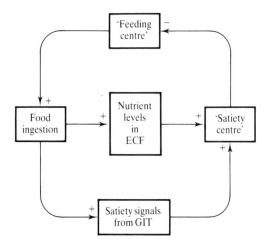

Fig. 1.3 A concept of food intake and its control. Food ingestion results from the loss of satiety signals from the gastrointestinal tract (GIT) and extracellular fluid (ECF)

from the hepatic vagus when a 5 per cent glucose solution is introduced into the duodenum and the hepatic portal glucose concentration rises.

Can nutrients act at sites other than the liver and contribute to satiety?

An attractive possible site clearly is the brain. Many have looked for a direct effect of nutrients on the hypothalamus. At first it was thought that low blood glucose levels might be recognized and associated with hunger. However, this concept could not be supported by the observations from subjects with diabetes mellitus where blood sugar concentrations and food intake are not inversely related. Then in 1953 Meyer proposed that it was not blood glucose concentrations that were detected but the availability of glucose to the tissues (the glucostatic hypothesis) (Fig. 1.4). It was suggested that satiety was maintained if glucose is utilized by cells of the VMH. Conversely hunger is experienced with decreased glucose availability. It was assumed that the hypothalamic cells required insulin in the same way as muscle cells.

Though rejected in its original form the glucostatic hypothesis introduces the concept that food intake is the result of the lack of a specific nutrient. It is thought that such mechanisms may well exist but do not contribute to the normal control of food intake. The stimuli necessary to activate them are believed to be produced only when there is a metabolic emergency.

Is insulin a satiety hormone?

Rather than describing it as a satiety hormone insulin should be regarded as a factor which promotes satiety by altering metabolism so that ingested carbohydrates can be utilized and stored. It should also be remembered that insulin release may be triggered, and perhaps contribute to satiety, before absorption occurs.

There is evidence that both oral and intestinal stimuli can modify insulin release. When rats were offered and ingested glucose solutions the plasma

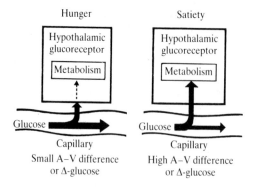

Fig. 1.4 The glucostatic hypothesis for the regulation of food intake. In hunger the difference in glucose concentration between arterial and venous blood (delta glucose) would be less than in satiety. An inverse relationship between delta glucose and hunger has been recognized both in normal and in diabetic subjects (Mayer, 1953)

insulin concentrations rose within minutes (after a short latency) while at the same time blood sugar concentrations actually fell. As this response could not be elicited in vagotomized animals or in diabetic rats with pancreatic transplants it has been concluded that the activation of oral receptors results in the vagal stimulation of pancreatic β-cells.

Factors from the small intestine are now known to provide an important mechanism for the control of insulin secretion. Thus if a test dose of glucose is given intravenously a higher level of blood glucose is detected than if the same amount is administered by mouth. In contrast, however, oral glucose evokes a greater release of insulin. Such an anticipatory secretion would prepare an individual for the rapid handling of glucose which would be absorbed. What factor(s) may be released from the small intestine to increase insulin release? Glucose-dependent insulinotrophic peptide (GIP) is considered to be at least one of the important factors in man. It has been shown that when hyperglycaemia is created and maintained by continuous intravenous glucose infusion (the glucose clamp technique) (Fig. 1.5) a typical biphasic insulin response is recorded. When endogenous GIP secretion is stimulated by oral glucose during a stable hyperglycaemia insulin release is greatly augmented. GIP contributes to an 'enteroinsular axis' in which 'incretins' liberated from the gastrointestinal tract potentiate insulin secretion. The peptide, however, is not an insulin secretagogue. It enhances insulin release only when the plasma glucose concentration is about 20 per cent above the fasting level.

One aspect that has not been considered so far is how pleasure derived from eating may contribute to the control of food intake. Certainly man does not have a constant reaction to a given stimulus experiencing more pleasure when a stimulus helps to correct an internal deficit. To illustrate this point studies have been performed in which volunteers introduced glucose solutions into their mouths. Subsequently these sweet fluids were either swallowed or expectorated. All enjoyed the sugar taste initially. Those expectorating the solutions found a subsequent identical stimulus pleasing. In contrast those who swallowed the fluids found the same stimulus given later to be unpleasant. A similar picture was observed with the smell of oranges. A fasting subject always found them agreeable but those who ingested sugar solutions found the smells progressively less pleasant. If a taste or a smell of a food is not enjoyed an individual will be less likely to eat to excess.

An internal deficit of an energy source is not the only factor that modifies the sensation of taste. Thus coal miners, working hard underground in hot conditions and losing large volumes of sweat, enjoy salty foods unpalatable to their wives or even to themselves after a short holiday. Interestingly, during pregnancy many women have increased salt taste thresholds, are unable to identify concentration differences and prefer more concentrated salt solutions.

The smells and tastes of foods may modify food intake in a different way. It has been proposed that these stimuli possibly promote a conditioned satiety response (as might the sight of food or even the physical presence of food in the mouth).

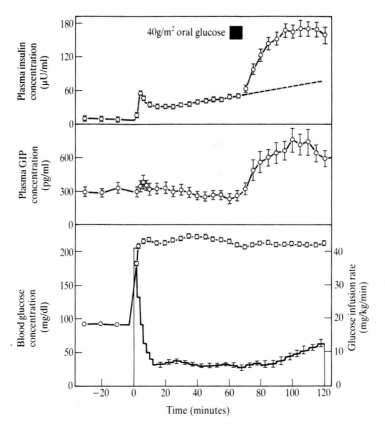

Fig. 1.5 The glucose clamp technique and GIP release. Plasma insulin, plasma GIP and blood glucose concentrations (o—o) are shown for 24 subjects. The infusion rates that were necessary to maintain the hypoglycaemia are also presented. (—) The dashes represent the expected plasma insulin concentrations for these subjects had oral glucose not been given. The vertical bars represent the SE of each mean value (From Anderson, D.K., Elahi, D., Brown, J.C., Tobin, J.D. and Andres, R. (1978). *Journal of Clinical Investigation* **62**, 152–61.)

Long-term control

Over long periods of time there must be relatively precise mechanisms which help to maintain body weight. Food intake and its control clearly have a role to play. This point is dramatically illustrated in *Human nutrition and dietetics* (Davidson *et al.*, 1975) where it was reported that one of the authors (R. Passmore) could still wear the tailcoat made for him four decades earlier despite having eaten subsequently some 20 tons of food.

In the non-growing adult changes in body weight are mainly due to changes in body fat (energy stores). Thus the regulation of body weight becomes equivalent to the regulation of body fat. How might body fat be monitored by the CNS? One possibility is that a metabolite could be released from adipocytes in amounts dependent on the total body fat. Its subsequent detection and measurement by the CNS is an attractive concept and forms the basis for the lipostatic hypothesis. However, so far, no satisfactory candidates have been discovered that could fulfil such a role. An alternative proposal is that the thickness of the fat might be detected by the different discharges of thermoreceptors located subcutaneously, subdermally and within muscles. This idea is incorporated into the thermolipostatic hypothesis. Nevertheless it would be difficult to envisage a system that could differentiate between, on the one hand, increased insulation which would decrease food intake, and on the other increased muscle temperature, due to shivering thermogenesis, which is accompanied by increased food intake.

The discovery of greater numbers of adipocytes in obese than in non-obese subjects is an interesting finding. Such cells can only be proliferated for a limited time after birth in response to genetic factors or as a result of increased fat deposition because of overfeeding. Subsequently the numbers of these cells are fixed for life. This has led to the proposal that depleted adipose cells 'scream' for food until replenished while overloaded fat cells reduce their ingestion until they reach their set point (equivalent to the body weight set point). How the CNS might be informed of the adipocytes contents remains a mystery. Whatever the mechanism it appears that no single point of energy stores is regulated. Rather there exists an acceptable range which changes in relation to diet, age, hormonal status and the activity of the autonomic nervous system.

Bibliography

Andersen, D.K. (1981). Physiological effects of GIP in man. In *Gut hormones*, 2nd edn., pp 256–63. Ed. by S.R. Bloom, and J.M. Polak. Churchill Livingstone, Edinburgh.

Bender, A.E. (1973). *Nutrition and Dietetic Foods*. Leonard Hill Books, Aylesbury.

Cabonac, M. (1971). Physiological role of pleasure. *Science* **173**, 1103–07.

Davidson, S., Passmore, R., Brock, J.T. and Truswell, A.S. (1975). *Human nutrition and dietetics*, 6th edn. Churchill Livingstone, Edinburgh.

Louis-Sylvestre, J. (1978). Relationship between two stages of prandial insulin release in rats. *Americal Journal of Physiology* **235**, E103–E111.

McHugh, P.A. and Moran, T.H. (1986). The stomach, cholecystokinin and satiety. *Federation Proceedings* **45**, 1384–90.

Mayer, J. (1953). *New England Journal of Medicine* **249**, 13–16.

Nicolaidis, S, and Even, P. (1985). Physiological determinant of hunger, satiation and satiety. *American Journal of Clinical Nutrition* **42**, 1083–92.

Paintal, A.S. (1980). Regulation of food intake. In *Scientific Foundations of Gastroenterology*, pp 123–29. Ed. by W. Sircusk and A.N. Smith. William Heinemann Medical Books, London.

Ramhamadany, E.M., Fowler, J. and Baird, I.M. (1989). Effect of the gastric balloon versus sham procedure on weight loss in obese subjects. *Gut* **30**, 1054–57.

Smith, G.P. (1982). The physiology of the meal. In *Drugs and Appetite*, pp 1–21. Ed. by T. Silverstone. Academic Press, London.

Stricker, E.M. (1984). Biological bases of hunger and satiety: therapeutic implications. *Nutrition Reviews* **42**, 333–40.

Welch, I.M., Sepple, C.P. and Read, N.W. (1988). Comparisons of the effects on satiety and eating behaviour of infusion of lipid into the different regions of the small intestine. *Gut* **29**, 306–11.

2

The mouth and the oesophagus

In this chapter consideration is given to mastication and swallowing, the secretion of the salivary glands and absorption through the oral mucosa. Finally a section is devoted to the forceful expulsion of gastric (and intestinal) contents, i.e. vomiting.

Mastication

During mastication food is broken down into small fragments which can be swallowed and mixed with saliva. In man the particle size is variable and depends on early training, the nature of the food, incidental conversation and habit. Normally, however, fragments of only a few cubic millimetres may be recovered. As food moves around the mouth taste buds are stimulated. Odours are released which activate the olfactory epithelium initiating the reflex secretions of saliva and gastric juice and contributing to the enjoyment of eating. Enjoyment is an important factor as shown by the frustration of those who fail to detect odours (anosmia gustatoria). Indeed it has been suggested that the inability to enjoy a meal diminishes the quality of life as greatly as deafness affects the classical music lover who can no longer listen to and appreciate Beethoven. Many hold the view that mastication does not have a great effect on the digestion of modern foods. However, utilization depends on the type of food eaten. This was observed by J. H. Farrell in 1956 who asked volunteers to swallow two cotton bags tied together. One contained masticated food (1 g). The food and its amount were the same in the other bag but it was not chewed. It was found that boiled eggs and cod were fully digested in both bags. However, the majority of the foods tested, including stewed beef and boiled potatoes, left a greater residue if not chewed. Thus insufficient chewing can be poor food economy, especially with vegetables having tough fibrous coverings not ruptured during their preparation.

Mastication is a complex process having both voluntary and reflex components. It can be initiated and modified voluntarily. Jaw opening and jaw closing are represented in the precentral and postcentral gyrus. Nevertheless a masticatory reflex has long been established as a result of the classical studies of C.S. Sherrington (1917) on decerebrate cats.

Several movements have to be recognized in mastication. For example, hinge-like opening and closing of the jaws result in biting by the incisors. If this is accompanied by protrusion and withdrawal of the mandible the cutting edges of the incisors are brought together. If associated with lateral movements the molars are able to grind food that is being eaten.

Both the tongue and the cheeks have important roles to play. Their movements keep the food between the masticatory surfaces. The tongue has the additional function of removing residues trapped between the cheeks and gingiva. It also provides information as to when the food is ready for swallowing. Occasionally the tongue even contributes to the breakdown of solids, as those who crush strawberries against their hard palates must readily admit.

A simple picture of jaw opening and closing can be presented. The jaws are normally closed against gravity by the contraction of the masseter, medial pterygoid and the temporalis muscles. However, the pressure of food against the gums, teeth, anterior hard palate and tongue results in the relaxation of the jaw closing muscles and the contraction of those producing jaw opening, the digastric and lateral pterygoid. The stimuli producing jaw opening are partially removed and the jaw closing muscles are stretched. As a result the jaw opening muscles relax while those closing the mouth undergo a rebound contraction. By repeating this process solid food particles are reduced in size. The mastication reflex is unilateral and directed to the side of the mouth that is full. The forces produced by 'young men eating civilized food' are 45 kg for the molars but only one-third of this value for the incisors. As 52–78 kg is sufficient to crack hazelnuts the forces that man can exert are undoubtedly greater than are normally required. Interestingly, isolated groups in North America obliged in the past to accept a diet requiring vigorous mastication have been found to produce 135 kg on their molars.

Teeth do not invariably make occlusal contact during mastication. The frequency of such contact depends on the food eaten. It is greater for bread and meat, where jaw movement can be relatively easily controlled, than for hard biscuits which suddenly break. Fortunately the teeth are not rigid structures. If they were they would be unable to withstand the sudden occlusal forces to which they are submitted without being damaged. They have slight mobility. With small forces teeth move as a result of stretching periodontal fibres. Greater forces produce small responses which depend on the deformation of alveolar bone.

Occlusal contact is frequently less violent than might be expected because of an unloading reflex. As brittle material breaks following powerful contractions of jaw closing muscles the digastric are quickly activated. At the same time electromyograms of jaw closing muscles show a rapid quietening.

Salivary secretion

More than 1 litre of saliva can be produced each day as a result of the activity of several glands. In man three pairs of glands – the parotid, submandibular and sublingual – have been recognized. These produce most of the saliva with the submandibular producing the greatest contribution at rest but with the parotid capable of increasing its flow rate the more dramatically when stimulated. Small volumes are also released from numerous other glands, e.g. the buccal glands of the cheeks and the lingual glands of the tongue.

In simple terms the secretion of saliva can be described as follows. A primary secretion is released into blind-ending acini. This fluid then flows through a series of converging ducts (intercalated, striated and excretory —) in which it is modified before passing into the oral cavity. The secretions produced by different glands vary considerably. Thus the parotid releases a watery (or serous) secretion of inconstant composition while a more viscous (or mucous) secretion, because of the presence of several mucopolysaccharides, is produced by the buccal glands. The submandibular and sublingual glands produce intermediate secretions and are described as mixed rather than mucous or serous glands. The secretions of the former are mainly serous while those of the latter are predominantly of the mucous type.

Collection of saliva

The secretions of the parotid gland can be collected using a simple device introduced by Carlsen and Crittenden (1910). This consists of a double cup now known as a Lashley cup. The inner vessel covers the opening to the gland (Stenson's duct). From it any collected saliva can be drained. Suction is applied to the outer cup so that the whole can be held against the cheek.

Secretions from the submandibular and sublingual glands are less easy to collect. Difficulties arise because of the proximity of the frenum and the root of the tongue to the sites at which the excretory ducts open. Furthermore, on the floor of the mouth the underlying bone limits the plasticity of the surface. Nevertheless appliances have been designed, some resembling artificial dentures, by which these specific secretions can be collected.

The electrolytes of saliva

The major electrolytes present in saliva are Na^+, K^+, Cl^- and HCO_3^- (Fig. 2.1). All these are present in the primary secretions. Usually their concentrations and the total osmolarity are similar to those found in the plasma, although a richer K^+-containing fluid may result in the primary secretion being slightly hypertonic. It has been suggested that Cl^- and perhaps HCO_3^- are actively transported by the acinar cells. Na^+ and water are passively transferred. Models for Na^+ movement via cation-selective channels (paracellular transfer around and not across cells) have been proposed. The processes involved in K^+ movement have not yet been determined (Fig. 2.2).

In the ducts sodium is reabsorbed by an active transport process. Possibly the whole of the duct system, including the main excretory ducts, are involved. Many are surprised to detect Na^+ concentrations as low as 1 mM in human parotid saliva collected from a subject at rest and using a Lashley cup. With the greater production of a primary secretion and a more rapid rate of flow along the ducts there is a shorter time for absorption to take place. The Na^+ concentration, therefore, rises although not to plasma levels as the ducts are relatively impermeable to water. The limited capacity of the ducts to absorb

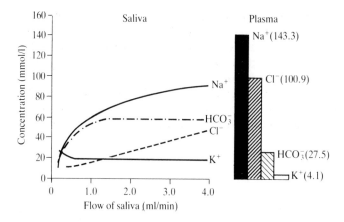

Fig. 2.1 The relationship between the concentration of sodium, potassium, chloride and bicarbonate in human parotid saliva and rate of salivary flow. Note the hypotonicity of the secretion released into the mouth (From Thaysen, J.H., Thorn, N.A. and Schwartz, I.L. (1954). *American Journal of Physiology* **178**, 155–9.)

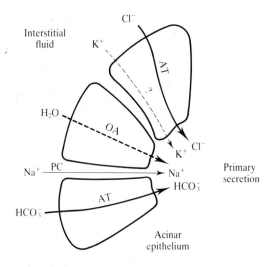

Fig. 2.2 The primary secretion of salivary glands. In this model Cl^- and HCO^-_3 are actively transported (AT). In contrast diffusion accounts for the paracellular (PC) movements of Na^+. Water is osmotically attracted (OA) by the solutes transferred to the acinar lumen. The mechanism by which K^+ is secreted has not been established

water but readily absorb Na^+ accounts for the finding that the saliva entering the oral cavity is always hypotonic. The ductal epithelia also secrete K^+. The mechanism has limited capacity so that high K^+ concentrations are only recorded when small volumes flow through the ducts. With increased flow rates the K^+ concentration falls towards that of the primary secretion.

No specific absorption of Cl^- is thought to occur. Changes in Cl^- concentration are regarded as due to the anion's movement in response to electrical gradients. The handling of HCO_3^- is more puzzling. The ducts of the various glands have different properties. However, an active transport process has been proposed whereby HCO_3^- can be secreted. To explain the finding that the HCO_3^- concentration increases as the salivary flow increases it has been postulated that the stimulation of salivary glands activates the HCO_3^- secretory process. One should always bear in mind that when a salivary gland is stimulated to release greater volumes of primary secretion the functions of the ducts may also be modified.

Organic components

Submandibular and parotid saliva contain only 0.1 and 0.5 g protein/100 ml, as compared with plasma concentrations of 7 g/100 ml. However, 25 per cent of protein in mixed saliva is amylase and this hydrolytic enzyme is present in much greater concentrations in saliva than in serum. It is derived from acini and granular cells of the proximal ducts. During the stimulation of salivary glands the intracellular stores are depleted and are rebuilt on removal of the stimulus. The secretory cycle includes synthesis of new enzymes on ribosomes of basally located rough endoplasmic reticulum, followed by intracisternal transport to the Golgi region where protein becomes encapsulated. Subsequently, fully formed zymogen granules accumulate in the apical regions of the cells, these being discharged when the gland is stimulated. How enzymes are released from cells is not well understood. Possibly the zymogen granule fuses with the intracellular surface of the cell membrane, followed by local dissolution and enzyme release.

Blood group substances possessing the same characteristics as agglutinogens on red blood cells are also found in submandibular saliva. Substances A, B, O (H) and Le^a have been identified as specific secretions of mucous cells.

Several other organic constituents should also be mentioned. One is mucus which consists of a whole family of proteins associated with different sugars or sugar derivatives. These substances contribute to the greater viscosity of the submandibular secretion as compared with parotid saliva. Another is lysozyme which is present in human parotid and submandibular saliva. It is capable of lysing certain bacteria, e.g. Staphylococcus and Streptococcus. Lysozyme acts by hydrolysing a component of the bacterial cell wall. A further enzyme in saliva is lingual lipase. This triglyceride-hydrolysing enzyme may be of value in the neonate and in situations where there are inadequate levels of pancreatic enzymes.

A 53 aminoacid polypeptide has been detected in human submandibular glands. This is epidermal growth factor (or EGF) found also in Brunner's glands and Paneth cells of the small intestine. Its biological actions include the stimulation of mitotic activity and an inhibition of gastric acid secretion. EGF is stable in acid and in the presence of pepsin. Thus EGF may have a role to play in the protection of the gastroduodenal mucosa. Whether it has in man is not known. In animal studies, however, it has been shown to prevent the development of ulcers (cysteamine-induced) and promote healing. Furthermore, while EGF binds readily to the surface of ulcers and even to the sites of small defects very little is attached to the normal mucosa.

Functions of saliva

1. General cleansing and protection of the masticatory apparatus.
2. Starting the digestion of carbohydrate.
3. Providing mucus.
4. Dissolving many components and contributing to taste.
5. By its absence, providing an urge to drink.
6. By keeping the mouth moist, helping speech, oral comfort, chewing and swallowing.
7. Contributing to the digestion of fat.

1. General cleansing and protection of the masticatory apparatus

Xerostomia (dry mouth) resulting from X-ray treatment has rapidly deleterious consequences. Saliva helps to protect the teeth and gums simply by washing them. The enzyme lysozyme is of value as it breaks down the cell walls of a number of potentially harmful bacteria. Saliva also has some acid neutralizing capacity. Bicarbonate is the most important factor. In addition to its effects in the oral cavity saliva serves to neutralize refluxed acid which oesophageal peristalsis has not returned to the stomach.

2. Starting the digestion of carbohydrate

Saliva contains an α-amylase produced by the cells of the acini. This enzyme breaks down $\alpha 1,4$ glucosidic linkages providing they are not terminal bonds. However, it is ineffective against $\alpha 1,6$ and $\beta 1,4$ linkages. It has a pH optimum of 6.9 although it is stable within the range 4–11.

The polysaccharides in the diet include starch, glycogen and cellulose. Starch is a mixture of two polymers. Approximately 20% is amylose, a glucose polymer in which all the glucose units are linked $\alpha 1,4$. The remainder is amylopectin where most are $\alpha 1,4$ but a small percentage of the bonds are $\alpha 1,6$. Glycogen is similar to amylopectin while cellulose is made up of thousands of glucose units all linked $\beta 1,4$. Thus as a result of amylase activity starch and glycogen can be hydrolysed to release maltose, the trisaccharide maltotriose and dextrins. Dextrins are molecules of variable structure containing about six glucose units linked by both $\alpha 1,4$ and $\alpha 1,6$ bonds. Initially salivary amylase was thought to be of little value and rapidly inactivated by the acid of the stomach. However, food is only slowly mixed with acid. The fundic region acts as a relatively quiescent food reservoir. It has been estimated that amylolytic activity may continue for 15–30 minutes and as much as 75 per cent of the starch in mashed potato and 60 per cent of that in bread may be converted to maltose before the enzyme is inactivated. Thus salivary amylase plays a not inconsiderable role in carbohydrate digestion.

Recently it has been suggested that some salivary amylase might even contribute to duodenal starch hydrolysis. This would be particularly useful for those with pancreatic insufficiency. For salivary amylase to function in the small intestine inactivation must be limited. How might the enzyme survive in the gastric lumen? It appears that starch and various glucose oligomers, ranging in length from two to seven glucose units protects amylase at pH3

(Table 2.1), possibly by binding to its active sites. Furthermore, starch protects amylase against pepsin. In contrast, lactose, sucrose and glucose are ineffective in sparing amylase.

3. Providing mucus which is strongly resistant to enzymic degradation and has a number of useful properties

Among these are the binding of small particles produced during mastication to form a bolus ready for swallowing. In addition, by forming a coating, mucus provides some protection for the delicate mucosal surface and lubricates the gastrointestinal tract allowing ease of movement of the bolus. A function unforeseen by nature is the fixation of dentures. For patients treated for hypertension with ganglion-blocking agents the resulting lack of saliva has been particularly inconvenient.

4. Dissolving many components and, therefore, contributing to the sensation of taste

Tastes are important for both the pleasure of eating and the stimulation of several gastrointestinal secretions. Four primary tastes are recognized. These are sweet, salt, sour and bitter. A sweet taste is the result of sugars and ketones stimulating taste buds on the anterior surface of the tongue. Sourness is detected particularly on the sides of the tongue and is dependent on hydrogen ions. However, other factors must play a role as all acids are not equally sour at the same pH. One possible explanation involves the binding of the anion. It is suggested that as hydrogen ions are absorbed to taste bud receptors the membrane becomes more positive so that other hydrogen ions which might contribute to the sour taste are repelled. By absorbing anions these electrical

Table 2.1 The protection of salivary amylase by starch and some of its hydrolytic products. The enzyme was incubated at 37°C and at pH3 for various time intervals in the presence of starch, its products of hydrolysis, glucose, lactose or sucrose. The values given are the percentages of the initial amylase activity remaining at a particular time (From Rosenblum, J.L., Irwin, C.L. and Alpers, D.H. (1988). *American Journal of Physiology* **254**, E775–E780.)

Carbohydrate added	Percentage amylase activity remaining at:			
	5 min	30 min	60 min	120 min
None	66	8	0	0
5% corn starch*	98	91	81	53
43 mmol/l maltoheptaose	95	92	78	51
43 mmol/l maltohexaose	98	94	83	57
43 mmol/l maltopentaose	100	94	87	66
43 mmol/l maltotetraose	94	80	61	32
43 mmol/l maltotriose	100	89	84	61
43 mmol/l maltose	82	36	13	1
43 mmol/l glucose	66	10	1	0
5% lactose	63	17	4	0
5% sucrose	65	17	4	0

* Partially digested.

changes can be limited and more hydrogen ions bound. As a result a more sour taste can be recognized.

A salty taste can be detected over the entire surface of the tongue. Both cations and anions contribute, the former stimulating the latter inhibiting the sensation. It is difficult to characterize those substances e.g quinine, producing the bitter taste recognized on the posterior surface of the tongue. No single structural component has been identified.

The picture presented above is an oversimplification. Taste buds, though concentrated on the tongue are found throughout the mouth and in the upper oesophagus. Furthermore they respond in varying degrees to three or all four of the primary taste sensations.

5. By its absence providing an urge to drink

When man becomes dehydrated his salivary secretions are reduced. This produces a dry mouth and results in the subject searching for fluids. Conversely wetting the buccal and pharyngeal surfaces can temporarily relieve thirst symptoms and help to prevent overdrinking. Wetting and gastric distension are two of the important signals which allow an animal to take almost exactly the volume of fluid it requires (Table 2.2). In man such signals may infrequently be generated as he drinks to excess to satisfy his social requirements.

6. By keeping the mouth moist it facilitates speech, promotes oral comfort and aids chewing and swallowing

This property of saliva is well known. For those patients producing too little saliva as the result of the radiotherapeutic treatment of tumours of the head and

Table 2.2   The wetting of the buccal and pharngeal surfaces as a means of temporarily relieving thirst symptoms. Dogs satisfy their thirst with a single draught of water in 5 min or less and they ingest accurately their water deficit. In the experiments below, a dog was made water-deficient and then allowed to drink. However, the water did not pass down the gastrointestinal tract to be absorbed because an oesophagostomy had been performed and the animal was obliged to sham drink. Under these conditions, the dog drank approximately 250% of its deficit. Artificially restoring the continuity of the oesophagus gave the dog the opportunity to replace its water losses. Subsequently, it showed no desire to sham drink (From Bellows, R. T. (1939). *American Journal of Physiology* **125**, 87–97.)

Experiment	Time in relation to real drinking period	Sham drinking (ml)	Real drinking (ml)	Percentage of real drinking	Percentage of body weight
1	3 h before	3920	–	240	–
	2 h before	3925	–	240	–
	1 h before	3800	–	232	–
	–	–	1635	–	11
	1 h after	0	–	–	–
2	2 h before	2100	–	220	–
	1 h before	2475	–	256	–
	–	–	960	–	6
	1 h after	0	–	–	–

neck a number of oral substitutes, based on mucus or carboxymethylcellulose have been developed.

7. Contributing to the digestion of fat

Located beneath the circumvallate papillae are the lingual glands. Initially their function was thought to be to produce a secretion washing the taste buds and preparing them for fresh stimuli. In addition, however, they produce a lipase which hydrolyses triglycerides containing longchain fatty acids. The enzyme is able to act in the absence of bile acids and at a low pH, i.e. the conditions that prevail in the stomach. How significant the enzyme is in fat digestion remains controversial. It may be important in patients with pancreatic deficiency, e.g. cystic fibrosis. In such patients the pH of the duodenal contents remains low after a test meal enabling lingual lipase to continue its action in the intestine. It may also be of value in the neonate, particularly when premature. These are normally lacking in pancreatic lipase and bile acids.

Another source of enzymes that enable neonates to digest lipid is human milk. Two lipases have been described. One, regarded as physiologically important, is a bile salt-stimulated lipase. The other, a lipoprotein lipase, is probably released from alveolar cells ruptured during lactation. The value of such enzymes is indicated by the finding that premature infants excrete less fat when fed mixtures of fresh breast milk and low birth weight infant formula than if fed the formula alone. Good fat absorption is essential for these infants not only because of the high calorie content of fat but also because of its role in brain development.

The control of salivary secretion

The resting flow of saliva in the absence of obvious stimuli is approximately 0.5 ml/min. Of this the submandibular, parotid and sublingual glands contribute approximately 69%, 26% and 5% respectively. Secretion is stimulated particularly by sapid substances and also by the smell of food and chewing. A maximal secretion of 7 ml/min can be induced by rinsing the mouth with 0.5 mol/litre citric acid (although experimenters should beware the effects of such a stimulus on their teeth). Perhaps a more attractive demonstration is that in which the chewing of lemon slices can be shown to increase by more than 100 times the flow of human parotid saliva into a Lashley cup.

The saliva produced by chewing has generally been attributed to information from masticatory muscle and joint receptors. Recently, however, a role for paradontal mechanoreceptors has been emphasized. The parotid saliva produced when a breakfast cereal is crushed between two teeth can be reduced by infiltration anaesthesia around one of the teeth.

There is not a continuous secretion of saliva into the mouth. A secretion must be stimulated. When man is asleep his parotid secretion is almost abolished and only small volumes of submandibular saliva are collected despite the bulky devices that need to be used.

At one time it was thought that conditioned reflexes modified salivary secretion in man and in dogs. Certainly in dogs such reflexes exist. Pavlov recognized that the ringing of church bells in St. Petersburg (Leningrad) at midday was associated by dogs with the arrival of food. As a result these animals salivated even when food was not available at that time. In man conditioned responses, if they exist, are not thought to be powerful. Thus volunteers, starved for several days, have had delicious meals prepared for them behind glass so that no smells could be detected. Their salivary flows were not greatly changed. Some even believed that their secretions had increased. It has been concluded that the thought of food made those subjects more conscious of the saliva in their mouths.

A number of factors reduce the resting flow of saliva. These include dehydration, hypnosis, severe mental effort and fear. In fact the reduction of salivary secretion as a result of fear has been used as a means of determining the guilt or innocence of a man in the Indian Rice Test. A person unable to swallow dried rice was thought to be guilty on the grounds that fear prevents secretions so that without the moistening and lubricating properties of saliva it was impossible to swallow. One might ask how many innocent people have been condemned after facing such an ordeal.

Salivary secretion is controlled from the medulla and both sympathetic and parasympathetic nerves have a role to play. Both branches of the autonomic nervous system contribute to the stimulation of a secretion. An inhibition of secretion can be regarded as the result of higher centres modifying medullary activity (Fig. 2.3).

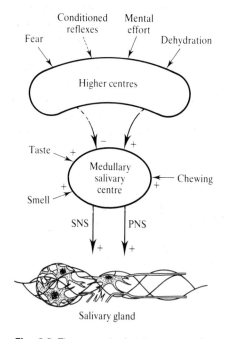

Fig. 2.3 The control of salivary secretion. When the medullary centre is stimulated both the parasympathetic (PNS) and sympathetic (SNS) branches of the autonomic nervous system contribute to increased salivary secretion (NB: All glands do not receive the same innervation.)

Sympathetic nerves leave the spinal cord from the upper three or four thoracic roots and terminate in the superior cervical ganglion. Postganglionic fibres leave the superior cervical ganglion to reach the salivary glands along the coats of blood vessels. It should be remembered that a characteristic of the sympathetic nervous system is the greater distances travelled by postganglionic neurons as compared with the parasympathetic postganglionic neurons which often originate close to or in the tissue they innervate.

Presynaptic parasympathetic neurons travel from the medullary inferior salivatory nucleus to the otic ganglion via the glossopharyngeal nerve. Postsynaptic fibres pass to the parotid gland. Nerves from the superior salivatory nucleus synapse in the submandibular ganglia with postganglionic neurons serving the submandibular and sublingual glands.

There are at least four sites (Fig. 2.4) at which the sympathetic and parasympathetic nerves could act to modify salivary secretion. These are:

1. The acini producing the primary secretion.
2. The ducts which modify it.
3. The blood vessels which provide the substrates necessary for secretion, satisfy the energy requirements of the gland and remove waste products.
4. The myoepithelial cells which surround the ducts and acini (Fig. 2.5).

The parasympathetic nervous system increases the secretion of acini and the activity of ducts. It produces contractions of myoepithelial cells. This response is thought to maintain the integrity of the gland and prevent the delicate epithelial cells from being stretched and disrupted. A leaky epithelial layer might not prevent salivary proteins passing from the ducts to the interstitial fluid in a concentrated form.

Parasympathetic nerves can also increase salivary gland bloodflow. This increase probably depends on more than one mechanism (Fig. 2.6). Unlike the secretory response the increase in bloodflow is resistant to atropine (the cholinergic muscarinic blocking agent). Initially it was thought that nerves stimulated the release of the enzyme kallikrein into the interstitial fluid from

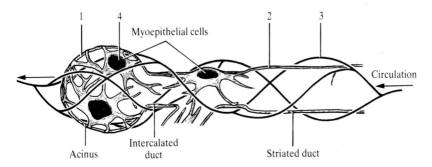

Fig. 2.4 Possible sites of action of the autonomic nervous system on salivary secretion. Remember that *both* branches, the sympathetic and the parasympathetic, are represented. These nerves may produce effects on those cells producing the primary secretion (1) or those modifying it (2). Alternatively, the circulation (3) or the activity of the myoepithelial cells (4) may be changed

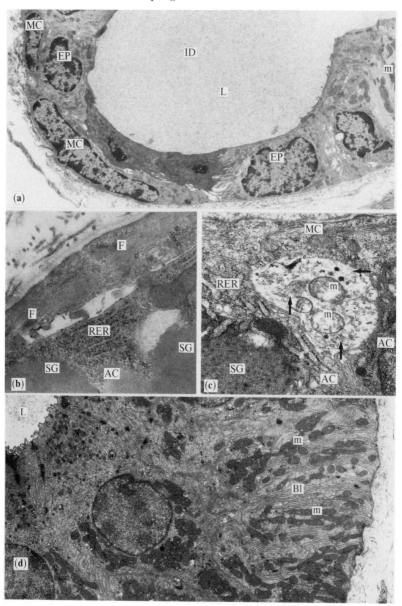

Fig. 2.5 Transmission electron micrographs of submandibular salivary gland. (**a**) The junction between an intercalated (ID) and a striated duct (SD). Despite marked distension of the lumen (L) epithelial cells (EP) are not disrupted because of the presence of closely associated, supporting myoepithelial cells (MC). Note the columns of mitochondria (m) at the beginning of the striated duct. (**b**) A myoepithelial cell process containing contractile filaments (F), enveloping an acinar cell (AC). Note the presence of secretory granules (SG) and a prominent rough endoplasmic reticulum (RER). (**c**) A cholinergic-type axon lying beneath a myoepithelial cell process (MC) and in close proximity to acinar cells (AC). Note the presence of both cholinergic agranular vesicles (↑) and dense core peptidergic vesicles (←) as well as mitochondria (m). Secretory granules (SG) and rough endoplasmic reticulum (RER) are evident in the acinar cells. (**d**) An epithelial cell of a striated duct. The basal membrane has extensive infolding (BL). As a result numerous mitochondria (m) are arranged in columns, giving the cell its well known striated appearance. L = Lumen. **a**, **b** and **d** are from rabbit; **c** is from baboon tissue (Kindly presented by Dr K. Kyriacou, College of Medicine, King Saud University, Riyadh, Saudi Arabia.)

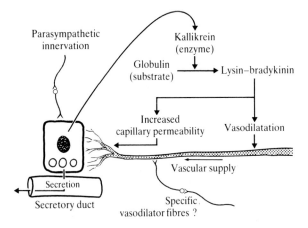

Parasympathetic
innervation

Kallikrein
(enzyme)

Globulin
(substrate) ⟶ Lysin–bradykinin

Increased
capillary permeability

Vasodilatation

Vascular supply

Secretion

Secretory duct

Specific
vasodilator fibres ?

Fig. 2.6 The influence of parasympathetic nerves on blood flow to salivary glands (based on Folkow, B. and Neil, E. (1971). *Circulation*. Oxford University Press, London.)

secretory cells. This proteolytic enzyme acts on a globulin to release the decapeptide kallidin (lysin–bradykinin) which is rapidly converted in plasma and tissue fluids to the nonapeptide bradykinin. Both peptides are powerful vasodilators. Furthermore they increase capillary permeability, allowing for the large movements of substances necessary when salivary secretion is stimulated. However, the importance of this mechanism has recently been challenged following the discovery that most of the kallikrein released appears in the saliva rather than the interstitial fluid.

A more direct control of the circulation has been sought. Nerve fibres releasing vasoactive intestinal polypeptide (VIP) are now thought to play an important role in vasodilatation. Thus the stimulation of parasympathetic nerves (chorda tympani) of anaesthetized cats results in an abrupt increase in the VIP concentration of submaxillary (submandibular) venous plasma accompanied by a substantially greater bloodflow both in the presence (Fig. 2.7) and absence of atropine. Furthermore intra-arterial infusions of VIP, which reproduce the venous plasma VIP levels, cause an increase in the bloodflow of the same order of magnitude as nerve stimulation.

Although a role for VIP in salivary secretion is probable a complete picture still has to emerge. Both VIP and acetylcholine coexist in the same neurons and modify each others functions. Thus while VIP does not act directly on secreting cells its presence greatly increases the affinity of cholinergic muscarinic receptors and so, may increase the responses of acini and ducts to parasympathetic nerve stimulation. How might this be brought about? It has been suggested that several interconvertible receptor populations exist with different affinities and that VIP might cause low-affinity receptors to adopt the high-affinity configuration. The question remains as to when are these different neurotransmitters released. The answers have yet to be found although the concept is slowly emerging that the release of specific neurotransmitters varies with frequency-dependent signals from the central nervous system. (To confuse

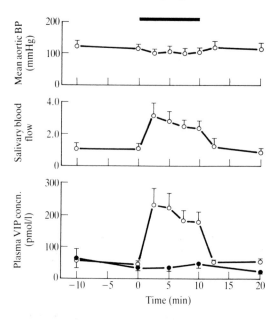

Fig. 2.7 Changes in mean aortic blood pressure (BP), submaxillary blood flow, arterial (●) and submaxillary venous (○) plasma VIP concentrations in cats (n = 5) given atropine (1 mg/kg) in response to stimulation of chorda tympani at 20 Hz for 10 min. The vertical bars represent the SE of each mean value (From Bloom, S.R. and Edwards, A.V. (1980). *Journal of Physiology* **300**, 41–53.)

the reader even more it must be recorded that yet another biologically active peptide is released with VIP from submandibular glands. This is PHI, peptide histidine isoleucine, a peptide with marked sequence homology and similar potency to VIP.)

The sympathetic nervous system also stimulates the epithelia concerned with secretion. However, the composition of the saliva produced is not identical to that stimulated by parasympathetic nerves. Parasympathetic nerves mainly control fluid and electrolyte secretion while protein secretion (e.g. amylase) is more dependent on sympathetic influences. Evidence is accumulating that food quality (taste and strain on the mandible during chewing) is assessed to subsequently modify the activities of sympathetic and parasympathetic nerves. The sympathetic nerves have vasoconstrictor activity on salivary gland blood vessels. However, if salivary secretion is reflexly stimulated vasoconstrictor tone is overwhelmed and vasodilatation occurs. Indeed noradrenaline, as well as causing vasoconstriction can also relax smooth muscle by releasing an endothelial derived relaxation factor (Fig. 2.8). Finally the sympathetic nerves may constrict myoepithelial cells. This is a similar response to that proposed for parasympathetic nerves. In summary the sympathetic and parasympathetic nerves function synergistically to produce salivary secretion. There appears to be no inhibitory influences on the secretion at the level of the gland. Secretion can be reduced only centrally.

A further example of the two branches of the autonomic nervous system

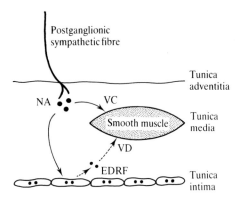

Fig. 2.8 Possible mechanisms of action of sympathetic nerves on salivary gland blood vessels. Nerves penetrate the arteriole wall and release noradrenaline (NA). This diffuses to (a) smooth muscle, causing vasoconstriction (VC); and (b) the endothelium, releasing endothelial derived relaxant factor (EDRF). EDRF causes vasodilatation (VD)

working together rather than antagonistically is provided from studies of the growth and biochemical development of salivary glands (Table 2.3 and Fig. 2.9). The parasympathetic nerves are important for growth. Thus 16 days after parasympathectomy the sizes and cell numbers of rat parotid gland cells are significantly reduced. The amylase levels are also much less than expected but may reflect changes in gland mass. In contrast sympathetic nerves make a valuable contribution to the biochemical development of the parotid gland. If the superior cervical gland is removed there is little effect on gland size but the amylase content is reduced by at least half.

Hormones and salivary secretion

No specific hormone is concerned with the stimulation of salivary secretion. This contrasts with the situation encountered in other gastrointestinal secretory glands. Some hormones, however, do modify the composition of saliva. Thus adrenal mineralocorticoids lower salivary $[Na^+]$ and raise $[K^+]$ and patients with adrenocortical insufficiency secrete a saliva with a high $[Na^+]:[K^+]$ ratio. A role for aldosterone in ductal transport has been suggested.

Oral absorption

The oral mucosa is a barrier across which a number of drugs can be transported. Such substances administered either sublingually (under the tongue) or bucally (between cheek and gingiva) may be rapidly absorbed by simple diffusion providing they have solubility in both the aqueous contents of the mouth and in the lipids of the epithelial membrane.

Although providing only a small surface for absorption the oral mucosa is highly vascular so that drugs absorbed are quickly removed and a concentration gradient between body fluids and the oral cavity maintained.

Table 2.3   The influence of the autonomic nervous system on the biochemical development of the parotid gland in rats (*see also* Fig. 2.9)

	Total amylase activity				*Percentage decrease in DNA content*	
Age (days)	*Px*	*Contralateral control*	*Sx*	*Contralateral control*	*Px*	*Sx*
16	418	411	345	207	16	0
23	3 654	11 083	9 324	12 712	22	0
32	15 763	34 522	17 400	35 498	34	0
49	31 000	75 556	25 190	56 829	34	0
64	36 000	83 000	38 850	75 629	43	0
86	26 101	82 000	28 000	86 000	46	0

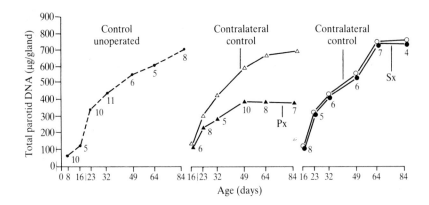

Fig. 2.9 and **Table 2.3** The influence of the autonomic nervous system on the growth (Fig. 2.9) and biochemical development (Table 2.3) of the parotid gland in rats. An index of growth was obtained by measuring the DNA content of the gland. Selective postganglionic denervation was performed under light ether anaesthesia on 8-day-old rats. Unilateral parasympathectomy (Px) was effected by removal of a section of the auriculotemporal nerve. Unilateral sympathectoy (Sx) involved the removal of the superior cervical ganglion. Subsequently at various times the parotid glands, both the denervated and the contralateral controls were removed and analysed for DNA. These DNA levels have been compared with those obtained from the glands of rats that had not been operated on.

In similar experiments amylase activity was measured in the parotid glands of fasted rats. Amylase activity is measured as mg reducing substance produced in 15 min per gland (From Schneyer, C.A. and Hall, H.D. (1970). *American Journal of Physiology* **219**, 1268–72; and (1972) *Proceedings of the Society for Experimental Biology and Medicine* **140**, 911–15.)

Rapidity of drug absorption is not the only advantage to be gained by oral absorption. Aseptic techniques are not required, and self administration is easy. Drugs are not broken down or otherwise structurally altered by the enzymes normally encountered in the stomach and intestines. Furthermore, once absorbed, they enter the systemic circulation from where they can be distributed to the various tissues of the body without first passing to the liver where they may be metabolized.

There are, however, disadvantages. The unpleasant taste of many drugs and the difficulty of guaranteeing predictable concentrations of them within the body limit the number of substances which can be recommended for oral absorption.

Of the drugs that can be absorbed organic nitrates have received considerable attention. Their value for the acute relief of angina pectoris or prophylactic management of situations likely to provoke angina attacks is well documented. The importance of the aqueous contents in providing a solvent to dissolve them has been stressed. Tachypnoea and a change from nasal to mouth breathing frequently accompany chest pain in those experiencing angina. The latter event can quickly dry the mucosa and result in patients who appear resistant to organic nitrates.

The oesophagus

The oesophagus is a hollow tube normally kept empty by waves of contraction passing along its length to the stomach (peristaltic waves). In man the proximal one-third is composed of striated muscle while the distal half to two-thirds contains only smooth muscle. Two layers of muscle are observed separated by a nerve network, the myenteric or Auerbach's plexus. There are no cytoplasmic differences between the outer longitudinal and inner circular muscles. Moreover, the muscle cells of both layers form a continuous syncitium or functional network where electrical activity passes from one cell to another through low resistance connections similar to the intercalated discs of cardiac muscle. At both ends muscular sphincters exist which are normally closed. The cricopharyngeal or upper oesophageal sphincter (UOS) prevents entry of air into the oesophagus during respiration while the gastro-oesophageal or lower oesophageal sphincter (LOS) prevents the reflux of gastric contents. This function of the LOS is particularly important as the oesophagus has virtually no tolerance to hydrochloric acid.

Both sphincters relax to permit the passage of the bolus from the mouth to the stomach. Controversy has surrounded the UOS. Although a zone of elevated pressure (ZEP) of 15–16 cm H_2O can be demonstrated complete agreement as to what and where the sphincter is has been difficult to obtain. Its closure at rest may depend on the elasticity of the surrounding tissues as no tonic electrical activity has been recorded in the muscles surrounding the pharyngo-oesophageal junction. The cricopharyngeus is the major contractile element of the UOS. This muscle relaxes immediately prior to sphincter opening.

The LOS is anatomically difficult to detect in man although it can be demonstrated physiologically. In the sloth, an animal more accustomed to being upside down, the sphincter is easily recognized. Evidence for the existence of a physiological sphincter is provided by manometric studies (Fig. 2.10). A ZEP, approximately 3 cm in length saddles the oesophageal foramen of the diaphragm. The resting pressures recorded (10–15 cm H_2O) are similar to those of the UOS.

The contraction of the sphincter at rest is to a large extent a myogenic response. This is not to say that the resting tone is exclusively myogenic and certainly the LOS can be influenced by a number of factors. However, some of the changes reported may be pharmacological rather than physiological. Two hormones should, at least, be considered. One is gastrin, released from the antrum, which increases gastric secretion and motility. In addition it increases the LOS pressure. Such a hormone could be valuable in reducing acid reflux. The other is progesterone which decreases LOS pressure. Thus in pregnant women and those practising birth control with progesterone-containing preparations acid reflux may be a problem.

Doubtlessly nerves also have a role to play in LOS control. The vagus is believed to contribute to the maintenance of resting tone and the rebound contraction that follows the opening of the sphincter during swallowing. Discharges from the vagus also produce sphincteric relaxation necessary for a bolus to enter the stomach. This process is abolished by cervical vagotomy. While the release of acetylcholine from postganglionic nerve fibres causes smooth muscle contraction the identity of the neurotransmitter(s) producing relaxation has been controversial. VIP is a strong candidate. The sphincter

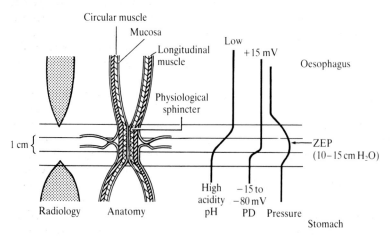

Fig. 2.10 Correlation of the radiological appearance with the anatomy of the physiological gastro-oesophageal sphincter and pH, potential difference (PD) and pressure measurements. The pH increases from the stomach to the oesophagus so that the mucosa of the latter is subjected to less acid conditions. Throughout the gastrointestinal tract there is a small PD across the mucosal epithelia. In the body of the stomach this is 15–80 mV with the lumen negative, while in the oesophagus it is 15 mV, lumen positive. The existence of a physiological sphincter is shown by the zone of elevated pressure (ZEP). This restricts acid reflux from the stomach. (From Earlam, R. (1975). *Clinical Tests of Oesophageal Function.* Crosby Lockwood Staples, London.)

region has a rich supply of VIPergic nerve fibres. When VIP is administered intravenously to man the increases in sphincteric pressure recorded in response to pentagastrin (a synthetic peptide simulating gastrin) are inhibited. Further support for VIP has been from studies of patients with achalasia. In these patients the sphincter fails to relax during swallowing and dysphagia is the consequence. Postmortem examinations have shown the degeneration of ganglion cells in the myenteric plexus and a reduced VIP content of the sphincter region.

Sympathetic nerves must not be ignored. In animal models the stimulation of such nerves induces rhythmic contractions that are suppressed by α-adrenergic antagonists (e.g. phentolamine) and greatly decreased by atropine. These observations suggest that noradrenaline might be released to act on myenteric cholinergic neurons to produce contractions of smooth muscle.

Finally the carminatives must be noted. These substances relieve the symptoms of postprandial bloating by producing belching. They relax the LOS, gastric and oesophageal smooth muscle. An example is peppermint. If taken after meals in solid form or in liqueurs peppermint permits excess gas in the stomach to be tolerated and released in a socially acceptable manner.

In considering the responses of the LOS one further question should be asked. If intragastric pressure increases what is the response of this antireflux barrier? To answer this it must be remembered that the intragastric pressure can be increased in two ways. One is by increasing the intra-abdominal pressure, a change that is transmitted to the stomach. This may result from coughing, changing position, straining or compressing the abdomen (e.g. a corset). The other way is by gastric distension, e.g. caused by delayed gastric emptying. When the intra-abdominal pressure of a cat is increased by abdominal compression the LOS pressure rises to a greater extent than the intragastric pressure. Thus the antireflux barrier is maintained. This contrasts with the significant decrease in the barrier when intragastric balloons are distended to produce consistent increases in pressure

The concept that the LOS (a) provides the ZEP and (b) is normally closed is perhaps too simple. A contribution from the crural diaphragm, unrelated to the control of ventilation, has been examined. When electromyographic activity of this muscle is measured it is found to be inhibited during both the primary and secondary peristaltic events associated with swallowing. Furthermore, the LOS is not always closed but shows transient relaxations. These relaxations account for the gastro-oesophageal reflux that occurs in normal subjects. Little is known as to what induces these events although their abruptness suggests that they are mediated by neural mechanisms. One potent stimulus is gastric distension. Their existence may help to account for the excessive reflux occurring in a substantial proportion of patients with reflux disease who have normal resting LOS pressures.

Swallowing or deglutition

Man swallows approximately seven times every hour while asleep, perhaps ten times more frequently during his hours awake and obviously more often when eating. The mechanism of swallowing has been divided into three phases. The first is the oral or voluntary phase in which the mouth is closed and the tongue pushes upwards and backwards against the hard palate forcing the bolus into the pharynx. The subsequent phases are involuntary. Some have suggested that a part, at least, of the oral phase is reflex as attempts to swallow voluntarily when the mouth is dry are ineffective.

The second or pharyngeal phase occurs when the bolus stimulates mechanoreceptors around the opening of the pharynx. Impulses are conducted via the glossopharyngeal and vagus nerves to the swallowing centre located in the medulla and pons which coordinate a subsequent complex sequence of events:

1. The superior constrictor muscle contracts and the soft palate is elevated towards the posterior pharyngeal wall to prevent the bolus entering the nasopharynx.

2. The palatopharyngeal folds are pulled medially to form a slit which impedes the movements of a large bolus.

3. The vocal cords come close together and muscles attached to the hyoid bone pull the larynx upwards and forwards. Thus the passage of the bolus into the trachea is unlikely and the entrance to the oesophagus is stretched.

4. The medullary respiratory region is inhibited to produce deglutition apnoea.

5. The UOS is relaxed and contraction of the superior constrictor muscle initiates a peristaltic wave which propels the bolus into the oesophagus. As the bolus enters the oesophagus the LOS, normally closed to prevent acid reflux, also relaxes.

The final or oesophageal phase of swallowing involves the coordinated waves of contraction that originated in the pharynx continuing along the length of the oesophagus. This peristaltic wave lasts for 7–10 seconds. Gravitational effects often result in the bolus descending more rapidly. On some occasions a peristaltic wave may fail to propel the bolus to the stomach. The resulting distension of the oesophagus is the stimulus for a vago-vagal reflex which produces secondary peristaltic waves. Clearly swallowing is a highly complex coordinated event. How might it be controlled? It has been proposed that the medulla possesses a central programme which, when initiated, is responsible for the entire motor sequence. It can operate without afferent nerve feedback. However, under physiological conditions the medulla receives information from pharyngeal and oesophageal receptors so that the central programme can be modified to adjust the motor sequence of the swallowed bolus.   Factors other than bolus size also modify the swallowing process. These include the temperature of the bolus and the frequency with which swallows are attempted. When very cold foods are swallowed (e.g. ice-cream at −5°C) the amplitudes of peristaltic contractions are considerably smaller than when the same foods are warmed to room temperature before eating.

The effect of swallowing frequency on peristalsis is interesting. A second swallow initiated (5 seconds after the first) while a peristaltic wave is still in the striated muscle results in the complete inhibition of contractile activity induced by the first swallow. This is known as deglutitive inhibition. It has been suggested that relaxation is the first event of the oesophageal phase of swallowing. As normally the oesophagus is relaxed no obvious response would be observed other than in the sphincters. A first swallow can also modify the oesophageal response to subsequent swallows. When swallows are about 10 seconds apart the frequency with which a peristaltic wave accompanies the second swallow or the amplitude of that wave is decreased. One explanation is that the second swallow occurs during the refractory period of the oesophageal muscle. Vanek and Diamant (1987) have recently challenged this interpretation suggesting that the modulation of neurogenic mechanisms is a more likely possibility.

Vomiting or emesis

Vomiting is the forceful expulsion of gastric and intestinal contents through the mouth. Preceding or accompanying vomiting are tachypnoea, copious salivation, pupil dilatation, sweating and pallor, and rapid or irregular heartbeat, all signs of widespread autonomic nervous system disturbance. The psychic experience of nausea is an indication of stimulation of the medulla.

The mechanism starts with a deep inspiration. The glottis is then closed to protect the respiratory passages and air, subsequently drawn into the oesophagus together with saliva, helps to distend the oesophageal tube. The soft palate is elevated to prevent vomit entering the nasopharynx. Expiration against a closed glottis with simultaneous contraction of abdominal muscles increases both intrathoracic and intra-abdominal pressures. The LOS and the body of the stomach relax and gastric contents are forced into the oesophagus where least resistance to flow is offered. Intragastric pressures of up to 850 mm Hg may be measured during vomiting. These could not be achieved by the contractions of the stomach alone. (The relative unimportance of the stomach can be demonstrated experimentally by replacing it with a bladder yet still inducing vomiting.) A number of cycles occur whereby the oesophagus is repeatedly filled and emptied, but as the cricopharyngeal sphincter is closed no gastric contents pass into the mouth. Indeed they flow back to the stomach with gravity. Finally, a violent expulsive effort forces the contents through the UOS and out of the mouth. If the stomach still contains a significant volume of fluid, a second filling and emptying of the oesophagus occurs culminating with a further expulsion. Subsequent massive contractions of the duodenum can force intestinal contents into the stomach with the appearance of bile in the vomit. This retrograde movement of intestinal contents is thought not to be due to reverse peristalsis, rather that the stomach relaxes and duodenal contractions reverse the normal pressure gradient.

Vomiting is governed by a centre in the medulla in close connection with respiratory and vasomotor regions (Fig 2.11). Vomiting is induced by many stimuli. Perhaps the most potent is the mechanical irritation of the pharynx. Distension of the stomach and the duodenum to a pressure of 20 mm Hg is sufficient to produce vomiting as is injury or distension of the renal pelvis, uterus or urinary bladder. A number of chemicals act on receptors in the GI

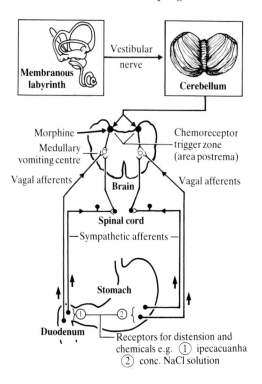

Fig. 2.11 Diagrammatic representation of some afferent pathways to the bilateral vomiting centre. Impulses from the stomach and duodenum are transmitted to the medulla via both vagal and sympathetic fibres

tract to cause vomiting e.g. strong salt solutions and ipecacuanha. However, the stomach is insensitive to some emetic agents. Thus ipecacuanha (emetine and cephaline) is ineffective in the stomach but is a powerful stimulus when it passes beyond the pylorus. Some substances e.g. morphine, induce vomiting by acting on the chemoreceptor trigger zone, a group of receptor cells in the area postrema on the floor of the 4th ventricle and connected with the true vomiting centre. The chemoreceptor trigger zone appears to be involved in the vomiting produced by radiation and by the excessive stimulation of labyrinths at a fairground or sometimes on board a ship.

Vomiting occurs in several other situations. For example, in the early weeks of pregnancy many women are affected. Presumably some metabolic change is brought about by the fetal or placental presence. The effects of nauseating smells and sickening sights need no comment. Psychological factors often aggravate the symptoms but an adjustment is usually quickly made. Finally, people locked in inescapable hostile relationships within the family may vomit when they think of disturbing experiences.

Bibliography

Boyle, J.T., Altschuler, S.M., Nixon, T.E., Pack, A.I. and Cohen, S. (1987). Responses of the feline gastroesophageal junction to changes in abdominal pressure. *American Journal of Physiology* **253**, G315–G322.

Burgen, A.S.V. and Emmelin, N.G. (1961). *Physiology of the Salivary Glands.* Edward Arnold, London.

Cook, I.J., Dodds, W.J., Dantas, R.O., *et al.* (1989). Opening mechanisms of the human upper esophageal sphincter. *American Journal of Physiology* **257**, G748–G759.

Dent, J., Holloway, R.H., Toouili, J, and Dodds, W.J. (1988). Mechanisms of lower oesophageal sphincter incompetence in patients with symptomatic gastrooesophageal reflux. *Gut* **29**, 1020–28.

Emmelin, N.G. (1987). Nerve interactions in salivary glands. *Journal of Dental Research* **66**, 509–17.

Farrell, J.H. (1956). The effect of mastication on the digestion of food. *British Dental Journal* **100**, 149–58.

Garrett, J.R. (1987). The proper role of nerves in salivary secretion: a review. *Journal of Dental Research* **66**, 387–97.

Griffith, T.N., Edwards, D.H., Collins, P., Lewis, M.J. and Henderson, A.H. (1985). Endothelial derived relaxant factor. *Journal of the Royal College of Physicians (London)* **19**, 74–9.

Hamosh, M. (1986). Lingual lipases. *Gastroenterology* **90**, 1290–92.

Jean, A. (1984). Control of the central swallowing programme by input from peripheral receptors. A review. *Journal of the Autonomic Nervous System* **10**, 225–33.

Lundberg, J.M. and Hokfelt, T. (1986). Multiple coexistence of peptides and classical transmitters in peripheral autonomic and sensory neurons – functional and pharmacological implications. In *Progress in Brain Research*, **68**, pp 241–62. Ed. by T. Hokfelt, K. Fuxe, and B. Pernow. Elsevier Science Publishers, Amsterdam.

Moffat, A.C. (1971). Absorption of drugs through the oral mucosa. In *Absorption phenomena*. Ed. by J.L. Rabinowitz and R.M. Myerson. *Topics in Medicinal Chemistry* **4**, 1–26.

Poulsen, S.S. (1987). On the role of epidermal growth factor in the defense of the gastroduodenal mucosa. *Scandinavian Journal of Gastroenterology* **22**, (S128), 20–1.

Roman, C. and Gonella, J. (1987). Extrinsic control of digestive tract motility. In *Physiology of the Gastrointestinal Tract*, 2nd edn., pp 507–53. Ed. by L.R. Johnson. Raven Press, New York.

Vanek, A.W. and Diamant, N.E. (1987). Responses of the human esophagus to paired swallows. *Gastroenterology* **92**, 643–50.

3

The Stomach

The stomach receives and can temporarily store ingested food. Acid and enzymes are secreted into its lumen. About 2 litres of gastric juice are produced daily. Muscular contractions result in the contents being mixed, partially digested and then emptied into the duodenum. The ingested material is modified in the stomach to produce a fairly uniform product as regards pH, osmolality, consistency and temperature, i.e. chyme.

Storage

The stomach can accommodate either very large or small volumes of material (5 or 0.5 litres). However, there is little change in intragastric pressure because the smooth muscle of the fundus and corpus (Fig. 3.1), those regions concerned with storage, adapt to the luminal contents. This is an example of receptive relaxation. At least two factors are involved in this response:

1. The plasticity of the smooth muscle fibres. When these fibres are stretched they either rearrange internally or slide past one another.
2. A reflex involving the vagus which produces an inhibition of smooth muscle tone in the corpus and fundus. A role for the vagus has been suggested because patients show early satiety following vagotomy.

When food is swallowed its weight is sufficient to overcome the resistance offered by the stomach wall and some passes rapidly to the antral region where mixing takes place. The remainder, in the corpus and fundus is relatively undisturbed. Salivary digestion continues, particularly at the centre of the mass. The luminal contents are arranged in layers in the order they are swallowed, the food taken first being closest to the stomach wall. This has been demonstrated by feeding rats three successive portions of bread, each differently coloured. Subsequently the animals were killed, their stomachs removed, frozen and sectioned. The coloured bread portions were distinctly separate.

(a)

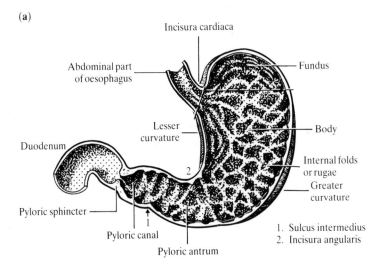

1. Sulcus intermedius
2. Incisura angularis

(b)

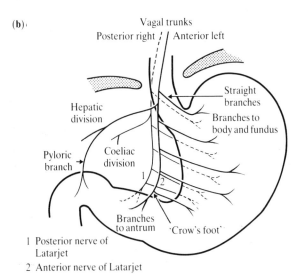

1 Posterior nerve of
  Latarjet
2 Anterior nerve of Latarjet

Fig. 3.1 Diagram showing (**a**) the regions of the stomach, its folds and its narrowing to form the pyloric sphincter; and (**b**) the vagal innervation of the stomach. The 'crow's foot' is a landmark of importance to the surgeon during operations to destroy the vagal innervation of parietal cells

Gastric secretion

The ability of the stomach to modify food was established long ago, in 1752 when Reaumur introduced tiny metal perforated containers holding food into the stomach of a tame kite. When these were regurgitated meat was found to be partially dissolved while starchy foods were unaffected.

The entire mucosal surface of the stomach is covered by columnar epithelial cells secreting an alkaline fluid containing mucus. Thus a tenacious slimy coat covers the mucosa. In the fundus, corpus and parts of the pylorus these epithelial cells extend into gastric pits, depressions into which 3–7 glands open. Several different cells can be recognized in these glands. At their opening are mucous neck cells secreting a mucus which is chemically and physically distinct from the secretion of the surface epithelial cells. The most numerous are the chief or peptic cells. These secrete pepsinogens, inactive precursors of pepsins, the first proteolytic enzymes to be encountered as food passes along the gastrointestinal tract. A third cell type, found particularly in the neck region of the gland is the oxyntic (Greek oxyntos = acid producing) or parietal cell (pertaining to a wall). Such cells contain many mitochondria, needed to provide the energy for acid secretion. The vast majority secrete no acid unless specifically stimulated. In the non-secreting state the cytoplasm is filled with tubulovesicular structures derived from the smooth endoplasmic reticulum. These elements contain the unique hydrogen ion pump and do not communicate with the relatively small apical surface membrane. However, when stimulated, parietal cells undergo remarkable structural changes (Fig. 3.2). The tubulovesicular structures coalesce and develop into deep trough-like invaginations of the apical surface, the secretory canaliculi. The surface areas of these canaliculi are increased by numerous microvilli (Fig. 3.3). When the stimulus is removed the microvilli recede, the canaliculi are less expanded and the tubulovesicular structures become more prominent. It has been calculated that in dogs the membrane surface of the parietal cells can increase ten fold when acid secretion is stimulated.

In man two other glands should be recognized. Cardiac glands, composed almost entirely of mucus-secreting cells are found in a small area surrounding the oesophagus (diameter up to 8 cm). Few chief cells can be detected. A mucus-containing secretion is also produced by the pyloric glands. This secretion also contains pepsinogens.

Hydrochloric acid

HCl is not essential for life or even adequate digestion. However, it helps in the breakdown of connective tissue and muscle fibres, activates pepsins and provides a medium of low pH in which pepsins can act. By forming soluble salts it also contributes to the absorption of calcium and iron.

Its most important role is in providing a non-specific defence mechanism. A reduction in acid secretion predisposes to infection with a variety of organisms including those responsible for typhoid and non-typhoid salmonellosis, cholera and bacillary dysentery. Furthermore, infection with the fish tapeworm, *Diphyllobothrium latum*, is more likely.

Large numbers of bacteria (over 10^6/ml as compared with considerably less than 10^5/ml) have been recorded in subjects with reduced gastric acidity. Such large numbers can increase the production of nitrites and N-nitroso-compounds. These substances may have carcinogenic potential and, therefore, increase the risk of gastric carcinoma with prolonged hyposecretion of acid.

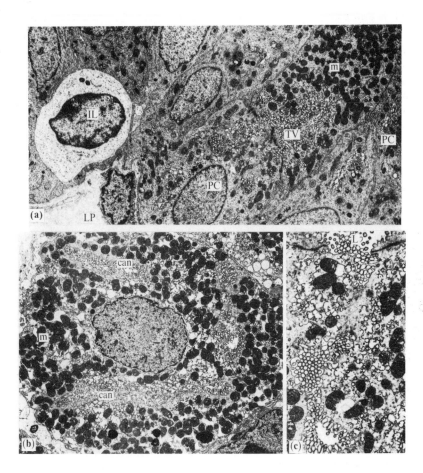

Fig. 3.2 Transmission electron micrographs of human stomach. (**a**) Unstimulated parietal cells (PC) in which tubulo-vesicular structures (TV) are prominent. An intraepithelial lymphocyte (IL), which has migrated from the lamina propria (LP), should be recognized. Lymphocytes are present throughout the gastrointestinal tract as part of the Gut Associated Lymphoid Tissue or GALT. m = mitochondria. (**b**) A stimulated parietal cell in which extensive membrane organization results in the production of canaliculi (can), a characteristic feature of the actively secreting cell. The great energy requirement of these cells is reflected by the abundant mitochondria (m) present. (**c**) A high-power micrograph of the canaliculus leading to the apical surface from which HCl is released into the lumen (L) (Kindly presented by Dr K. Kyriacou, College of Medicine, King Saud University, Riyadh, Saudi Arabia.)

At the luminal face of the secreting cells the pH measured is 0.8–1.0. No fluids of similar acidity are known in mammalian systems. The concentration of HCl produced is about 150–160 mmol/l. This represents an increase in the $[H^+]$ of more than 10^6-fold when compared with plasma. The $[Cl^-]$ gradient is smaller. Nevertheless this anion moves from a plasma concentration of 108 mmol/l to 160 mmol/l in gastric juice. In addition the mucosal surface is electrically negative with respect to the serosal surface so that energy expenditure is required to account for chloride as well as hydrogen ion transport. The two systems are

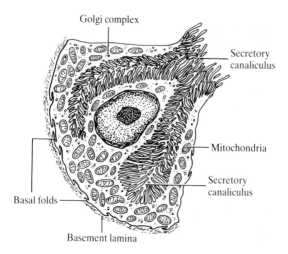

Fig. 3.3 The parietal or oxyntic cell of the gastric gland. Note the abundance of mitochondria and the deep, trough-like invaginations of the apical surface

closely coupled. The main force attracting water to the lumen is the osmotic gradient created by the active transport of hydrogen and chloride ions. A simple hypothesis of HCl secretion is presented in Fig 3.4(a).

1. Hydrogen ions derived from oxidative processes are actively secreted. Their origin is not carbonic acid.
2. At the same time hydroxyl ions are produced.
3. Carbon dioxide, derived from plasma or cellular metabolism, reacts with water to form carbonic acid. The reaction is accelerated by carbonic anhydrase, an enzyme found in abundance in the parietal cell.
4. The resulting bicarbonate is exchanged for chloride, and water is formed from interactions of protons and hydroxyl ions.

The pH of the plasma can be described by the Henderson–Hasselbalch equation:-

$$pH = 6.10 + \log_{10}[HCO_3^-]/[CO_2]$$

As carbon dioxide is removed from the plasma and bicarbonate added to it during acid secretion it follows that the gastric venous blood will be more alkaline than the arterial blood. This 'alkaline tide' may be detected by a rise in the urinary pH.

Considerable progress has been made in recent years following the discovery of a unique H^+:K^+ exchange system driven by a H^+,K^+-ATPase. This system provides a proton pump which uses the energy from ATP hydrolysis to carry out the vectorial transport of H^+ in one direction in exchange for K^+ in the reverse direction. In the secretory canaliculus there is a Cl^- channel and a KCl cotransport pathway which allows K^+ and Cl^- to leave the cell (Fig. 3.4(b)). The K^+ is recycled back into the cell by the proton pump and hydrogen secretion occurs into the canalicular space. The H^+, K^+-ATPase is in an

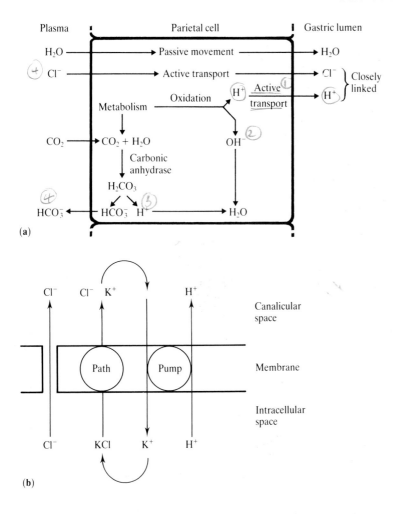

Fig. 3.4 Hydrochloric acid secretion by the parietal or oxyntic cell. (**a**) A simple hypothesis for acid secretion. (**b**) A model for HCl secretion at the canalicular membrane. The proton pump exchanges H^+ for K^+. A KCl pathway provides K^+ for this exchange. Cl^- can also reach the canalicular fluid via a separate channel

active form in both the resting and the stimulated parietal cells. Vesicles formed from membranes of resting cells do not readily transport hydrogen ions. It appears that the resting membrane lacks the carrier for KCl and that the stimulation of hydrogen transport occurs when the cotransporter is inserted into the canalicular membrane. This delivers K^+ to the apical surface for exchange.

Enzymes in gastric juice

Several enzymes hydrolysing protein are detected in gastric juice. These are the pepsins, released as inactive pepsinogens, primarily from the chief cells of the main gastric glands. Some can also be derived from the pyloric and Brunner's glands. The pepsinogens are converted to active enzymes in one of two ways. As HCl mixes with the precursors and the pH falls below 5.0, enzyme activation is initiated. In addition small amounts of pepsin act autocatalytically. The result is that several peptides are cleaved from the pepsinogen molecules (mol. wt. 42 500) to produce enzymes (mol. wt. about 35 000) with pH optima varying between 1.8 and 3.5. Human pepsins are endopeptidases. They hydrolyse several peptide bonds within the interior of ingested protein molecules to form polypeptides but little free amino acid. They have powerful milk clotting activities and take over this role from rennin, present in the calf's stomach but absent in man. Pepsins are stable only in an acid environment and are inactivated when they reach the duodenum.

A gastric lipase is also released by the stomach. It has a pH optimum between 4.5 and 5.5. Its activity decreases sharply when the pH rises above 6.5, conditions which are found in the lumen of the small intestine. Though more active against triglycerides containing short chain fatty acids, e.g. the tributyrin of butter fat contains butyric acid, it causes some hydrolysis of lipids with longer chain fatty acids. By releasing fatty acids and monoglycerides it facilitates the subsequent hydrolysis by pancreatic lipases. Furthermore when pancreatic function is compromised, e.g. in cystic fibrosis or chronic alcoholism, the gastric enzyme may contribute more significantly. Pancreatic deficiency will result in a slower neutralization of acidic intestinal contents so that the lipase remains active for a greater length of time.

Intrinsic factor

Another protein component of gastric juice is intrinsic factor. It is produced in man by parietal cells and is important because:

1. It combines with and protects vitamin B_{12} as it passes along the small intestine.
2. It adheres to ileal epithelial cells and plays a part in the absorption of the vitamin.

If vitamin B_{12} is unavailable, pernicious anaemia develops, a condition characterized by the formation of fewer but excessively large erythrocytes (macrocytic anaemia). Dietary B_{12} is protein-bound and there is sufficient to satisfy requirements, unless the individual eats no food of animal origin. The vitamin is released by cooking, gastric and pancreatic digestion and then becomes bound to intrinsic factor. Although vitamin B_{12}-intrinsic factor complex is relatively resistant to digestion, it can be utilized by some parasites, e.g. the tapeworm *Diphyllobothrium latum*, which infests fish, and by bacteria, thus producing vitamin B_{12} malabsorption and anaemia. Normally the bacterial population of the small intestine is scanty. Their numbers, however, can dramatically increase when anatomical abnormalities exist, e.g. diverticula, which produce stasis.

Stimulation of gastric secretion

Many factors influence the secretion of gastric juice. Some stimulate while others inhibit its production. Indeed, unless specifically stimulated most parietal cells are inactive. Gastric secretion may be divided into three phases depending on the region in which factors act to produce a response:

1. Cephalic phase.
2. Gastric phase.
3. Intestinal phase.

Cephalic phase

The thought or expectation of food, its sight or taste, chewing and swallowing all contribute to the cephalic phase. Thus before food reaches the stomach some fluid is secreted. The contribution of the cephalic phase was originally studied in dogs by Pavlov. The oesophagus was divided and the two ends brought to the surface of the neck (oesophagostomy). A fistula was made into the stomach so that gastric juice could be collected. Such animals could eat food but that swallowed was removed from the oesophageal fistula in the neck instead of passing to the stomach. This procedure is known as 'sham feeding' and allows the collection of pure gastric juice uncontaminated by food. The introduction of disagreeable or inert material into the mouth does not induce a secretion. Hence the cephalic phase secretion has been called 'appetite juice'.

The relative contribution of the cephalic phase total acid output must vary but in general it accounts for a significant proportion (one-third to one-half) of the acid secretion in man. Recently the role of the thought of food has been studied in human volunteers. A 30-minute intense discussion on the variety of foods preferred by the subjects, the means of their preparation and the restaurants serving these dishes caused greater acid release than the sight and smell of appetizing food.

The production of gastric juice during the cephalic phase depends on the activity of the vagus. However, the parasympathetic nerve influences gastric secretion in more than one way (Fig. 3.5):

1. Postganglionic fibres exerting a direct effect.
2. Vagal activity causing gastrin release.

Postganglionic fibres – Postganglionic fibres in the myenteric plexus innervate the gastric glands. When activated these fibres release acetylcholine which stimulates directly the secretion of pepsinogens and acid. The vagus also causes the release of the potent secretagogue histamine. It is assumed that the mast cells are, at least, one source of this histamine although endocrine-like cells have been described in the gastric mucosa which could also contribute. How might the vagus release histamine from mast cells? Are such cells innervated? The situation in the stomach is not clear although a large proportion of mucosal mast cells in the human gastrointestinal tract are closely apposed to nerves. Such a relationship may not be necessary. It has been suggested that even without true synapses autonomic nerves can exert their actions on effector cells

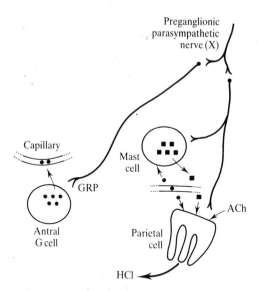

Fig. 3.5 The parasympathetic control of HCl secretion. Postganglionic fibres directly innervate parietal cells and acetylcholine (ACh) induces a secretion. They also innervate mast cells (and endocrine-like cells) releasing histamine (■), a powerful secretagogue. Furthermore antral G cells are activated to release gastrin (●). The neurotransmitter is GRP. Gastrin can act either directly on parietal cells or on those cells releasing histamine

providing the distance across which the neurotransmitter must diffuse does not exceed 100 nm.

Vagal activity – Vagal activity also causes the release of the hormone gastrin from antral G cells. (The gastrointestinal mucosa is the largest and most diverse endocrine gland in the body. However, unlike most hormone-secreting tissues the endocrine cells are not grouped together but are scattered as single cells amongst the other mucosal cells. The G cells in the antrum are concerned with the elaboration and release of gastrin.) This hormone is carried by the bloodstream to the gastric glands where it produces a direct effect on secretory cells. Like acetylcholine, it also stimulates the release of histamine. Gastrin-releasing peptide (GRP) is a strong candidate to be the neurotransmitter involved. Its discovery is an interesting story. In 1971 the tetradecapeptide bombesin was isolated from frog skin. Surprisingly, it was found to be a powerful stimulant of gastric acid secretion. Subsequently bombesin-like immunoreactivity was discovered throughout the human gastrointestinal tract and a peptide chemically and biologically homologous to bombesin was identified and named GRP. Bombesin antiserum inhibits neurally mediated gastrin release.

GRP may increase gastrin release in two ways (Fig. 3.6). A direct stimulation of the G cells has been proposed. GRP may also act indirectly by inhibiting the release of a local agent (a paracrine) thought to exert a continuous restraint on the G cell. This paracrine is somatostatin, a peptide originally isolated from the hypothalamus and recognized as a potent inhibitor of growth hormone release from the adenohypophysis (hence its name). Subsequently somatostatin has

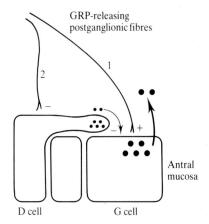

GRP-releasing
postganglionic fibres

2

1

Antral
mucosa

D cell

G cell

Fig. 3.6 Two mechanisms by which GRP may stimulate gastrin release. (1) A direct effect on antral G cells. (2) A reduction of somatostatin release. This peptide is a paracrine which exerts a continuous inhibitory effect on the G cell

been found in substantial amounts in endocrine-like cells of the gut and pancreas (D cells) and in peripheral nerves. In the stomach D cells give off long cytoplasmic processes which end on antral G cells.

Gastric secretions are increased by at least three stimuli, i.e. acetylcho- line, gastrin and histamine (Fig. 3.7). Receptors have now been described on the basolateral membranes of parietal cells for all these substances. Once the agonists binds to their receptor sites cells are activated as the result of increased intracellular concentrations of cytosolic free calcium or cyclic $3'5'$-adenosine monophosphate (cAMP). All three stimuli elevate $[Ca^{2+}]$, although whether this is due to the opening of membrane calcium channels and/or the alteration of phospholipid metabolism continues to be debated. In a variety of cells activation of membrane receptors results in the stimulation of phospholipase C and the generation of a pair of intracellular messengers. The two products are a diacylglycerol and inositol 1,4,5- triphosphate (IP_3) derived from the hydrolysis of phosphatidylinositol 4,5-bisphosphate (see page 85). The diacylglycerol remains in the membrane activating a protein kinase. As a result of this action specific proteins are phosphorylated, some of which may regulate ion channels. The IP_3 is released into the cytoplasm and liberates calcium from the endoplasmic reticulum. A number of phosphatases and kinases within the cell convert the IP_3 to additional inositol phosphates. This terminates the signalling activities of IP_3 and salvages 1D—myo-inositol for lipid resynthesis. Intracellular calcium concentrations are lowered as the ion is pumped back into the endoplasmic reticulum. The other intracellular messenger, cAMP, is released by histamine but not by gastrin or acetylcholine. Binding of histamine to its receptor activates adenylate cyclase which accelerates the conversion of ATP to cAMP. This in turn activates a protein kinase which promotes HCl secretion. The time during which cAMP can exert its effects is limited by a phosphodiesterase. This enzyme converts cAMP to $5'$-adenosine monophosphate, a product that can be metabolized to reform ATP.

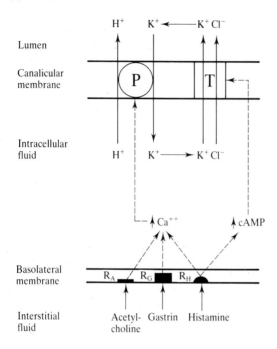

Fig. 3.7 A simple model for the control of gastric acid secretion. Acetylcholine, gastrin and histamine bind to specific receptors (R_A, R_G, and R_H) on the basolateral membranes of parietal cells. All three agonists cause $[Ca^{++}]_i$ to rise. Only histamine inceases the cellular levels of cAMP. Ca^{++} is important for the incorporation of the proton pump (P) into the canalicular membrane. The availability of the KCl pathway (T) depends on cAMP

In recent years our understanding of the processes controlling cAMP production has been advanced. The subunit catalysing cAMP production is linked to the histamine receptor by a stimulatory G protein (G_s). Binding of histamine to its receptor causes G_s to 'switch on' the adenylate cyclase activity. In contrast other receptors e.g. those recognizing prostaglandins of the E group, are linked by an inhibitory G protein (G_i) to the cAMP producing mechanism. When these are activated the adenylate cyclase is 'switched off'.

Prostaglandins of the E group are derived from polyunsaturated fatty acids, e.g. arachidonic acid, and are synthesized in the stomach. It has been suggested that such substances are released on feeding and may contribute to a feedback inhibition of acid secretion. The question remains as to how the two intracellular messengers contribute to acid secretion. Both are important. The increased $[Ca^{++}]$ allows the migration of the proton pump from cytoplasmic vesicles to the canalicular membrane. The cAMP, on the other hand, is necessary for the provision of the KCl pathway without which a supply of K^+ at the luminal surface is not available for $H^+:K^+$ exchange.

Gastric phase

The presence of food in the stomach produces an increase in gastric juice secretion both chemically and mechanically (by distension). The latter was described by William Beaumont, an American army surgeon. He was the first to study adequately human gastric secretion. His subject was Alexis St. Martin, an employee of a fur-trading company, who had suffered an accidental shotgun wound and subsequently presented a permanent gastric fistula. Contributions of both nervous and hormonal systems have been established using stomach pouches (Fig. 3.8).

The Heidenhain pouch. – This is produced from the midportion of the greater curvature of the stomach. The vagal branches to it were severed. Many have considered it, therefore, a vagally denervated pouch and used it to determine the contribution of the hormonal component of gastric secretion. However, this assumption is not strictly valid, as some vagal input remains from those branches accompanying the sympathetic nerves along the blood vessels.

The Pavlov pouch. – In this preparation a more complete vagal innervation is preserved. The same region of the stomach was used as in the Heidenhain preparation. However, the pouch was in nervous and vascular continuity with the remainder of the stomach, as the two regions were separated only by a surgically introduced double mucosal septum.

Farrel and Ivy pouch. – A completely denervated preparation was introduced in 1926 by transplanting a pouch into the mammary gland region of the abdominal wall.

At least four components of the gastric phase have now been described.

1. A local reflex in response to distension and not involving the central nervous system.
2. A vago-vagal reflex produced by mechanical stimulation. A significant contribution of this mechanism to gastric secretion is indicated by the finding that vagotomy decreases the acid output in response to distension by more than 80 per cent.
3. A second local reflex, the result of which is that gastrin is released.
4. The chemical stimulation of gastrin release. Many substances produce a secretory response when introduced into the stomach. Proteins are among

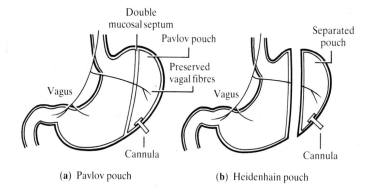

(a) Pavlov pouch　　　　　(b) Heidenhain pouch

Fig. 3.8 Types of gastric pouch. (**a**) Pavlov pouch, in which a vagal innervation is preserved. By forming a double mucosal septum to separate the pouch from the remainder of the stomach, vagal fibres running deep to the mucosa are not destroyed. (**b**) Heidenhain pouch, in which all vagal fibres were thought to be severed

the most effective. However, their potency may be partially explained in terms of their ability to buffer the gastric contents. Proteins themselves are poor stimulants although peptic hydrolysates of these macromolecules and individual amino acids are potent secretagogues. Bile acids, short chain fatty acids and ethanol also increase gastrin release.

Recently the effects of alcohol on acid secretion and gastrin release have been questioned. High concentrations of alcohol, as found in French cognac and scotch whisky had no stimulatory effects on the secretions of heathy volunteers. On the other hand, more dilute alcoholic beverages (beer and white wine) were powerful stimulants, producing greater responses than those observed with ethanol alone (under 4 per cent v/v). It has been concluded that non-alcoholic constituents, as yet unidentified, of beer and white wine must contribute appreciably.

Intestinal phase

Approximately 5 per cent of the acid secreted in the response to a meal is accounted for by the intestinal phase of secretion. Its existence has been demonstrated by introducing food directly into the duodenum and measuring the secretions of denervated pouches. The precise mechanism is unknown although gastrin, detected in the duodenal wall in concentrations almost as high as those in the stomach, may have a role to play. Gastric secretion observed when food has been emptied from the stomach may be largely dependent on the effects of absorbed amino acids on parietal cells. Certainly intravenously infused amino acids provide a potent stimulus for acid production.

The action of nerves and hormones on gastric secretion

More information has been available on the mechanisms controlling acid secretion presumably because of the relative ease with which measurements could be made. It has been noted that acetylcholine and gastrin act directly on parietal cells and indirectly by releasing histamine to increase acid secretion. One should ask whether:

1. Other cells contributing to gastric secretions are similarly affected.
2. The blood supply to the mucosa is altered. This circulation is so important for the provision of nutrients and secretory components and for the removal of waste products.

As regards pepsinogen secretion cholinergic agents, histamine and gastrin are all effective. Not all agents, however, modify enzyme and acid secretion in parallel. Thus CCK has been shown to be a potent pepsigogue despite its inability to alter acid secretion.

Less than 0.5 per cent of the cardiac output flows to the non-secreting stomach. In contrast up to 20 per cent is supplied to the active organ. Doubtlessly several mechanisms contribute to this huge increase in bloodflow including VIP released from postganglionic parasympathetic fibres and local metabolites accumulating in the secreting tissues.

Histamine and acid secretion

Whatever its physiological role histamine has been a valuable tool for assessing the capacity of the stomach to secrete acid. In 1953 Kay realized that although histamine has several actions its effects on gastric secretion were unopposed by the then available antihistamines and introduced the augmented histamine test. Patients were given antihistamines to protect them against the distressing side-effects of histamine (e.g. severe headache, bronchospasm and shock) and then given histamine in doses sufficient to produce a maximum secretory response. The histamine-related substance betazole avoids the need for antihistamines, which may have their own undesirable side-effects, by having a more pronounced effect on gastric secretion. Since 1966 pentagastrin, a synthetic derivative of gastrin containing the active C-terminal tetrapeptide of pig gastrin, has been used as an alternative to histamine or betazole.

The question must be asked as to why gastric secretion is unaffected by many antihistamines. It has now been established that histamine receptors in various tissues fall into two categories. Those involved in smooth muscle contractions, e.g. bronchi and gut, are classified as H-1, whereas H-2 receptors, insensitive to H-1 antagonists, are concerned with gastric secretion.

A number of disorders are associated with abnormally high acid secretion rates. One of these is the Zollinger–Ellison syndrome where non β-islet cell tumours release gastrin. A considerable proportion of those with duodenal ulcer also have greater than normal secretory rates. Clearly it would be an advantage for patients with these conditions if acid secretions could be effectively suppressed (or alternatively if the resistance of the gastrointestinal mucosa to acid could be improved). To do this several different approaches have been tried. Specific H-2 receptor antagonists, such as cimetidine and ranitidine, have been made available which significantly reduce the secretions stimulated by gastrin and cholinergic mechanisms. These agents act by blocking the H-2 receptors on the basolateral membranes of parietal cells.

A more recent approach has been to antagonise the proton pump on the apical membrane. This can be done with substituted benzimidazoles, e.g. omeprazole. These are weak bases with pKa values of approximately 4. In relatively neutral environments omeprazole can readily cross cell membranes but is inactive. When the parietal cell is stimulated to secrete HCl the pH of the canalicular fluid is about 1.0. The omeprazole is trapped and accumulates, therefore, in this fluid. Furthermore, it is activated by acid and as a result inhibits the proton pump. When the canalicular fluid loses its acidity omeprazole no longer specifically accumulates at that site and any omeprazole which is there is inactivated. Thus substituted benzimidazoles have their own negative feedback mechanism.

Insulin and acid secretion

Over 50 years ago intravenous insulin was found to be a stimulus for gastric secretion. The response to insulin is not a simple one (Fig. 3.9). Hypoglycaemia results in changes in hypothalamic activities and effects mediated by the parasympathetic and sympathetic nervous systems and the adrenal cortex.

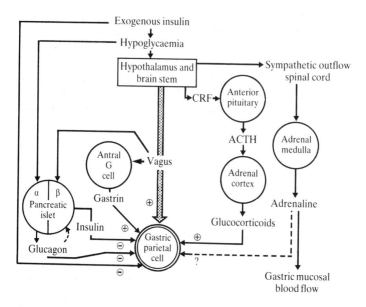

Fig. 3.9 Pathways by which insulin may exert an influence on acid secretion by the stomach. CRF = Corticotrophin-releasing factor; ACTH = Adrenocorticotrophic hormone; + and − = stimulation and inhibition respectively (From Hodge, A.J., Masarei, J.R. and Catchpole, B.N. (1972). *Gut* **13**, 341–5.)

Nevertheless, after vagotomy gastric secretion is markedly reduced and insulin tests have been devised to assess the completeness of vagal denervation after surgery.

Inhibition of gastric secretion.

One can describe cephalic, gastric and intestinal phases for the inhibition as well as the stimulation of acid and pepsinogen release.

Cephalic inhibition

Our understanding of cephalic inhibition in man has been influenced by observations on those patients with a gastric fistula. Perhaps the most famous patient was Tom. As a 9 year old, Tom swallowed scolding hot clam chowder after guessing incorrectly the contents of a cooled beer pail. The resulting burned surfaces of his oesophagus could not be prevented from growing together. It became necessary, therefore, to create an opening through the abdominal wall to his stomach so that he could be fed. Subsequently, observations were made of the mucosa and it was found that its colour, wetness and turgidity were correlated to Tom's mood. The mucosa appeared pale, dry and thin (gastric hypoactivity) when Tom was depressed or frightened. This contrasted with a scarlet, turgid mucosa (hyperactivity) associated with excitement and anger.

If thinking about food significantly increases gastric secretion then by encouraging different thoughts it would seem possible that acid secretion could be reduced. A non-pharmacological, self-induced altered state of consciousness lowering acid secretion would be an advantage for those hypersecreting and, therefore, at greater risk of ulcer formation. Recently, Klein and Spiegal (1989) have reported that when highly hypnotizable volunteers are instructed to experience deep relaxation their acid secretions were inhibited. Would similar responses have been achieved with yoga or with religious practices that include meditative prayer.

Gastric inhibition

A mechanism exists whereby excessive acid secretion is prevented. As the intragastric pH falls below 2.5 the release of gastrin is reduced. It is thought that acid acts directly on the G-cells and terminates the gastric phase of gastric secretion. A second mechanism has been proposed. Acid produced by parietal cells stimulates the release of somatostatin from nearby cells in the gland. The peptide acts as a paracrine to inhibit further acid formation. This concept is supported by the finding that gastric acid secretion stimulated by pentagastrin is inhibited by the somatostatin analogue SMS 201-995 in man (Fig. 3.10).

During the interdigestive period the volume of the stomach contents is small but acidic. Little further secretion occurs. The introduction of more food into the stomach dilutes and neutralizes the acid present, thus removing the inhibition and allowing the cephalic and gastric phases of secretion to operate.

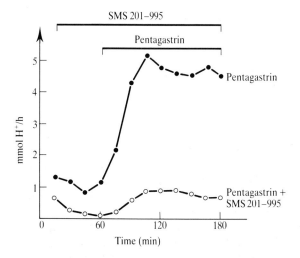

Fig. 3.10 Basal and pentagastrin (150 ng/kg/h) stimulated gastric acid secretion without and during the infusion of the somatostatin analogue SMS 201-995 (50 pmol/kg/h). These studies were conducted with healthy volunteers (From Olsen, J.A., Loud, F.B. and Christiansen, J. (1987). *Gut* **28**, 464-7.)

Intestinal inhibition

When chyme appears in the duodenum acid secretion decreases. Thus a negative feedback system is available which helps to prevent overloading of the small intestine with acid contents. Hypertonic solutions and fats introduced intraluminally also inhibit acid secretions. As secretory activity of denervated pouches is modified by these factors a hormonal mechanism is thought to be involved. The term enterogastrone was introduced to describe a hypothetical hormone released from the small intestine. Several hormones including secretin, CCK, GIP and VIP, when given in pharmacological doses, inhibit gastric secretion. Perhaps a combination of these will be a 'physiological enterogastrone'.

The question remains as to how a 'physiological enterogastrone' might produce its effects. One possibility is that the hormone releases somatostatin, a powerful inhibitor of acid secretion, from gastric glands. Of the putative enterogastrones listed above CCK, at least, has receptors on fundic mucosal cells and stimulates somatostatin release from the stomach.

Protection of the gastric mucosa

The stomach frequently contains a potentially corrosive mixture of HCl and pepsins. Clearly mechanisms must be available to prevent the destruction of the mucosa (Fig. 3.11). Some protection is afforded against endogenous aggressors by the mucus and bicarbonate released from mucosal cells. In the stomach an electroneutral $Cl^-:HCO_3^-$ exchange mechanism accounts for bicarbonate secretion. Mucus forms a water-insoluble gel that adheres to the

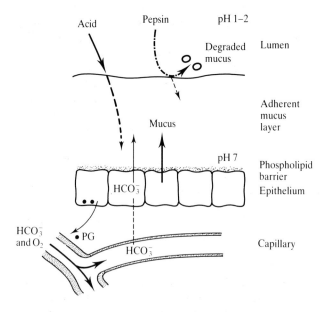

Fig. 3.11 The mucus–bicarbonate barrier for the protection of the gastric mucosa against acid and pepsins

luminal surface. In man this layer is of variable thickness (5–200 μm). It significantly reduces the flow of hydrogen ions and provides a permeability barrier to pepsins. The bicarbonate would be ineffective against the larger volumes of acid in the lumen. Nevertheless, small volumes within the mucous layer have buffering capacity against the luminal acid and create a more neutral environment at the cell surface. Mucus can be degraded by pepsins. However, the bicarbonate in the mucous gel raises the pH and so produces an environment in which the proteolytic enzymes are less active.

Even if agents penetrate the surface gel and damage the underlying epithelium mucus still has a role to play. It acts as a template for the conversion of fibrinogen with the result that a fibrin gel coat containing mucus and necrotic cells can be formed. This layer is approximately ten times thicker than the one normally measured. Under such a barrier repair is possible providing the vasculature is intact and epithelial cells have retained their capacity to migrate to the damaged areas.

Bicarbonate and mucus release are controlled, in part, by factors that normally control gastric secretion. Thus:

1. Sham feeding (cephalic phase) activates the vagus and elicits both an acid secretion and an increased release of mucus and bicarbonate.
2. Local nerve reflexes (cholinergic) contribute to an increased bicarbonate output following gastric distension.

In addition other local control mechanisms are involved, e.g. luminal acidity markedly accelerates (although bile acids inhibit) bicarbonate secretion. Perhaps luminal acid induces the synthesis and release of prostaglandins from the gastric mucosa. These paracrines are potent stimulants of bicarbonate release. However, prostaglandins have a number of other roles, an important one being to preserve microvascular continuity. By causing vasodilatation prostaglandins not only enhance the supply of essential nutrients but also provide bicarbonate to neutralize temporarily any damaged mucosa and allow time for repair.

Mucus and bicarbonate are not the only factors protecting the gastric mucosa. While these agents offer a first line of defence against gastric juice their contribution is thought to be overwhelmed when the luminal pH falls below 1.5. This frequently occurs. Furthermore mucus and bicarbonate provide little defence against exogenous factors such as ethanol and non-steroidal anti-inflammatory drugs (NSAIDs). The latter are of considerable value for patients with arthritis. So what are these other factors? One that has received attention are the mucosal phospholipids. These are hydrophobic and contribute to the low permeability of the epithelium to hydrogen ions. Indeed it has been suggested that complete neutralization at the cell membrane may be unnecessary, and that the main function of bicarbonate is probably the maintenance of intracellular pH. If these phospholipids are of such value it may be that natural foods containing similar substances can be identified. Their ingestion might provide valuable additional protection particularly for subjects with gastric ulcers. These patients often do not secrete acid excessively. A potentially useful fruit is the banana which offers substantial protection, in the rat stomach, at least, by forming an adsorbed layer of surface active phospholipid.

Absorption

The rapidity with which hydrocyanic acid produces its effects in animal experiments, even when the pylorus is obstructed, indicates that some absorption can take place from the stomach. In general it is thought that the gastric absorption of water-soluble substances is unimportant. An exception is ethyl alcohol, although its movement to the blood stream depends on its lipid solubility, which allows it to diffuse rapidly through the lipoprotein membranes of the mucosal cells.

Several organic substances can be absorbed, depending on the pH of the luminal contents. Such substances are un-ionized, fat-soluble and absorbable at one pH but ionized, water-soluble and virtually unabsorbed at another. Take as an example aspirin or acetylsalicylic acid (Fig 3.12). The dissociation constant (pKa) of the acid group is 3.5. Thus in highly acid intraluminal contents the aspirin molecules are mainly in the un-ionized, fat-soluble form and these can diffuse across the mucosal membrane. The pH of the environment beyond this barrier is nearly neutral. Thus most aspirin molecules are converted to the ionized form which is unable to diffuse back to the lumen. Furthermore, this conversion allows the concentration gradient between the lumen and the cell to be maintained and aspirin can continue to be absorbed.

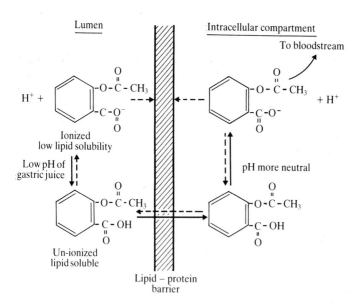

Fig. 3.12 The absorption of aspirin (acetylsalicyclic acid) from the lumen of the stomach. At low pH aspirin is present mainly in the un-ionized lipid-soluble form and it can penetrate the lipid membranes of the lining cells. Inside the cells where pH is closer to neutral, the ionized water-soluble form is produced which is trapped and not able to pass back towards the lumen. (After Davenport, H,W. (1977). *Physiology of the Digestive Tract*, 4th Edn. Year Book Medical Publishers, Chicago.)

Gastric motility

The stomach grinds food, mixes it with gastric juice and then empties it into the duodenum at a suitable rate. This organ can be divided conveniently into two parts:

1. The cephalad region or proximal stomach = corpus + fundus.
2. The caudad region or distal stomach = distal corpus + antrum.

There is little mixing in the former, this being the storage region. Mixing requires the contractions of the caudad region. Such contractions contribute to gastric emptying but are only one of the factors involved. Emptying also depends on the viscosity of the gastric contents, the tone of the gastric muscle in the proximal stomach, the patency of the pyloroduodenal region and the vigour of the duodenal contractions.

When the stomach is empty it is small and relaxed and only feeble muscle contractions occur. If the subject becomes hungry, waves of contraction can be detected and pangs of hunger are often experienced. The correlation of hunger with stomach contractions is, however, poor.

When the stomach is full, peristaltic waves begin high on the greater curvature and spread towards the antrum at the rate of 3 per minute. During the first hour of digestion these waves are shallow over both corpus and antrum. Subsequently some waves deepen near the incisura angularis and the gastric contents are pushed ahead. The pressure in the antrum increases as more of the viscous contents are pushed into it by the peristaltic wave. As a result some of the antral content is squirted into the duodenum beyond the pyloric sphincter.

The antral lumen is not occluded by the peristaltic wave, so that some contents are propelled back into the proximal stomach (Fig. 3.13) and more effectively mixed. The terminal parts of the pylorus and antrum contract almost simultaneously, an event known as 'the systolic contraction of the terminal segment'. The result is that expulsion of more antral content into the duodenum is prevented. The terminal segment subsequently relaxes until the next peristaltic wave arrives.

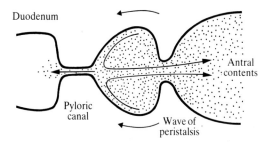

Fig. 3.13 The concept of antral mixing. The antral lumen is not occluded by peristaltic waves and some contents are propelled back towards the body of the stomach and are more effectively mixed

Control of gastric motility

Gastric motility results from the coordinated contractions of smooth muscle cells arranged in three layers – the outer longitudinal, the middle circular and the inner oblique – none of which completely overlap. The stomach is richly innervated with both intrinsic and extrinsic nerves. Cell bodies of the former lie in plexuses, the most prominent of which is the myenteric plexus present within the circular muscle layer. Intrinsic nerve cells synapse with other intrinsic neurons and with extrinsic fibres. The extrinsic innervation includes postganglionic sympathetic fibres originating in the coeliac plexus and preganglionic parasympathetic fibres of the vagus. Four factors may alter the force and frequency of muscle contractions :

1. Myogenic properties of smooth muscles themselves.
2. Neural activity of intrinsic nerves.
3. Neural activity of extrinsic nerves.
4. Chemical properties of locally released agents or hormones from more distant sites.

The frequency of peristalic contractions depends on an electrical event originating in the cells of the longitudinal muscle layer. The event, a rhythmical depolarization and repolarization of the resting membrane potential (5–15 mV), does not occur simultaneously over the caudad stomach (Fig. 3.14). Rather, it seems to pass from a point on the greater curvature towards both the lesser curvature and the pyloric region. The terms basic electrical rhythm (BER), slow wave and pacesetter potential have been used to describe it. The BER is always measured whether or not peristaltic waves can be detected. There is, however, a relationship between BER and peristalsis in that action potentials correlating

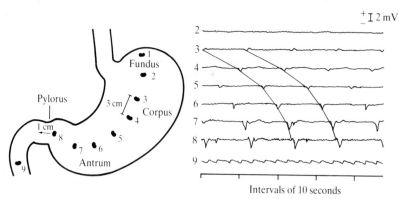

Intervals of 10 seconds

Fig. 3.14 Recordings of gastric and duodenal electrical activity from electrodes placed at equal intervals on the surface of the stomach of a dog. The pacesetter potential is detected by an electrode on the corpus and by all others cauded to it. The amplitude was greater in the antrum but the frequency was the same at the different sites. The velocity of the pacesetter potential (as indicated by the slope of the lines connecting a cycle) increased as it approached the pylorus (From Kelly, K.A., Code, C.F. and Elveback, L.R. (1969). *American Journal of Physiology* **217**, 461–70.)

with peristalsis coincide with the maximum depolarization of the BER, i.e. when the smooth muscle is at its most excitable. Thus the BER sets the frequency of peristalsis. This is fairly constant, although it can be increased by gastrin. The force of contraction depends on both hormonal and neural mechanisms. Gastrin, motilin (a polypeptide isolated from the small intestine) and vagal activity all increase this force while other hormones, e.g. secretin, inhibit contractions.

Control of gastric motility – relaxation and inhibition

Neural mechanisms have been described which when stimulated result in responses other than an increased force of contraction of gastric smooth muscle. Thus there exist :

1. Vagal relaxatory fibres which induce profound muscle relaxation and increase the volume of the corpus and fundus. Oesophageal and gastric distension and swallowing produce this relaxation. The identity of the neurotransmitter involved has been controversial. Evidence supporting a role for VIP (peptidergic) and ATP (purinergic) has been presented. Perhaps multiple mechanisms rather than a single process are involved.

2. Sympathetic adrenergic fibres which inhibit gastric motility. Initially it was thought that such fibres acted directly on the stomach muscle. However, if vagal cholinergic fibres are inactive the adrenergic fibres have little effect. Nevertheless motility induced by the vagus is inhibited by the stimulation of splanchnic nerves. These observations have led to the view that adrenergic nerve fibres have a ganglionic site of action.

What is the significance of these two mechanisms? When gastric distension results in the activation of vagal afferent and efferent fibres gastric smooth muscle can elongate. Thus food can be accommodated without increasing the intragastric pressure. At the same time vagal cholinergic fibres induce mixing and some emptying. In contrast the adrenergic mechanism inhibits gastric motility. Distension of the small intestine is one of the stimuli which reflexly activates the mechanism. Thus there is slowing down of the mixing process and inhibition of emptying. Such an inhibitory reflex prevents even greater intestinal distension.

Gastric emptying

The rate at which gastric contents pass into the duodenum depends on their chemical and physical characteristics. The following should be noted.

Contractions of the proximal stomach

For the emptying of liquids the slow sustained contractions of the proximal stomach make an important contribution. These contractions are reduced by swallowing and the gastric distension resulting from food ingestion. Nevertheless they provide gastric tone which can increase the pressure gradient between the stomach and the duodenum. If the pyloric sphincter is not closed liquids may be propelled from the stomach.

A basal tone of the proximal stomach, dependent on vagal cholinergic activity has been described. It is not constant. Changes are recorded which correlate with the cyclical electrical events occurring during fasting. Two hormones, gastrin and CCK, inhibit the contractions of the proximal stomach and the gastric emptying of liquids. The effect of gastrin may not be physiological. Nevertheless, it is interesting that gastrin can promote relaxation of proximal gastric smooth muscle while increasing the rate and force of contraction of the antral region and contribute to the production of chyme. A role for CCK can be readily conceived. This peptide is released from the small intestine by the products of fat and protein digestion. The inhibitory effects of intraluminal lipid on gastric emptying are well established.

Gastric tone is not easy to monitor but recently has been cleverly assessed in man using a 'gastric barostat'. This instrument measures the change in volume of the proximal stomach by determining the volume of air that has to be withdrawn or introduced into an intragastric ultrathin polythene bag to maintain the pressure within the bag at a constant preselected level. Withdrawal of air and a reduction in bag volume reflects an increase in tone, i.e. a contraction of the proximal stomach. While gastric tone is important for the emptying of liquids it has but a minor role for the emptying of solids. Indeed, digestible solids are normally not emptied at all. The contractions of the distal stomach are designed to titurate solid contents thoroughly. The solid fragments of food are reduced in size to a diameter of less than 1 mm. These become suspended in the liquid phase of the gastric contents and emptied as part of this phase. This would suggest that solid indigestible materials are not readily emptied from the stomach. Evidence supporting this concept has been obtained from studies in which small plastic spheres, 7 mm diameter and with a specific gravity similar to that of gastric juice, were introduced into the stomach of fasting dogs. The spheres remained quiescent in the stomach for 1–2 hours. Subsequently within a short time (20 minutes) all the plastic spheres were emptied. The removal of the spheres from the stomach could be correlated with the intense bursts of action potentials and contractions that form a part of the cycle of mechanical and electrical events repeated during the interdigestive period (see page 195).

To summarize: if digestible and indigestible foods are ingested fasting patterns of gastric motility are abolished. Liquids are emptied along with digestible solids which have been reduced in size so that they form a suspension. When this has been completed a fasting pattern of contractions is again introduced and the stomach rids itself of the indigestible debris left over from the meal.

Gastric volume

The greater the volume of the gastric contents the faster the rate of emptying. If one plots the logarithm of the volume of stomach contents remaining against time, an approximately linear relationship can be seen. In other words the stomach pumps into the duodenum a volume that is a relatively constant proportion of the contents remaining.

Osmolarity of chyme

The osmolarity of chyme entering the duodenum has a marked effect on subsequent gastric emptying. Sodium chloride solution (200 mosmol/kg) is the most rapidly emptied and solutions of greater or reduced osmolality remain in the stomach for a longer period. It has been suggested that osmoreceptors, shrinking and swelling to hyper- and hypotonicity, exist in the proximal small intestine. They must be localized deep to the brush border, because on a molar basis disaccharides are twice as effective as monosaccharides. The inhibitory effects of several amino acids have been explained in terms of their osmotic properties. This may not be the complete story, however, as tryptophan, at concentrations which may occur under physiological conditions (2–5 mmol/l), delays emptying.

Fats in the upper intestine

The presence of fats and their digestive products in the upper small intestine inhibits gastric emptying. Fatty acids are more potent than triglycerides, and myristic acid (C–14) was the most effective of the range tested (C–2 to C–18).

Acid in the small intestine

Acid in the small intestine delays gastric emptying. NB. The acidity of the duodenal contents depends not only on the acid released from the stomach but also on the secretions of the liver and the pancreas which have neutralizing effects. A receptor has been envisaged (Fig. 3.15) which is capable of detecting acid at pH under 6.5. It is proposed that:

1. Acid enters a titration chamber and the pH is maintained at 6.5 by chloride and bicarbonate exchange.

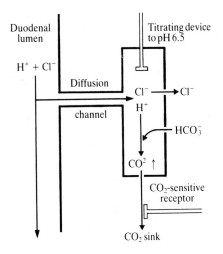

Fig. 3.15 A duodenal receptor sensitive to the acidification of the luminal contents (From Hunt, J.N. and Knox, M.T. (1972). *Journal of Physiology* **222**, 187–208.)

2. The resultant increase in the partial pressure of CO_2 is detected as it diffuses out of the titration chamber and into a CO_2 sink.

Cold liquids

Very cold liquids (4°C) in the form of isosmotic orange juice are emptied more slowly than the same fluids as 37°C. This can be demonstrated during the first half hour after drinking cold fluids during which time the temperature of the intragastric contents warms to body temperature. These findings point to a possible role for the puzzling thermoreceptors detected in the antrum and duodenum the stimulation of which results in greater activity of vagal afferent fibres.

Clearly many substances present in the duodenal contents inhibit gastric emptying. In some instances sectioning the vagi reduces the response. The term enterogastric reflex has been used to describe these events. Several substances, particularly fat, still exert an effect following vagotomy and a hormonal mechanism is considered likely. The inhibitors released have been described as enterogastrones. Whether they represent a mixture of the hormones already discovered or new ones yet to be chemically identified is not known. A putative list includes secretin, somatostatin, gastrin and CCK.

Other factors

Gastric contractions are not the only factors important in the control of gastric emptying. Others that must be considered are as follows.

The sphincteric activity of the gastroduodenal junction

During fasting pyloric tone is either absent or detected only intermittently in man. However, the direct infusion of a lipid emulsion into the duodenum stimulates basal tone and induces phasic pyloric contractions (isolated pyloric pressure waves or IPPWs). These events obstruct transpyloric flow and so delay gastric emptying. Hypertonic glucose solutions also modify pyloric motility. An intraduodenal delivery of glucose at rates exceeding 2.1 kcal/min (8.8 kJ/min) stimulates both phasic and tonic contractions in dose dependent manners. These findings may help to explain why glucose solutions in the range 5–25 g/100ml (0.28–1.39 mmol/l) are emptied from the human stomach at a constant caloric rate (2.1 kcal/minute (8.8 kJ/min)).

The neural mechanisms controlling pyloric motility are not well understood. Basal tone and phasic contractions persist after treatment with tetrodotoxin (TTX – the puffer fish poison which selectively blocks the increase in sodium permeability associated with the depolarization phase of the action potential). They may, therefore, be predominantly myogenic in origin.

Neural mechanisms can alter pyloric motility. The vagi contain fibres which can both excite and inhibit the pylorus. Intrinsic pathways have also been described. One may involve cholinergic neurons from the duodenum. The activation of the pylorus by the intraduodenal infusion of HCl is completely abolished by atropine. In contrast stimulation of antral intramural nerves by antral contractions elicits a very powerful inhibitory effect on pyloric motor function.

Contractions of the proximal duodenum and their relationship with those of the stomach

Gastrointestinal contents are likely to move from a region of contractile activity to an inactive zone. Thus liquid test meals which empty rapidly have been found to increase gastric contractions while having little effect on duodenal activity. On the other hand, those meals that only slowly leave the stomach have the opposite effects (Fig. 3.16). Increased intestinal motility could result in the reflux of duodenal contents. Even the simplest meals taken probably induce duodenal motor responses by stimulating duodenal osmoreceptors. As the osmolalities of some foods, e.g. seasoned soups and stews, may exceed 1500 mosmol/kg the motor responses may make an important contribution to the postpyloric resistance controlling normal gastric emptying.

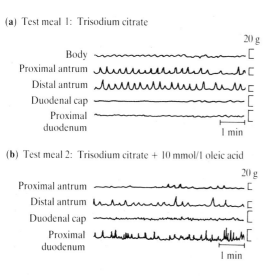

(a) Test meal 1: Trisodium citrate

Body
Proximal antrum
Distal antrum
Duodenal cap
Proximal duodenum

1 min

(b) Test meal 2: Trisodium citrate + 10 mmol/l oleic acid

Proximal antrum
Distal antrum
Duodenal cap
Proximal duodenum

1 min

Fig. 3.16 Contractile patterns of the stomach and duodenum elicited by two test meals. (**a**) Test meal 1, trisodium citrate; (**b**) test meal 2, trisodium citrate plus 10 mmol/l oleic acid. Measurements were made on unanaesthetized dogs (beagles). 300 ml test meal (200 mosmol/l)were administered by stomach pump and contractile activity was measured using extraluminal strain gauge force transducers. Note the relatively high antral and low duodenal activity elicited by the citrate test meal and the opposite relationship induced by the addition of fatty acid (From Weisbrodt, N.W., Wiley, J.N., Overholt, B.F. and Bass, P. (1969). *Gut* **10**, 543–8.)

Bibliography

Allen, A., Hutton, D.A., Leonard, A.J., Pearson, J.P. and Sellers, L.A. (1986). The role of mucus in the protection of the gastric mucosa. *Scandinavian Journal of Gastroenterology* **21 (S125)**, 71–7.

Aspiroz, F. and Malagelada, J.R. (1987). Gastric tone measured by electronic barostat in health and postsurgical gastroparesis. *Gastroenterology* **92**, 934–43.

Bengtsson, P., Lundqvist, G. and Nilsson, G. (1989). Inhibition of acid formation and stimulation of somatostatin release by cholecystokinin–related peptides in rabbit gastric glands. *Journal of Physiology* **419**, 765–74.

Berridge, M.J. (1984). Inositol triphosphate, a novel second messenger in cellular signal transduction. *Nature (London)* **312**, 315–21.

Crampton, J.R. (1988). Gastroduodenal mucus and bicarbonate: the defensive zone. *Quarterly Journal of Medicine* **67**, 269–72.

Feldman, M. and Richardson, C.T. (1986). Role of thought, sight, smell and taste of food in the cephalic phase of gastric acid secretion in humans. *Gastroenterology* **90**, 428–33.

Heddle, R., Fone, D., Dent, J. and Horowitz, M. (1988). Stimulation of pyloric motility by intraduodenal dextrose in normal subjects. *Gut* **29**, 1349–57.

Hills, B.A. and Kirkwood, C.A. (1989). Surfactant approach to the gastric mucosal barrier: protection of rats by banana even when acidified. *Gastroenterology* **97** 294–303.

Howden, C.W. and Hunt, R.N. (1987). Gastric secretion and infection. *Gut* **28**, 96–107.

Kay, A.W. (1953). Effect of large doses of histamine on gastric secretion of HCl: the augmented histamine test. *British Medical Journal* ii, 77–80.

Kelly, K.A. (1984). Gastric emptying of liquids and solids: roles of proximal and distal stomach. *American Journal of Physiology* **239**, G71–G76.

Klein, K.B. and Spiegal, D. (1989). Modulation of gastric acid secretion by hypnosis. *Gastroenterology* **96**, 1383–7.

Minami, H. and McCallum, R.W. (1984). The physiology and pathophysiology of gastric emptying in humans. *Gastroenterology* **86**, 1592–1610.

Sachs, G. and Wallmark, B. (1989). The gastric H^+, K^+, ATPase: the site of action of omeprazole. *Scandinavian Journal of Gastroenterology* **24 (S166)**, 3–11.

Schubert, M.L., Edwards, N.F. and Makhlouf, G.M. (1988). Regulation of gastric somatostatin secretion in the mouse by luminal acidity. *Gastroenterology* **94**, 317–22.

Starlinger, M. and Schiessel, R. (1988). Bicarbonate (HCO_3) delivery to the gastroduodenal mucosa by the blood: its importance for mucosal integrity. *Gut* **29**, 647–54.

Thompson, D.G. and Wingate, D.L. (1988). Effects of osmoreceptor stimulation on human duodenal motor activity. *Gut* **29**, 173–80.

Tovey, P. (1979). Peptic ulcer in India and Bangladesh. *Gut* **20**, 329–47.

Wolf, S. (1965). *The Stomach*. Oxford University Press, New York.

Wolfe, M.M. and Soll, A.H. (1988). The physiology of gastric acid secretion. *New England Journal of Medicine*, **319**, 1707–15.

4

Liver and secretions of pancreas and duodenum

Chyme is emptied into the small intestine and secretions from the liver and pancreas are mixed with it. In this chapter these secretions are described. In addition, a short and incomplete account of other liver functions is presented. No space is given to the secretions of the small intestine at this stage other than those of the glands of Brunner. At one time this would have been thought strange as the succus entericus was thought to contain many of the enzymes involved in the final stages of digestion. That this is not so will become apparent, and intestinal secretion will be considered while discussing the handling of water and electrolytes by the small intestine (see Chapter 5).

The glands of Brunner

These duodenal glands are detected at various distances from the pylorus. In the young they can extend into the jejunum. They are usually located submucosally beneath the muscularis mucosa. However, they can be observed in the lamina propria near the pylorus. Their secretion has been described as a viscous, mucus-rich, alkaline fluid probably containing epidermal growth factor. Such a fluid could make a valuable contribution by protecting the duodenum from the actions of gastric acid and pepsins. The glands do secrete mucus. Whether they are the source of the bicarbonate giving duodenal secretions their alkalinity is less certain. Bicarbonate can be released from the surface epithelium.

A spontaneous secretion is thought to be produced. The release of bicarbonate is increased by the introduction of gastric juice into the duodenum. Part of this response is humorally mediated. Secretin is a strong candidate, being an effective stimulant of duodenal secretions. Endogenous prostaglandins also play a role, particularly when the intraduodenal contents are highly acidic (e.g. pH = 2.0). The large bicarbonate secretion induced under these conditions is reduced by aspirin.

Neural mechanisms have also been reported. When the vagus nerves of a cat are electrically stimulated gastric acid secretion is increased. This is accompanied by a greater duodenal bicarbonate release, an event only partially inhibited by atropine (VIP may be the non-cholinergic transmitter). These observations suggest the existence of an anticipatory response before acid reaches the duodenum.

The effects of circulating catecholamines and sympathetic nerves must also be considered. Electrical stimulation of splanchnic nerves or the elicitation of sympathetic reflexes (e.g. by bleeding) powerfully inhibits duodenal bicarbonate secretions in cats. In unanaesthetized volunteers an intravenous injection of the alpha$_2$-adrenoceptor agonist clonidine decreases the bicarbonate secretion resulting from intraduodenal acid perfusion. This indicates that increased sympathetic activity may decrease the degree of protection afforded the proximal duodenum and facilitate ulceration. Interestingly, in duodenal ulcer patients the plasma concentrations of catecholamines and the urinary output of their metabolites are increased.

Pancreas

The human pancreas is a large gland, often more than 20 cm long, its head lying within the curve of the duodenum. Most of the pancreatic cells are arrayed in acini as single layers of pyramidal cells containing zymogen granules (Fig 4.1). The acini are connected to the main excretory ducts via intercalary, intra- and interlobular ducts. The terminal portions of the duct system extend into the acini so that flattened duct cells are interposed between acinar cells and the lumen. These duct cells are known as centroacinar cells. The main excretory channel (or duct of Wirsung) runs close to the ductus choledochus. In some 50 per cent of the cases examined these two ducts join to form an ampulla. An accessory pancreatic duct, the duct of Santorini, is located cranially to the main pancreatic duct.

Composition of pancreatic juice

The pancreatic juice has two major components.

1. An alkaline fluid

A bicarbonate-rich fluid helps to neutralize acid entering the duodenum and provide a medium in which pancreatic enzymes can exert their effects. The major cations are Na^+ and K^+, both present in concentrations similar to those recorded in plasma. The major anions are Cl^- and HCO_3^-. Their concentrations depend on the rates of secretion (Fig. 4.2). At the slowest flow rates the $[HCO_3^-]$ may be as low as 25 mmol/l. However, as the flow rates increase the $[HCO_3^-]$ rises to 140–150 mmol/l. The sum of the $[HCO_3^-]$ and $[Cl^-]$ is constant with the result that as the $[HCO_3^-]$ increases the $[Cl^-]$ is reduced.

The exact mechanisms by which this alkaline fluid is produced have not been completely defined. Electrolytes are secreted by both ductal and centroacinar cells. However, the chloride-rich fluid released by the latter makes only a minor contribution. Ductal cells (intra- and interlobular) have a greater role to play. The simplest model that can explain ductal secretion is presented in Fig. 4.3.

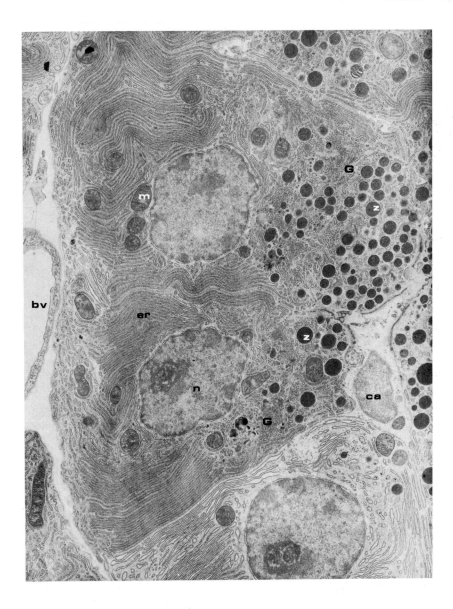

Fig. 4.1 An electron micrograph of pancreatic acinar cells. The extensive endoplasmic reticulum (er) and a few mitochondria (m) occupy the cytoplasm parallel and basal to the nuclei (n). It is within the endoplasmic reticulum, assembled in lateral arrays, that the secretory product (enzymes) is segregated following its synthesis. The product then finds its way via the endoplasmic reticulum to the Golgi complex (G). There the protein is packaged into granules to become the zymogen granules (z) of the apical regions. The cells lining the duct seem relatively inactive compared with their secretory relatives. One such centro acinar cell (ca) is shown containing only a few organelles and no complex membranous system. The close proximity of the acinar cells to the circulation (bv) is easily observed (Kindly presented by Professor K.R. Porter, University of Colorado.)

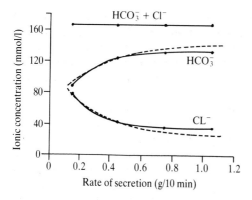

Fig. 4.2 The bicarbonate and chloride concentrations of pancreatic juice secreted by the glands of the anaesthetized cat (- - -), and by isolated glands perfused with a fluid isotonic with cat plasma at pH 7.6, maintained at 38°C and a pressure of 30 mm Hg (—) (From Case, R.M., Harper, A.E. and Scratcherd, T. (1968). *Journal of Physiology* **196**, 133–49.)

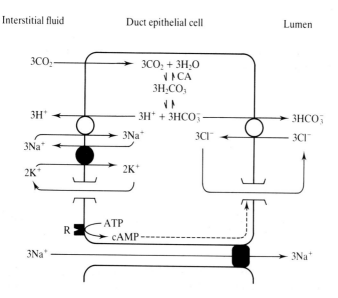

Fig. 4.3 A simple model for the secretin of $NaHCO_3$ by epithelial cells of pancreatic ducts. ○ = Exchange mechanism; ● = Na^+,K^+–pump; ⊣ = ion channel; CA = carbonic anhydrase; R = receptor for agonist, e.g. secretin

A low intracellular [Na^+] is maintained by the energy-dependent Na^+,K^+-pump located in the basolateral membrane. The luminal membrane possesses a Cl^-: HCO_3^- exchange mechanism and a Cl^- channel. A paracellular route has been proposed for the movement of Na^+ from the interstitial fluid to the ductal fluid.

HCO_3^- and H^+ are produced intracellularly from CO_2 and water, the reaction being catalyzed by carbonic anhydrase. Most of the CO_2 is derived from the plasma. It diffuses down its concentration gradient through the lipid of the basolateral membrane. H^+ is removed from the cell to the interstitial fluid via the $Na^+:H^+$ exchange process. The Na^+,K^+-pump expels Na^+ entering this way and replaces it with K^+ ($3:2 = Na^+:K^+$) which had diffused through the basolateral K^+ channel.

The HCO_3^- is transferred across the luminal membrane by the $HCO_3^-:Cl^-$ exchange system. Cl^- presumably is available either from the Cl^--rich fluid secreted by the acinar cells or as the result of the opening of luminal membrane Cl^- channels. Finally Na^+ diffuses from the interstitial fluid to the lumen via a paracellular pathway and maintains electrical neutrality. Water is attracted osmotically either trans- or paracellularly. Agents increasing HCO_3^- secretion stimulate the production of cAMP. One of the functions of this intracellular messenger is to regulate (open) the luminal Cl^- channel. Whether this is its only action remains to be determined.

2. Enzymes

In human pancreatic juice a versatile mixture of enzymes or their precursors are encountered. Their active forms are capable of hydrolysing all the major classes of nutrients. They include:

1. Trypsin.
2. Chymotrypsin.
3. Carboxypeptidase.
4. Pancreatic amylase.
5. Lipolytic enzymes.
6. Other enzymes.

Trypsin.

This proteolytic enzyme is released as inactive trypsinogen (there are several forms). It changes spontaneously to the active form in solution. This change can be accelerated by:

1. Enterokinase, secreted by the enterocytes of the proximal small intestine and resistant to proteolytic digestion. Trypsin activation appears to be the only function of enterokinase, a process enhanced by low concentrations of bile acids.
2. Activated trypsin which converts more precursor into the active form (autocatalysis).

Trypsin hydrolyses peptide bonds within the protein molecule. The linkages particularly affected are those in which the carboxyl group is provided by an amino acid with a positively charged side chain e.g. lysine or arginine.

Chymotrypsin

A second endopolypeptidase detected in pancreatic juice is chymotrypsin. This enzyme is also released in an inactive form, i.e. as chymotrypsinogen. Its activation is trypsin dependent. Unlike trypsin it is incapable of autocatalysis. Chymotrypsin acts preferentially on peptide bonds in which the carboxyl groups are provided by tyrosine or phenylalanine.

Carboxypeptidase

As the result of the action of pepsin, trypsin and chymotrypsin peptides of various sizes are produced. These can be further digested by carboxypeptidase which removes the amino acid with the free carboxyl group from the end of the peptide chain. As with other proteolytic enzymes carboxypeptidase is released in an inactive form (procarboxypeptidase). For its activation trypsin is required.

Clearly the activation of trypsin in either the acinar cells which elaborate the pancreatic enzymes, or the ducts that convey pancreatic juice to the duodenum must be avoided. The alternative is autodigestion, a feature of acute necrotizing pancreatitis. A number of mechanisms have been proposed which prevent the formation of trypsin in its active form. One of these, in the rat pancreas at least, involves the acidification of intracellular zymogen granules in which digestive enzymes or their precursors are stored. An ATP-dependent active proton transport process provides an environment in which trypsin is inactive.

Other mechanisms suppressing trypsin activation are encountered in the ducts. A trypsin inhibitor (the Kazal inhibitor, a small protein of mol. wt. 6000 daltons) is released in pancreatic juice and rapidly forms a complex with trypsin accidentally activated. Furthermore, the high pH (8–9.5) and the low calcium concentrations (less than 1 mmol/l) of pancreatic secretions promote the degradation rather than the activation of trypsinogen.

Recently evidence has been obtained for another mechanism protecting the pancreas against digestion by its own enzymes. The factor involved, described as enzyme Y, may be a product of trypsinogen digestion or a previously unrecognized proteolytic enzyme activated by traces of trypsin. However, its properties are very different from those of trypsin and include the rapid destruction of zymogens. Thus in an environment likely to trigger the activation of proteolytic enzymes there may be a valuable self-destruct system making such an event less likely.

Pancreatic amylase

Pancreatic juice contains an endoamylase which like that enzyme found in saliva hydrolyses 1,4 glucosidic bonds. Its action results in the formation of maltose and maltotriose from amylose, the straight chain polysaccharide. When amylopectin or glycogen are the substrates the di- and trisaccharides are again formed in addition to a mixture of dextrins with both $\alpha 1,6$ and $\alpha 1,4$ branches. The pH optimum of the enzyme is 6.9 although it is stable between pH 4 and 11. Unlike salivary amylase the pancreatic enzyme has activity against uncooked starch. Unlike pancreatic proteolytic enzymes amylase is secreted in its active form.

Lipolytic enzymes

Several enzymes concerned with the breakdown of lipids are detected in pancreatic juice. One of these is pancreatic lipase which acts on water-insoluble triglycerides to release fatty acids and 2-monoglycerides. If the lipase was to be adsorbed to the oil:water interface it would be denatured as the result of its loss of ternary structure. Such adsorption is prevented by a colipase. This is a small protein secreted by the pancreas which anchors lipase sufficiently close to the interface for the enzyme to exert its effects. Bile acids also have a role to play. When they are adsorbed to the interface they provide a negative charge which attracts lipase and colipase. Lipase has an isoelectric pH of 6.8 so that in the more acid contents of the proximal small intestine it will have a net positive charge.

Two other lipolytic enzymes are secreted by the pancreas. One is a carboxyl ester lipase which probably acts in the aqueous phase following the transfer of its lipid substrates to bile acid aggregates (see page 138). The other is a phospholipase (A_2) which releases fatty acids from phosphate containing lipids, e.g. lecithin is converted to lysolecithin.

Other enzymes

Numerous other enzymes have also been detected in pancreatic juice. These include :

1. Ribonuclease and deoxyribonuclease which partially hydrolyse nucleic acids to mononucleotides.
2. Elastases which have been described as proteolytic enzymes adsorbing to elastin and exhibiting specificity to amino acids with short aliphatic side chains, the predominant species in elastin. They could contribute to the hydrolysis of haemoglobin, albumin, fibrin and casein. As with other proteolytic enzymes elastases are released as inactive precursors and activated by trypsin.

The fate of pancreatic enzymes in the small intestine

Several questions should at least be asked even though complete answers to them are not available.

1. How quickly are digestive enzymes inactivated in the intestines?

Amylase and trypsin survive the journey from the duodenum to the ileum to a far greater extent than lipase. It has been estimated that only 1 per cent of the lipase secreted could be accounted for when the luminal contents reached the distal ileum. In contrast 22 per cent and 74 per cent respectively of the trypsin and amylase could be detected. These observations may help to explain why progressive pancreatic atrophy leads first to fat malabsorption. The loss of lipase activity could reflect lipase absorption. However, digestion of the lipolytic enzyme has been considered a more likely possibility. *In vitro* studies support this view. Lipase activity has been monitored in duodenal contents incubated at 37°C. Only 25 per cent of that initially present could be detected after 2 hours. Chymotrypsin exerted greater effects on lipase activity than trypsin.

2. What happens to pancreatic enzymes? Are they excreted or is there some capacity for their absorption and re-use?

Evidence has been presented suggesting the existence of an enteropancreatic circulation analogous to the enterohepatic circulation of bile acids. Thus it has been found that the small intestine is permeable to several digestive enzymes. Furthermore chymotrypsinogen and amylase can cross the basolateral membranes of pancreatic cells. This has been demonstrated with an *in vitro* technique. The whole pancreas (rabbit) was bathed in a physiological saline. The pancreatic duct was cannulated so that uncontaminated secretions could be collected. Labelled chymotrypsinogen and albumin were added to the bathing fluid. When subsequently a steady state was produced the labelled trypsinogen:labelled albumin ratio in the secreted fluid was 20:1. If unlabelled chymotrypsinogen was added to the bathing medium a decreased secretion of the labelled form was observed suggesting that competition had occurred. A similar experiment was conducted with labelled amylase. The secretion of this labelled enzyme into the pancreatic duct could be greatly increased by CCK (see page 83).

3. What is the influence of dietary components on pancreatic enzymes?

Inhibitors of the proteolytic enzymes are widely distributed in many food items commonly consumed by man. Although the physiological consequences of chronic ingestion of such inhibitors has not been established their immediate influence on pancreatic secretions has been recognized. Pure secretions have been collected from healthy volunteers by endoscopic retrograde cannulation of the pancreatic duct. At the same time the duodenum was perfused with pancreatic juice containing either (a) the Bowman–Birk inhibitor of soybeans in which 90 per cent of the trypsin and chymotrypsin activities had been abolished, or (b) heat-inactivated inhibitor and, therefore, simulating more normal conditions where the duodenum is exposed to its own secretions. The secretions of trypsin, chymotrypsin, elastase and amylase were considerably greater in the presence than the absence of the active inhibitor. It has been concluded that a feedback control exists in man so that when the levels of trypsin and chymotrypsin in the duodenum are diminished CCK can be released from the duodenal mucosa and further enzymes secreted.

The question remains as to how intraduodenal trypsin might interfere with CCK release. It has recently been proposed that the proximal small intestine secretes a CCK-releasing peptide into the lumen. This peptide is trypsin sensitive. As a result it is immediately inactivated when pancreatic juice is present in the absence of food. On the other hand, it is capable of inducing pancreatic hypersecretion when trypsin is inhibited, removed or involved in the digestion of protein. Such a peptide has been isolated. It is referred to as the monitor peptide because it 'monitors' the intraduodenal environment (Fig. 4.4).

Control of pancreatic secretion

Pancreatic secretion, like gastric secretion, can conveniently be classified into the cephalic, gastric and intestinal phases.

1. Cephalic phase

A secretion is evoked by both conditioned and unconditioned reflexes. Thus the sight, smell and taste of food all combine to excite vagal efferent fibres. At one time it was thought that this phase was of little consequence. However, the finding that protein output from the pancreas was greatly increased by sham feeding has led to this view being altered.

Parasympathetic postganglionic neurons to exocrine glands release both acetylcholine and VIP. These neurotransmitters act synergistically (Fig. 4.5). Thus when VIP is infused intra-arterially it causes the exocrine pancreas to secrete a fluid containing bicarbonate and protein. Blood flow is also increased. Both secretory and vascular responses are potentiated by acetylcholine. The neurotransmitters exert their effects on acinar cells via different intracellular messengers. Acetylcholine stimulates membrane phospholipid hydrolysis and the formation of IP_3 (see page 85). In contrast VIP (and the hormone secretin) increase cAMP production.

2. Gastric phase

Food distending the stomach results in a small contribution to the total pancreatic secretion. The response to distension can be blocked by atropine and vagotomy suggesting the existence of a gastropancreatic vago-vagal reflex.

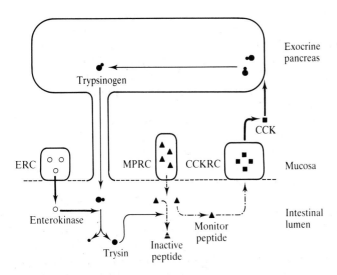

Fig. 4.4 Feedback inhibition of pancreatic secretion. ERC = enterokinase releasing cell; MPRC = monitor peptide releasing cell; CCKRC = CCK releasing cell

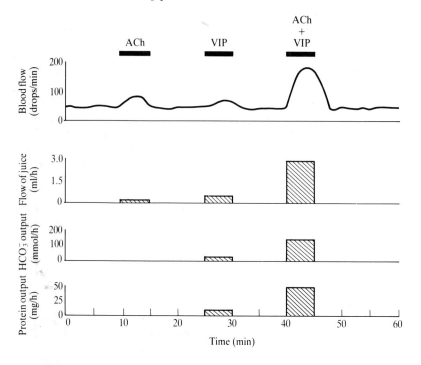

Fig. 4.5 Effects of intra-arterial infusions of acetylcholine (50 μg/min) and VIP (0.1 μg/min) alone and in combination on pancreatic secretion and blood flow in the cat (From Fahrenkrug, J. and Emson, P.C. (1982). *British Medical Bulletin* **38**, 265–70.)

In addition peptides and amino acids in the stomach have also been regarded as initiators of pancreatic secretion perhaps by stimulating the release of the antral hormone gastrin. Gastrin has structural similarity to, and a wide range of biological actions that overlap with, CCK. However, a more important role for the stomach in contributing to pancreatic secretion may be in the digestion of protein and lipid to produce factors that initiate the intestinal phase.

3. Intestinal phase

The major secretions of electrolytes and enzymes occur after chyme enters the duodenum. Several factors increase pancreatic secretions when present within the lumen of the small intestine. Among the most powerful stimuli are the products of protein and fat digestion. Thus monoglycerides and fatty acids with chain lengths of more than eight carbon atoms are effective although intact triglycerides are not. Similarly peptides and amino acids resulting from the breakdown of proteins by pepsins in the stomach and proteolytic enzymes from the pancreas elicit further secretions. It is thought that only very low concentrations of amino acids are necessary to stimulate intestinal mucosal receptors and that the length of the intestine exposed to these products is the important determinant of the total secretory response.

A third major stimulant of pancreatic juice in the intestinal phase may be gastric acid. Intraluminal acid causes the release of large volumes of a bicarbonate-rich solution. There is, however, a pH threshold above which acid does not stimulate. In man the threshold may be lower than 3.0. This finding raises the question as to whether acid is normally an important factor. There is general agreement that the intraluminal pH of the duodenum beyond the pancreatic duct does not fall below 5.0 in either the interdigestive or postprandial states. Only the proximal duodenum is even potentially acidified to the levels required to stimulate a secretion. What is the situation in the first few centimetres of the duodenum? During the interdigestive period the intraluminal pH is nearly neutral although it decreases to values as low as 2.0 transiently.

After a test meal transient decreases continue to be detected although pH values of less than 3.0 are recorded for only 2–3 per cent of the time. Thus there are few occasions when the pH falls below the threshold needed to stimulate the pancreas. However, these occasions may be of more importance than at first they appear. This is because there are significant interactions between acid and the products of fat and protein digestion resulting in the potentiation of bicarbonate secretion.

What processes do these stimuli initiate? Certainly the hormones CCK and secretin have roles to play. However, the following concepts are a gross oversimplification of what is thought to occur:

1. Secretin released by acid in the duodenum provides a bicarbonate-rich secretion.
2. CCK released by the products of protein and fat digestion stimulates the production of an enzyme-rich fluid.

The importance of secretin has been recognised for many years. Indeed it was the first hormone to be discovered giving rise to the science of endocrinology. Bayliss and Starling (1902) had investigated alimentary tract reflexes in dogs and observed that even when all accessible nerve connections had been severed, the introduction of acid into the duodenum produced a secretion by the pancreas. Acid given via the blood stream did not elicit such a response. They realized that some substance must have been released from the intestine by the action of the intraluminal acid. Their next step was to cut out a loop of jejunum and scrape off the mucosal layer. This they rubbed with sand and dilute HCl in a mortar and then filtered it through cotton wool to get rid of the lumps. They injected the product intravenously and were able to observe a copious pancreatic secretion.

Secretin is also released by intraduodenal fatty acids. The process involved is not dependent on a low pH. This may explain why bicarbonate-rich secretions can be produced even though the acidity of the duodenal contents has not risen to the threshold previously thought necessary to induce secretin release.

The actions of secretin are potentiated by both nerves and other hormones. Thus atropine inhibits pancreatic bicarbonate release in response to low (physiological?) doses of secretin. This can be demonstrated both before and after extrinsic denervation of the pancreas. Furthermore, truncal vagotomy or atropine also decrease the intestinal response to HCl although neither procedure affects secretin release. Such observations suggest that acetylcholine liberated as a result of (a) the activity of intrinsic nerves of the pancreas, or (b) HCl activating an enteropancreatic vago-vagal reflex interacts with secretin to produce a bicarbonate secretion.

A vago-vagal reflex in response to acid is not difficult to appreciate. The concept of an intrinsic nervous system providing 'pancreatic tone' and capable of interacting with and potentiating the actions of circulating peptides is, perhaps, more difficult to imagine. Such a system, however, might explain why only small amounts of secretin, released during the digestion of a meal, are necessary to stimulate pancreatic bicarbonate output.

CCK is at least one of the hormones modifying the effects of secretin on bicarbonate secretion. This has been demonstrated in man (Fig. 4.6). Physiological doses of secretin have been administered intravenously with varied amounts of CCK to healthy volunteers. The bicarbonate outputs observed were significantly greater than those achieved by secretin or CCK alone or the sum of the outputs produced by each hormone. Thus CCK potentiates the actions of secretin on bicarbonate secretion. (NB. Pancreatic enzyme secretion does not appear to be potentiated by the combined actions of these two hormones.)

The release of enzymes

For many years the hormone CCK has been thought to exert two major effects. One was to cause gall-bladder contractions, the other to produce pancreatic secretions rich in enzymes. The concept of a hormone changing

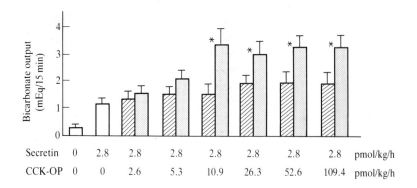

Fig. 4.6 The potentiation of pancreatic bicarbonate secretion in man. Secretions were measured after an overnight fast in five healthy volunteers. Collections were made under basal conditions and while giving intravenous infusions of secretin (2.8 pmol/kg/h) and/or graded doses of cholecystokinin octapeptide (CCK-OP, 2.6–109.4 pmol/kg/h). The data presented are of (**a**) the basal and that produced while infusing secretin alone (unshaded bars); (**b**) the sums of the bicarbonate outputs produced when the two hormones were administered separately (striped bars); and (**c**) the bicarbonate secretion resulting from the simultaneous infusion of CCK-OP and secretin (shaded bars). Each bar represents the mean ± SE of mean for the five subjects. * Differences between (b) and (c) are significant ($p < 0.05$). (From Yai, C.H., Rominger, J.M. and Chey, W.Y. (1983) *Gastroenterology*; **85**; 40–5.

gall-bladder motility was proposed by Ivy and Goldberg in 1928 to account for the contractions observed in response to fat in the lumen of the small intestine. The name cholecystokinin was given to the agent involved.

Fifteen years later Harper and Raper described a process in which the introduction of polypeptides into the duodenal lumen elicited the secretion of pancreatic enzymes. The factor mediating this response was named pancreozymin. As attempts were made to purify cholecystokinin and pancreozymin it was unexpectedly found that they were chemically identical. The name cholecystokinin (or CCK) has been retained. The most potent stimuli for its release include (a) amino acids, particularly the essential amino acids e.g. phenylalanine and methionine, and (b) long chain fatty acids, e.g. palmitic, stearic and oleic acids.

The physiological importance of CCK in the control of enzyme release has been a controversial topic. It would appear that the hormone can provide a major contribution when there are large loads of fatty acids within the duodenum. If only small amounts are present enteropancreatic vago-vagal cholinergic reflexes are thought to be quantitatively more important. Such reflexes would provide rapid responses as chyme flows into the duodenum from the stomach.

CCK exerts a further influence on the pancreas. The peptide is probably the most powerful stimulator of pancreatic growth. Increases in pancreatic weight, DNA and enzyme content in response to CCK have been reported and the possibility recognized that CCK might be used in the treatment of patients with chronic pancreatitis.

The action of acetylcholine and CCK on pancreatic acinar cells.

When acetylcholine and CCK bind to their appropriate receptors membrane-bound phospholipid is hydrolysed to produce IP_3 and a diacylglycerol (Fig. 4.7). IP_3 is released intracellularly where its major function is to mobilize calcium stores. These are thought to be held in the endoplasmic reticulum. In the absence of a stimulus these membranes are relatively impermeable to calcium. However, IP_3 opens a calcium channel and the cation is released. Calcium probably initiates secretion by activating a calmodulin-dependent protein kinase, an enzyme phosphorylating specific cellular proteins. Secretion can also be the result of the activation of protein kinase c by the diacylglycerol. Thus both products of phospholipid hydrolysis have a role to play in pancreatic secretion.

The picture presented above is, perhaps, too simple. IP_3 is not the only possible product of phospholipid hydrolysis. Another is inositol 1:2,4,5 triphosphate in which the 1-phosphate is linked between the 1- and 2-hydroxyl groups. This cyclic compound can also mobilize calcium. Indeed, it has a similar potency to IP_3. However, the intracellular concentration of the cyclic derivative rises much more slowly than IP_3 so that it may contribute less to the initial response.

The question should be raised as to why two second messengers are formed. They certainly provide an exceptionally versatile signalling system which is adapted to control a host of processes in many different cells. A role has been proposed for them in the control of several secretions, muscle contractions and metabolism and even in the longer term control of growth. In many cases the two appear to act synergistically. Their relative contributions are, however, unknown, although the IP_3 pathway is thought to play the major role in initiating cellular responses. The diglyceride pathway may contribute to the final response but its predominant role may be to modulate the calcium signalling pathway (homologous interactions) or other signalling mechanisms, e.g. those dependent on cAMP (heterologous interactions).

One way in which the diglyceride pathway could modulate the calcium signalling pathway would be to alter the intracellular calcium levels (Fig. 4.8).

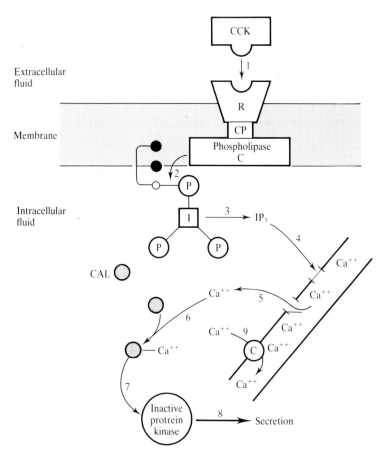

Fig. 4.7 A model for the action of CCK on acinar cells. When CCK reacts with its receptor (1) phospholipase C is activated. As a result membrane phospholipids are hyrolysed (2) and IP_3 is released (3). This intracellular messenger opens calcium channels in the endoplasmic reticulum (4). The released calcium (5) binds to calmodulin (6) which subsequently activates a protein kinase (7) necessary for inducing pancreatic enzyme secretion (8). Free calcium within the intracellular fluid can rapidly be removed and stored in the endoplasmic reticulum by active transport (9). R = CCK receptor; C = calcium carrier; CAL = calmodulin; CP = coupling protein

When calcium is released from its stores as a result of an external stimulus there is often an explosive increase in the intracellular calcium concentration, exceeding that necessary to activate the cell. If unchecked the cell could be damaged. The diglyceride, by activating protein kinase c, limits the increase. The enzyme acts in two ways. It inhibits the hydrolysis of membrane phospholipid (PtdIns 4,5P_2) and removes calcium from the cells by stimulating plasma membrane calcium pumps (NB. calcium can also be pumped back into the endoplasmic reticulum store).

Two other questions remain. If calcium is removed from cells following their activation how are the stores replenished? One suggestion is that when the acinar cell is activated a calcium channel in the plasma membrane is opened. Both this channel and the calcium pump in the endoplasmic reticulum remain active following agonist removal until the stores have again been filled. Secondly, what happens to the CCK? After its binding CCK is taken into acinar cells by receptor mediated endocytosis. It is degraded intracellularly. Breakdown can be inhibited by chloroquine, a lysosomotropic agent that blocks intracellular proteolysis. Although a complete picture cannot be presented the concept is, at least, introduced of the removal and intracellular processing of peptide hormones by target tissues.

Heterogeneity of the exocrine pancreas

It has generally been assumed that the anatomical and functional characteristics of all the pancreatic acini are equivalent. Thus the amounts of enzymes released from the pancreas should depend on the intensity of the stimulus applied and the composition of the enzyme mixture should not readily be varied. This

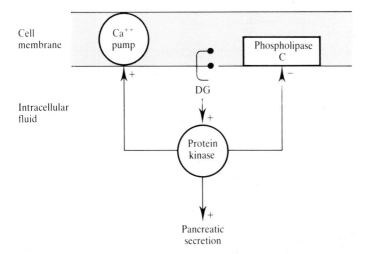

Fig. 4.8 Possible roles for diglyceride (DG) in pancreatic secretion. By activating protein kinase C which phosphorylates specific cellular proteins it is thought to stimulate a secretion. Protein kinase C also inhibits phospholipase C and stimulates membrane calcium pumps. As a result potentially damaging rises in intracellular calcium concentrations may be avoided.

view is no longer held. Morphologically differences in cell size and digestive enzyme content can be demonstrated. Cells of acini close to the pancreatic islets (peri-insular) are usually larger and contain more digestive enzymes than those more distant (tele-insular). The latter are relatively enriched with lipase rather than amylase and chymotrypsinogen. The reverse is true in peri-insular cells. This raises the possibility that the proportions of different enzymes secreted could be rapidly altered by stimulating specific pancreatic regions.

Evidence is available to show that specific secretagogues may act on only a limited number of acini. Pancreatic lobules have been incubated *in vitro* with maximal concentrations of caerulein (a CCK analogue isolated from the skin of the frog *Hyla caerulea*), carbachol (a synthetic choline derivative) or secretin. Their acinar secretory activities were estimated by following the loss of zymogen granules or estimating the residual amylase. If only one secretagogue was used approximately one-third of the amylase was released from the tissue but only some of the acini were degranulated. If lobules were incubated with secretin and either caerulein or carbachol additional acini lost their zymogen granules. To explain these observations it has been proposed that at least two groups of acini exist. One reacts to a single secretagogue the other requires a combination of such agents. The variable enzyme content of the acinar cells and the differences of sensitivity of acini to specific secretagogues leads to the concept of a non-parallel secretion. With such a secretion the relative proportions of digestive enzymes could be rapidly altered by neural or hormonal stimuli or even recently absorbed nutrients.

The release of pancreatic enzymes

Most people support the view that exocytosis is the major mechanism by which digestive enzymes are secreted. Specific proteins are synthesized in the rough endoplasmic reticulum, sorted and directed to their destinations in the Golgi complex and then packaged and stored in zymogen granules. When the acinar cell is stimulated zymogen granules move towards the apical membrane. Recognition by the zymogen granule of an appropriate site is then followed by fusion and fission with the apical plasmalemma and the release of enzymes. The pancreatic enzymes are exposed within the ducts to a bicarbonate-rich fluid. This is probably necessary for the final dissolution of the zymogen granule contents. Subsequently the zymogen granule membrane is rapidly internalized by endocytosis and can be re-used for the storage of newly synthesized digestive enzymes.

The process described above has been called the regulated (or stimulated) secretion. It may occur under resting conditions but can be greatly accelerated by secretagogues. Not all proteins, however, are released in this way. Some may be secreted by an alternative route involving neither storage in, nor exocytosis from zymogen granules. This process is known as the constitutive (or basal) secretion. The composition of the constitutive secretion differs from that of the regulated secretion in that the former is particularly rich in amylase. The availability of these two systems may be yet another factor that contributes to the variable enzyme content of pancreatic secretions.

Though endocytosis is thought to be the process by which pancreatic enzymes are released S.S. Rothman (1980) reminded everyone that it was not the only possibility. His alternative proposal became known as the equilibrium hypothesis. In it proteins are transferred across cell membranes by diffusion. For diffusion to occur interactions must take place between enzymes and either protein or lipid components of the acinar cell membranes. Interactions with the membrane might (a) lead to the formation of a fugacious or fleeting pore allowing the enzyme to enter the membrane, or (b) provide a carrier-mediated system analogous to the facilitated diffusion processes transferring the water-soluble products of digestion from the lumen of the small intestine (see Chapter 5). The equilibrium hypothesis has been regarded as too radical, unlikely with respect to known existing mechanisms of protein secretion and never proven. Two important concepts emerge, however, from a consideration of it. These are that (a) the simplest hypothesis (i.e. diffusion not exocytosis) should be favoured until it is explicitly excluded by the weight of evidence against it, and (b) very large molecules such as proteins could conceivably diffuse across cell membranes. The latter comes as quite a shock to those of us who have observed that small water-soluble molecules such as disaccharides are not readily transferred across cell membranes.

Pancreatic adaptation

The proportions of enzymes released in pancreatic juice depend on the food eaten. Thus high carbohydrate, fat and protein diets fed repeatedly to rats over a period of time lead to increases in amylase, lipase and protease activities respectively. Premature babies fed soy-based formula diets have greater secretions of lipase and trypsin than those provided with a milk-based formula diet. These changes are ascribed to alterations in the rates of synthesis of different enzymes so that what is eaten one day helps to determine the mixture of enzymes released in response to future meals. Clearly such a mechanism would not be of great value if the composition of meals taken were to vary markedly.

How might enzyme synthesis and secretion be altered? One suggestion has been that specific hormones are released by digestive products which modify protease, lipase or amylase syntheses. Several hormones may have roles to play. One is insulin which is presented to the acini in relatively high concentrations. This is the result of a significant proportion (11–23 per cent) of the total pancreatic blood flow passing initially through the islets before the rest of the pancreas. Amylase synthesis can be controlled by insulin. Two other hormones influencing enzyme synthesis are secretin and CCK. The former, released by fatty acids (as well as HCl) in the intestinal lumen stimulates lipase secretion. CCK, on the other hand, released by the products of protein digestion and by the protease inhibitor camostate increases protease synthesis.

So far emphasis has been placed on what happens if the diet contains different quantities of particular nutrients. Changes also occur when there is a lack of a specific requirement. For example during total protein deprivation the protein synthetic activity of acinar cells is directed almost exclusively to the production of proteolytic enzymes. This has been regarded as a 'last chance mechanism' enabling the body to digest what limited amounts of protein are available in the intestinal lumen e.g. from sloughed epithelial cells. In this way those amino acids necessary for survival may be made available.

One should also recognize that large amounts of some dietary components reduce the release of enzymes. When carbohydrate or lipid meals are infused directly into the jejuna of healthy volunteers pancreatic secretions are inhibited. This 'jejunal brake' appears to depend on the jejunal caloric load. The mechanisms involved in this inhibition are unknown but might explain why pancreatic insufficiency can result from gastrectomy or gastroduodenal anastomosis. Furthermore in malabsorption (see Chapter 5) unabsorbed nutrients in the jejunum would inhibit pancreatic secretions and contribute to an even greater loss of nutrients from the gastrointestinal tract.

The liver

The liver is the largest gland of the body and has many functions. Approximately 25 per cent of the cardiac output is supplied to the liver by one of two routes. The portal vein carries blood that has already been transferred through the intestinal capillary beds and is, therefore, rich in absorbed nutrients but relatively poor in oxygen. This vessel contributes some 80% of the hepatic blood flow. The remaining 20% is provided by the hepatic artery, which carries a more oxygenated blood. The portal vein branches repeatedly within the liver lobes to produce vessels which lead directly to sinusoids. The argument continues as to whether or not arterial blood passes directly to the sinusoids. Many believe that most of the arterial component mixes with venous blood before reaching the sinusoids. The latter form a rich anastomosing network which converges towards a central vein. The contents of the central veins drain into hepatic veins and finally into the inferior vena cava.

Two types of cell are found in the sinusoid. These are:

1. lining endothelial cells,
2. phagocytic Kupffer cells.

The endothelial cells lie close to the sinusoidal surfaces of the functional cells of the liver, the hepatocytes or liver parenchyma (Fig. 4.9). No basal lamina separates the sinusoidal endothelia and hepatocytes. Further, the endothelial cytoplasm is fenestrated by numerous openings forming clusters or sieve plates. With such a structure, there is no significant barrier to exchange between blood and hepatocytes, even for large molecules (mol. wt. under 250 000). The surface area of the hepatocyte membrane facing the sinusoid is increased by its foldings.

The region between the hepatocyte and the sinusoidal wall is the perisinusoidal space of Disse (Fig. 4.10). This contains a delicate but structurally important frame of collagen fibres to support the hepatocytes. These hepatocytes contribute 60% of the total liver cells and are stacked to form continuous plates one cell thick. The space of Disse continues a variable distance between hepatocytes as the perisinusoidal recess. This terminates at the tight junction. Between two continuous tight junctions is the bile canaliculus, the

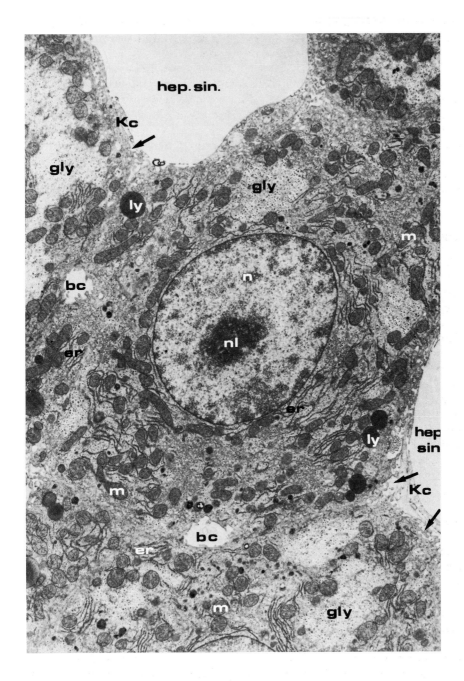

Fig. 4.9 A low-power electron micrograph of rat liver cells showing their relationship to the hepatic sinusoids (hep. sin.) and bile canaliculi (bc). The space of Disse (↑) separates the Kupffer cells (Kc) from the liver cells. Within the hepatocytes are the nucleus (n) and nucleolus (nl), mitochondria (m), rough endoplasmic reticulum (er), lysosomes (ly) and areas of glycogen (gly) (Kindly presented by Mr R.P. Gould, The Middlesex Hospital Medical School, London.)

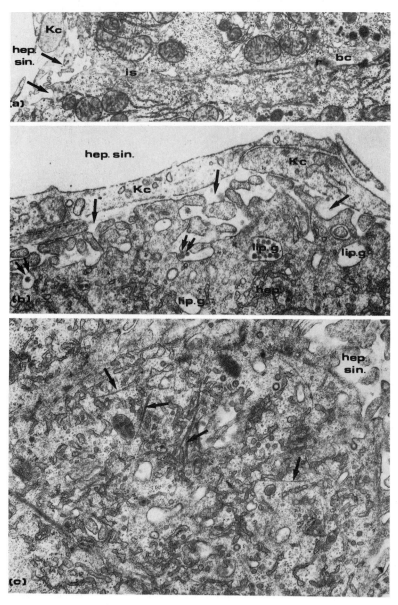

Fig. 4.10 Electron micrographs of liver cells. (**a**) Shows part of two hepatocytes as well as the hepatic sinusoid (hep. sin.) Kupffer cell (Kc) and space of Disse (↑). The space of Disse is in continuity with the intercellular space (is) but is sealed off from the bile canaliculus (bc) by the tight junction (in region r). (**b**) Illustrates the relationship between the vascular pole of the hepatocyte (hep), the space of Disse (↑), Kupffer cell (Kc) and the lumen of the sinusoid (hep. sin.). Note the cytoplasmic vacuoles containing dense lipoprotein granules (lip. g), some of which appear to be discharging (↑ ↑) into the space of Disse. (**c**) Hepatocyte cytoplasm adjacent to a sinusoid (hep. sin.). Bundles of microfilaments (↑), probably composed of actin, form an anapical network. Such filaments may form a contractile system which could ruffle the vascular surface of the liver cell and so aid the movement of materials between the cell and its blood supply (Kindly presented by Mr R.P. Gould, The Middlesex Hospital Medical School, London.)

smallest component of the biliary duct system. Thus every facet of the hepatocyte not in contact with a sinusoid is occupied by a canaliculus. The smaller ducts collecting the bile converge to form larger but fewer ducts, until two main ducts, the right and left hepatic ducts, emerge from the definite hilus or porta hepatis, the point where blood vessels also enter and leave the liver. These unite to form the common hepatic duct and then receive the cystic duct from the gall-bladder to become the bile duct passing to the duodenum. Separating the bile duct from the duodenum is a muscular apparatus which has the double function of (a) providing a resistance to the evacuation of bile, and (b) preventing reflux. This is the sphincter of Oddi.

For many years it has been recognized that the liver occupies a central position in metabolism. It has been referred to as 'the kitchen of the body', a description readily appreciated when the liver is extirpated in animals or when its functions are seriously compromised by disease. Disturbances of essential functions may not, however, be detected until the liver is severely damaged, because of its large reserves of metabolic capacity. Then changes rapidly take place leading to imbalances incompatible with life.

In this section on the physiology of liver only a glimpse is given of many of the processes occurring. Emphasis is placed on the secretion and functions of bile acids and the excretion of bile pigments. Before considering these events, I shall refer to some of the many other activities of the liver. Perhaps sufficient will be presented to whet the appetites of readers so that they delve deeper into the subject.

The handling of drugs and hormones

To be therapeutically useful, drugs must be eliminated from the body so that their effects will be limited. The kidney is the route for the removal of the majority of drugs from the body. The parent drug or its metabolites enter the renal tubule either by filtration at the glomerulus or by active secretion across the renal tubular epithelia. The lipid solubility of the drug is then the major determinant as to whether reabsorption from the tubular fluid takes place or the substance is excreted in the urine. Those substances that are highly water soluble remain in the tubular fluid and thus are removed from the body. On the other hand, drugs with lipid solubility can be reabsorbed by diffusion across the tubular membranes.

To convert lipid-soluble to water-soluble substances two enzyme systems have been described which are found predominantly, but not exclusively, in the liver. The first system, organized within the smooth endoplasmic reticulum, brings about hydroxylation. The second group of enzymes is involved in conjugation reactions. Lipid-soluble substances with readily available -OH, -COOH, $-NH_2$ or SH_2 groups are modified by the removal of a hydrogen atom and its replacement by a large water soluble moiety. These mechanisms tend to abolish the pharmacological actions of drugs and render them more water soluble. Glucuronic acid is the substance most commonly conjugating with drugs. Others include sulphates and various amino acids e.g. glycine. In addition acetylation and methylation reactions and the formation of mercaptopurates from glutathione contribute to drug elimination.

It is hardly surprising that the capacity of the liver to excrete a number of dyes has been used to assess hepatic function. One dye that has been used extensively is sulphobromphthalein. A dose of 5 mg/kg body weight is administered intravenously. The dye is removed from the blood and conjugated, mainly with glutathione, and excreted in the bile. With normal liver function not more than 5% of the dye should remain in the plasma after it is injected. Retention of 15% or more has often been recorded in cirrhotic patients. The greatest value of the test is in non-jaundiced patients (bilirubin may interfere with the uptake of the dye) where abnormal results may reflect impairment of the hepatic circulation and the resultant collateral blood flow.

Several enzyme systems have been described in the liver which can modify and inactivate naturally occurring steroid hormones. The physiologically inactive products are then conjugated and excreted in the urine, e.g. progesterone is reduced to pregnanediol and then excreted as a sulphate or a glucuronide.

Carbohydrate metabolism

Blood glucose levels are held within reasonably narrow limits considering the large variations in supply from the small intestine and the utilization by tissues. Glucose levels fall below 60 mg/100 ml (3.3 mmol/l) only during severe exercise or a prolonged fast. In contrast, blood glucose levels may rise as high as 130–140 mg/100 ml (7.2–7.8 mmol/l) after the ingestion of a carbohydrate meal.

Glucose is essential for the adequate provision of energy in the brain, muscle and cellular components of the blood. The liver has a central role in maintaining blood sugar levels and is able to introduce glucose into or remove it from the circulation, depending on the requirements of the body. The liver acts as a storage tissue for glucose, the hexose being held in the form of the polysaccharide glycogen. Glucose can be made available from this store by glycogenolysis or added to it by glycogenesis. The latter process, the synthesis of glycogen from glucose, does not depend significantly on blood glucose unless sugar levels are very high. Glycogen is synthesized largely from lactate (e.g. derived from muscle metabolism during exercise) and other non-carbohydrate sources, such as fatty acids and amino acids.

The question remains as to what controls the liver as it functions to maintain blood glucose levels. Both humoral and nervous mechanisms are involved. Glycogenolysis may be regarded as an emergency reaction to meet the extra metabolic requirements of tissues. It is hardly surprising that the sympathetic branch of the autonomic nervous system and the hormones of the adrenal medulla exert a considerable influence on glycogen breakdown leading to a rise in blood glucose.

A hyperglycaemic stimulus, on the other hand, activates the release of insulin from the pancreas. This hormone accelerates movement of glucose into most cells of the body from the blood. Liver cells (and brain) appear to be exceptions. The permeability of liver cells to glucose is normally very high. However, insulin does promote glycogen synthesis in liver cells so that the liver contributes to the powerful hypoglycaemic action of the pancreatic hormone.

From the above discussion it would be expected that disturbances of carbohydrate metabolism accompany hepatic dysfunction. Indeed, severe hypoglycaemia has been described in massive liver cell necrosis, a condition fatal unless treated with intravenous glucose. The importance of the liver can be demonstrated experimentally in hepatectomized dogs. Such animals rapidly recover from the operation and, to all outward appearances, seem relatively normal for a few hours. However, there is a progressive fall in blood glucose producing marked muscular weakness, followed by convulsions, coma and death. If glucose (0.25–0.5 g (1.39–2.78 mmol) /kg body weight) is administered to a comatose, hepatectomized dog, the results are remarkable. Within 30 seconds the animal can walk and respond to a call. The heart beats more strongly. Subsequently, as the blood glucose concentrations fall again, the symptoms reappear.

The development of fatal hypoglycaemia following the removal of the liver shows that this organ is of cardinal importance in maintaining normal blood sugar levels. Intravenous injections of maltose, fructose and mannose into hypoglycaemic, liverless animals have similar effects to glucose. In contrast, galactose administration is not effective. The liver is the site at which galactose is converted to glucose.

Protein metabolism

The liver is active in three areas of protein metabolism:

1. Protein synthesis.
2. Formation of urea as the main nitrogenous end product of amino acid metabolism.
3. Interconversions of amino acids. Such changes, involving e.g. phenylalanine and tyrosine, methionine and cysteine, are not exclusive to the liver.

Many of the plasma proteins are synthesized in the liver. Quantitatively the most important is albumin. It has been calculated that the liver synthesizes de novo some 3 g each day. Albumin in the plasma provides a large colloid osmotic pressure and is concerned with the maintenance of plasma volume and tissue fluid balance. In addition, this protein contributes to the buffering capacity of blood and transports several substances, e.g. bilirubin and free fatty acids. A number of agents that are used therapeutically also bind to albumin. These include penicillin, chlorothiazide and salicylates. Competition may result between these different substances for binding sites on albumin, resulting in toxic substances, e.g. bilirubin, being present in the unbound form. This must be remembered if antibiotic treatment of neonates is considered.

Other proteins synthesized by the liver include components of the complement system and several concerned with blood coagulation. Fibrinogen is formed only in the liver. Additional clotting factors probably exclusively synthesized in the liver are prothrombin, and factors V, VII, IX and X. Thus in liver disease the coagulability of blood is decreased. Globulins (α and β but not γ) concerned with the transport of iron, copper and fat also have their origins in liver cells. As regards iron transport, three proteins synthesized by the liver have been described. These are transferrin, haptoglobin and haemopoxin which combine with iron, haemoglobin and haem respectively.

The liver is of importance in the degradation of proteins and amino acids as well as in their synthesis. All the enzymes necessary for the production of urea from nitrogen obtained as a result of amino acid metabolism are present in this organ. Thus instead of the accumulation of toxic amounts of ammonia in the body, urea is formed, which can be tolerated even at high concentrations. The series of reactions whereby urea formation occurs is known as the Krebs' urea cycle.

Fat metabolism

The liver is important in the handling of fat by the body. Its role in bile acid metabolism is considered elsewhere (see page 99). In addition, it removes (as does adipose tissue) the chylomicrons resulting from fat digestion and absorption that pass into the lymphatics. In the liver the triglycerides are again hydrolysed and some of the released fatty acids are incorporated into phospholipids and cholesterol esters or used again for triglyceride synthesis.

Lipids synthesized in the liver are released in association with a protein fraction (apoprotein) as lipoproteins. Depending on the protein fraction and the proportions of lipid present, the lipoproteins have different densities and electrophoretic mobilities. They are divided into chylomicrons, very low (VDLD), low (LDL) and high (HDL) density lipoproteins.

Some fatty acid is metabolized in the liver to provide energy. This occurs predominantly in mitochondria by the process of -oxidation. A high energy yielding series of reactions oxidizes fatty acids to produce 2-carbon units. However, the liver has limited capacity to oxidize fatty acids completely to carbon dioxide and water, with the result that the acetyl-coenzyme A formed is readily converted to the ketone bodies acetoacetic acid and -hydroxybutyric acid. These bodies may accumulate in the blood stream if produced in excess, with the resultant problems of ketosis.

A fatty liver is one of the most frequently seen abnormalities in liver morphology, accompanying excessive alcohol consumption and protein-calorie malnutrition. The fat that accumulates in the hepatocytes is mainly triglyceride. Remember, however, that several mechanisms may contribute to a fatty liver. These include:

1. A decreased synthesis or impaired secretion of lipoprotein.
2. An increased synthesis of triglyceride due to reduced fatty acid oxidation or reduced incorporation into phospholipid or cholesterol.
3. An increased supply of fatty acids to the liver because of mobilization from fat depots.

The handling of vitamins

The liver plays a prominent role. It is regarded as the main store of fat-soluble vitamins (A, D, E and K). Some water-soluble vitamins, particularly B_{12}, are also stored. Furthermore, the liver contributes to the absorption of fat-soluble vitamins by the small intestine. Bile acids maintain these substances in the micellar phase.

Hepatocellular heterogeneity

Evidence has accumulated to support the view that hepatocytes along the sinusoids are not functionally identical. Perhaps hepatocellular heterogeneity should have been anticipated. As blood flows along the sinusoid from the terminal portal venules and hepatic arterioles towards the hepatic venules numerous substances are removed or added. This creates a different microenvironment for the hepatocytes found close to the hepatic venule (arbitrarily said to be in zone 3) than that to which cells located around the portal venules are exposed. The latter hepatocytes are regarded as being in zone 1. An intermediate zone 2 accommodates those cells between zones 1 and 3. One example of heterogeneity is provided by the enzymes concerned with carbohydrate metabolism. Those involved in gluconeogenesis and glycolysis are present in both zones 1 and 3 but in different proportions. Thus phosphoenolpyruvate carboxykinase, presumably the rate-limiting enzyme of gluconeogenesis, fructose 1,6 diphosphatase and glycogen synthetase are located predominantly in zone 1 hepatocytes. In contrast, pyruvate kinase and glycogen phosphorylase, enzymes contributing to glycolysis and glycogen breakdown respectively, have greater activities in zone 3. It has been proposed that hepatocytes in zone 1 participate mainly in gluconeogenesis while cells in zone 3 are concerned more with glycolysis. Such an arrangement would permit shifts of carbohydrate metabolism without reversing the metabolic machinery of individual hepatocytes. For example, in the postabsorptive state glucose formation by zone 1 hepatocytes would increase whereas glucose utilization by zone 3 cells would decrease. The net result would be a change from hepatic glucose uptake to glucose production and release.

The handling of ammonia by the liver provides another example of heterogeneity (Fig. 4.11). The liver possesses two pathways for ammonia removal, one involving the production of urea, the other the formation of glutamine. Urea synthesis occurs in zone 1 (and some hepatocytes in zone 2) by a low-affinity, high-capacity mechanism. This results in decreasing concentrations of ammonia

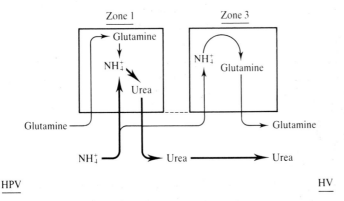

Fig. 4.11 Hepatocellular heterogeneity. The two major pathways for ammonia removal, i.e. urea and glutamine synthesis, occur in hepatocytes located in different zones along the sinusoid. HPV = hepatic portal vein; HV = hepatic vein

in sinusoidal blood as the hepatic vein is approached. Glutamine production takes place only in zone 3. However, because of the high affinity of this system more ammonia can be removed. Glutamine synthetase is exclusively detected in a 1–3 cell thick layer of hepatocytes surrounding hepatic venules. It is the only enzyme so far so specifically localized.

An alteration in hepatic ammonia metabolism between urea and glutamine synthesis may help to correct imbalances of systemic pH. Urea production utilizes bicarbonate and ammonia and may provide a mechanism for buffering base generated by catabolism after a protein-rich meal. In contrast, decreased urea production during acidosis accompanied by increased glutamine formation leads to less base removal by the liver. Furthermore the glutamine produced can be metabolized by the kidney to produce ammonia which contributes to the excretion of the acid load.

Hepatocyte volume regulation

Many cells exposed to changes in the tonicity of the fluids surrounding them endeavour to keep a constant volume. The mechanisms by which they achieve this are not identical in all cell types. When rat hepatocytes are exposed to a hypotonic stress *in vitro* a large increase in K^+ permeability and, therefore, K^+ efflux is triggered. On restoring the tonicity to normal values a net K^+ influx is recorded. This is thought to be accomplished by (a) a decrease in the passive conductance of the cell membrane to K^+, and (b) an activation of a $Na^+:H^+$ transfer system whereby the intracellular $[Na^+]$ is raised. Na^+ is subsequently exchanged for K^+ via the active Na^+,K^+-pump.

The secretion of bile

Bile, the secretion of the liver, is a variable complex mixture of organic and inorganic solutes. The daily output is 700–1200 ml. The major organic solutes are bile acids, phospholipids (particularly lecithin), cholesterol and bilirubin. The bile acids exist in the ionic form rather than as undissociated acids because their pK values are well below the pH encountered in the bile ducts. Bile acids have the tendency to form large polyionic aggregates (micelles, see page 138) so that their osmotic activity may be much less than that anticipated from measurements of their concentrations. Proteins, in small amounts, are also detected in bile. They include immunoglobulin A (IgA) formed when antigens are sampled by the intestines (see page 150). Secreting cells absorb circulating IgA by receptor-mediated endocytosis and transport it to the bile along a vesicular pathway.

As regards electrolytes Na^+ and K^+ are found in concentrations similar to those in plasma. The levels of the major anions in bile, Cl^- and HCO_3^-, however, are often less because of the presence of bile acid anions which contribute significantly to the total anion concentration. An important constituent of bile is calcium. It crosses the hepatocyte barrier by a paracellular route and achieves concentrations between 0.6 and 2.4 mmol/l. However, in the gall-bladder, bile becomes supersaturated with calcium as a result of water reabsorption.

When this occurs calcium precipitation and gallstone formation are more likely. Certainly many stones contain a central core of insoluble calcium salts around which are deposited layers of cholesterol or pigment (bilirubin). Different calcium concentrations in bile may help to explain why cholesterol stones are only found in some people with cholesterol-saturated bile. Many normal individuals produce secretions with similar cholesterol contents.

A number of gall-bladder defence mechanisms lessen the risk of stone formation. Among them are:

1. The secretion of hydrogen ions by the mucosa which lessens the likelihood of calcium precipitation.
2. The absorption of large amounts of calcium (about 50%). As a result the concentration of free calcium is lowered.
3. The release of potent antinucleating factors which inhibit cholesterol and calcium precipitation. The existence of these factors is recognized but what they are and from where they originate is unknown and a subject of current research.
4. The secretion of water and electrolytes during digestion which inter-mittently dilutes the gall-bladder contents. A stimulatory role for secretin has been proposed. Such a process may also help to wash out any particulate matter which could act as a nidus for stone formation.

Bile acids

These acids are water-soluble derivatives of cholesterol. The cholesterol is obtained from high density lipoproteins (HDL) taken up by membrane mediated endocytosis and directed into the bile acid synthesis pathway. Two primary bile acids are produced in the liver. These are cholic acid and chenodeoxycholic (chenic) acid (Fig. 4.12). The former is produced at twice the rate of chenic acid synthesis. Both acids are conjugated completely with glycine or taurine. This process has functional significance in that the conjugated acids are less likely to be precipitated by acid and Ca^{++} and, therefore, are able to produce their physiological effects. In addition, the conjugated form is more slowly absorbed by passive non-ionic diffusion in the proximal small intestine than the unconjugated acid. Nevertheless, a significant proportion is absorbed by passive diffusion because (a) the luminal contents are only slowly propelled towards the colon, and (b) bile acid concentrations rise following water absorption. Bile acids reaching the terminal ileum are absorbed by an active transport process. Such bile acids and those absorbed by diffusion are returned via the portal circulation to the liver.

Approximately 75% of the conjugated primary bile acids are unaltered as they pass along the small intestine. When bile acids reach the liver they are immediately removed by the hepatocytes from the sinusoids and resecreted into the bile. In this way the bile acids are made available again to aid digestive and absorptive processes taking place in the jejunum.

Of the 25 per cent of the primary bile acids deconjugated by bacteria, the greatest proportion is also absorbed and reconjugated in the liver. However, each day, one-quarter to one-third of the primary bile acids are lost or converted by intestinal bacteria into secondary bile acids, e.g. deoxycholic acid and lithocholic acid. A proportion of the deoxycholic acid formed follows the same route as the primary bile acids, i.e. intestinal absorption, passage back to the liver in the bloodstream and conjugation. Lithocholic acid is insoluble at body temperature and only a small proportion is absorbed, the remainder excreted. The cycle whereby bile acids are secreted by hepatocytes, pass through the lumen of the small intestine to be absorbed specifically in the ileum (but also by non-ionic diffusion in the small intestine and colon), and subsequently returned to the liver to be secreted again is the enterohepatic circulation (Fig. 4.13). A particular bile acid molecule must cycle many times per day. The total bile acid pool is of the order of 1.8–3.2 g, but the bile acid secretion by the liver can be 19–72 g per day.

Bile acids have several functions.

1. Triglyceride assimilation.
2. Induction of bile flow.
3. Lipid transport.
4. Bile acid synthesis.
5. Water and electrolyte secretion.

1. Triglyceride assimilation.

Bile acids are concerned with the final stages of digestion and absorption of triglycerides (see Chapter 5).

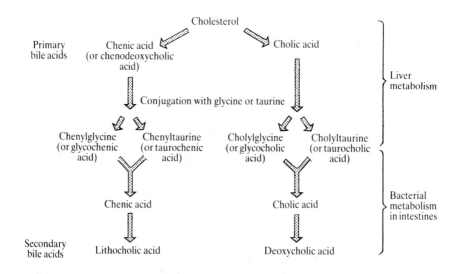

Fig. 4.12 The major primary and secondary bile acids in man. A further bile acid, ursodeoxycholic acid, has been classified as a tertiary bile acid. This substance is formed as a result of the liver modifying a bacterial metabolite of chenic acid and is detected in patients ingesting chenic acid for the dissolution of gallstones. In this case the liver is producing a bile acid which is not a primary bile acid.

2. Bile flow induction

Bile acids are choleretics, i.e. they induce the flow of bile. Bile acids osmotically attract water, and its dissolved electrolytes, as they are transported.

Some bile acids stimulate much greater bile flows than expected. They are said to be hypercholeretic. How could they produce their effects? One proposal has been that some bile acids may not be conjugated before being transported into the bile canaliculi. This would result in lipophilic unconjugated bile acids being absorbed from the bile ducts (but not water and electrolytes) and quickly carried to the liver sinusoids to be resecreted.

Normally less than 1 per cent of the bile acids secreted are unconjugated. These include the nor-bile acids which have one less carbon atom (23) than the major acids. Some of them, in rats at least, have remarkable choleretic properties.

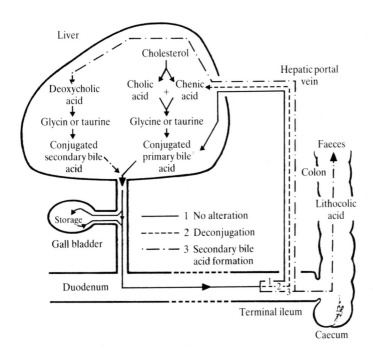

Fig. 4.13 The enterohepatic circulation. In this diagram bile acids in the intestinal lumen are shown to follow one of three pathways. 1. Absorption unaltered and return to the liver to be recycled. 2. Deconjugation, absorption and return to the liver to be reconjugated and recycled. 3. Deconjugation and further modification by intestinal bacteria to produce secondary bile acids. Some of these are absorbed and conjugated in the liver and secreted in the bile. Others, e.g. lithocholic acid, are relatively insoluble and are excreted in the faeces. A special mechanism for bile acid absorption is located in the distal ileum. However, bile acids can also be absorbed by non-ionic diffusion both at this site and at others in the small intestine and colon

3. Lipid transport

Bile acids contribute to the transport and elimination of lipid, e.g. cholesterol. Most body tissues continually synthesize cholesterol which is a major component of cell membranes. However, excessive cholesterol retention is associated with elevated serum cholesterol levels and arterial disease so that a means of removing this lipid is necessary. The liver secretes 1–2 g cholesterol per day, some of which is excreted from the body.

Hepatocytes secrete phospholipid and cholesterol into the bile as vesicles produced from microtubules close to the Golgi apparatus. Bile acids may induce vesicle formation and indeed be secreted to a limited extent with them. However, bile acids have further roles to play. Remember that conjugated bile acids are water-soluble substances derived from cholesterol. A proportion of them are lost each day and are replaced. Thus when bile acids are synthesized some cholesterol is also eliminated. Furthermore, when bile acids are present above a minimal concentration they form polymolecular aggregates known as micelles (see page 138). The minimal concentration necessary for micellar formation (the critical micellar concentration) is lower when the aggregates include lecithins (mixed micelles). Micelles provide a shell in the core of which cholesterol can be carried in a non-precipitated state from the liver to the small intestine.

4. Bile acid synthesis

Bile acids regulate their own synthesis. An interruption of the enterohepatic circulation, e.g. by the administration of cholestyramine (which has a marked affinity for bile acids) or choledocho-ureteral anastomosis, results in increased bile acid production. This finding has led intuitively to the view that normal absorption of bile acids from the intestines resulted in an inhibition of hepatic synthesis. However, all bile acids are not equally effective. Thus in the rabbit neither cholic acid nor its conjugates down regulated bile acid synthesis even though glycocholate makes up more than 90% of the total bile acid formed. In contrast the administration of chenic acid or its derivatives e.g. lithocholic acid, significantly inhibited cholic acid formation, perhaps by reducing the activity of cholesterol 7α-hydroxylase, the rate limiting enzyme for synthesis.

5. Water and electrolyte secretion

When present in high concentrations in the colon, bile acids stimulate the secretion of water and electrolytes, which may result in diarrhoea.

Mechanism of transport of bile acids across hepatocytes

One has to remember that bile acids in the plasma must traverse two membranes in series to appear in bile. The processes used are complex and, as yet, incompletely defined. One mechanism for uptake across the sinusoidal membrane is via a carrier whch requires and cotransports Na^+ ions simultaneously. The cation can be removed from the cell by a Na^+, K^+-pump into the space of Disse. A second system by which bile acids enter hepatocytes involves a carrier which recognizes other organic anions. This carrier should be regarded as a multispecific, rather than a non-specific carrier which is capable of recognizing different substrates at a series of different binding sites.

The means by which the bile acids are transferred from the sinusoidal to the canalicular membrane is poorly understood. It has been proposed that bile acids interact with cytoplasmic proteins and that the resulting complex moves across the hepatocytes. Such protein binding could diminish the potentially damaging effects of free bile acids on intracellular organelles. On reaching the canalicular membrane bile acids are secreted by a sodium-independent carrier mechanism. This is the rate limiting step of the hepatocyte transport process. It is sensitive to the potential difference across the canalicular membrane (35 mV, inside the cell negative) which provides a major driving force for organic anion transport.

Bile pigments

The major pigment of bile is bilirubin. Its formation is of considerable biological significance as it is the most important means by which haem, produced during the breakdown of haemoglobin, is eliminated. The conversion to bilirubin takes place in the reticuloendothelial system (mainly in the spleen and bone marrow but also in the liver). Not all the bilirubin produced is derived from haemoglobin. Up to 20 per cent of that present in bile is synthesized from other sources, e. g. myoglobin and cytochromes. Bilirubin has limited solubility in aqueous solutions at physiological pH and is carried in the blood bound mainly to albumin with only a small amount present as the free diffusible anion. Drugs such as salicylates and sulphonamides compete with bilirubin sites on proteins and increase the 'free bilirubin' in the plasma. As (a) the blood–brain barrier appears to be more permeable in neonates than in the adult, and (b) the liver has not attained full enzymatic maturation and has limited capacity to modify and secrete bilirubin, it follows that these drugs may increase the risk of kernicterus in the jaundiced infant.

The liver removes bilirubin rapidly from the plasma. At the hepatocytes' sinusoidal membrane bilirubin becomes dissociated from albumin and passes into the cell (Fig. 4.14). Two intracellular cytoplasmic proteins (Y and Z) bind most of the pigment. It is then transferred to the endoplasmic reticulum where it is converted to a glucuronide. Bilirubin must be converted to a polar compound before it can be excreted by a carrier-mediated, energy-dependent process. The conjugated bilirubin is not absorbed appreciably by the small intestine. However, in the colon bacterial enzymes partially hydrolyse it to release the pigment which is then reduced to non-pigmented metabolites, the urobilinogens, the form excreted in the faeces. Urobilinogens can be absorbed and either excreted by the liver or eliminated from the body via the kidney. The remaining non-hydrolysed pigment in the stools is responsible for their colour. If bile cannot reach the intestine (complete obstructive jaundice) the faeces are colourless and there is no urobilinogen in the urine.

In the past bilirubin has been regarded as a potentially toxic but otherwise useless waste product. However, recently it has been shown that bilirubin has antioxidant activities. Bilirubin suppresses the formation of lipid peroxides and limits the harmful alterations to hepatocyte membranes that such agents produce. It has been proposed that bilirubin might be added to the growing list of antioxidant defence systems which includes superoxide dismutase, glutathione and vitamin C.

Control of bile secretion

Bile secretion has often been thought to be made up of three fractions.

1. A bile acid-dependent part in which water and electrolytes move passively as the result of the active transport of bile acids. Water follows bile acids because of solute drag and creates a diffusion gradient for inorganic ions. Water and electrolytes are transferred probably both transcellularly and paracellularly from the space of Disse.

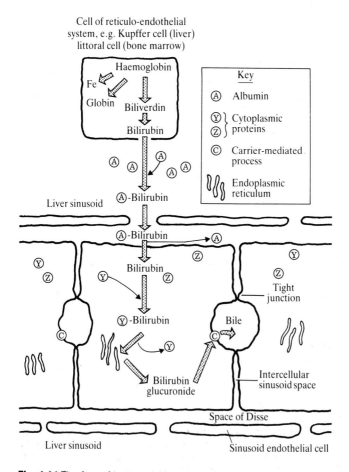

Fig. 4.14 The fate of haemoglobin

Paracellular movement of water and electrolytes between cells depends on the permeability of the 'not so' tight junctions. These junctions can no longer be regarded as static barriers with fixed pores and charges allowing the selective sieving of molecules. Indeed, they provide a dynamic barrier the permeability of which can be increased by some bile acids (e.g. taurocholate) and hormones (e.g. vasopressin, adrenaline and angiotensin II).

2. A bile acid-independent system involving the active transport of electrolytes across hepatocytes has been proposed from data collected in animal studies. Such a process does not occur in man.

3. The intrahepatic bile ducts have structural characteristics (microvilli and enlarged subcellular or intercellular spaces) which are hardly consistent with the view that they are simple conduits. It is thought that these ducts are the sites at which a significant proportion of the water and electrolytes in bile are secreted (Fig 4.15). A mechanism for HCO_3^- secretion and one of coupled

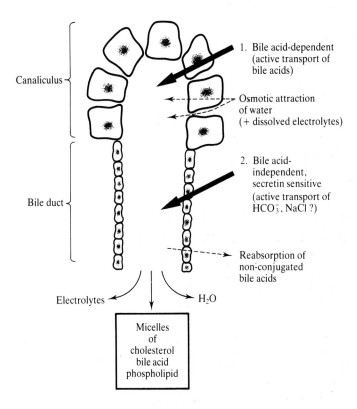

Fig. 4.15 Bile entering the duodenum is a fluid which although modified by the gall bladder is produced at two sites. 1. A bile acid-dependent secretion. This is derived from hepatocytes. Water (containing dissolved electrolytes) follows the transported bile acids passively into the canaliculi. 2. A bile acid-independent secretion formed by duct cells which is sensitive to secretin. Roles for HCO_3^- and NaCl secretory processes have been suggested. Reabsorption of non-conjugated bile acids from the ducts, their rapid return to hepatocytes and resecretion contribute to the hypercholeretic effects of some bile acids.

Na$^+$ and Cl$^-$ movement have been proposed. Injections of the hormone secretin increase bile flow to twice the basal rate. The concentration of the HCO$_3^-$ in this fluid is high although the bile acid content is not increased. It appears that those stimuli releasing secretin cause a HCO$_3^-$-rich fluid to be produced by both the liver and the pancreas.

The gall-bladder

In man the gall-bladder is a readily distensible bag with a capacity of about 30–50 ml. It performs two functions.

1. Water and electrolyte absorption.
2. Contraction to deliver bile.

Water and electrolyte absorption

The gall-bladder absorbs most of the water and electrolytes from dilute hepatic bile to produce a concentrated fluid rich in Na$^+$ and bile acids. A Na$^+$-rich fluid seems an unlikely event until one remembers that bile acids are mainly in the anionic form and the volume remaining is small. The fluid absorbed from the gall-bladder is isotonic with respect to plasma. The primary process involved is the active transport of Na$^+$ accompanied by Cl$^-$ with water following passively. NaCl movement across the apical membrane is partly due to:

1. Coupled Na$^+$: proton and Cl$^-$: HCO$_3^-$ exchange
2. NaCl symport on a single carrier.

However, the passive permeability of the gall-bladder to water is too low to account for the observed isotonic fluid absorption. To explain it, a barrier must be present that will prevent these solutes, which have been actively transported across the epithelia, from diffusing away until sufficient water has followed. An involvement of the long spaces between the epithelial cells, the lateral spaces, was suggested by the finding that these became widely dilated during fluid absorption and collapsed when no fluid transfer was taking place. The question remained as to how an isotonic fluid was being absorbed. Two theories have been put forward. The concepts presented in both are important. Each of the mechanisms proposed makes a contribution:

1. *The serial membrane model (Fig 4.16)* – In this theory solute is actively transported across the lateral cell walls into the intercellular spaces. Water then passes into these spaces and an osmotic equilibrium is reached. A non-specific barrier provided by the basal clefts and lamina propria is overcome when the hydrostatic pressure developed within the intercellular spaces increases and drives the isotonic solution out.

2. *The standing gradient model (Fig 4.17)* – As in the above model solute (NaCl) is transported into the intercellular spaces. This causes an increase in the local osmotic pressure. The fluid in these channels is not stirred and solute moves out of them by diffusion and in the water stream that is attracted from the lumen. The result is that when fluid absorption is in a steady state an

osmotic gradient exists along the length of the intercellular spaces. At the apical region, close to the tight junction, the tonicity is high. Where the fluid crosses the basement membrane to the interstitial space the fluid is isotonic.

When these theories were first proposed, it was thought that the luminal and intercellular space fluids were separated by tight junctions (and tight meant exactly that) and exchanges of water between these compartments were via an intracellular pathway. It is now clear that the tight junctions of gall-bladder epithelia are leaky and that water and solutes can be exchanged across them. Thus the osmotic gradients anticipated in the second model are not produced. Nevertheless the concept of electrolytes accumulating in the intercellular spaces and osmotically attracting water with the result that an isotonic fluid is produced at the level of the basement membrane is a useful and appealing one.

Contraction to deliver bile

The gall-bladder contracts to deliver concentrated bile to the small intestine. Even during the interdigestive period the gall-bladder is not quiescent. It has tone which reflects the inherent compliance of smooth muscle and fibroelastic tissue within its walls. This tone is modulated by hormones and autonomic mechanisms. Thus, for example, loxiglumide (a potent CCK-receptor antagonist) increases the volume of the unstimulated gall-bladder in fasting man. In addition bile is delivered intermittently into the duodenum. Gall-bladder contractions producing this can be correlated with the migrating myoelectric complexes which characteristically can be recorded in the stomach, gall-bladder and small intestine during fasting (see page 195). Such contractions eliminating bile would prevent the accumulation of microcrystals

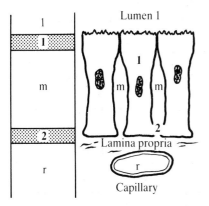

Fig. 4.16 The serial membrane model to explain isotonic fluid absorption. The Curran and MacIntosh model has three compartments (l, m and r) separated by a semipermeable membrane (**1**) and a non-selective barrier (**2**). Solute is actively pumped from space l to m across barrier **1**. This creates an osmotic gradient which causes water to move from **1** to m. Hydrostatic pressure then forces the fluid out across barrier **2**. In the gall bladder **1** is analogous to the lumen, **1** to the cell membranes, m to the lateral intercellular spaces, **2** to the basal clefts and lamina propria and r to the bloodstream (From Curran, P. and MacIntosh, J.R. (1962). *Nature* **193**, 347–8.)

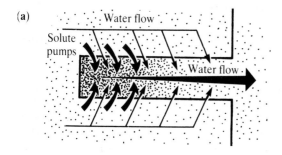

(a)

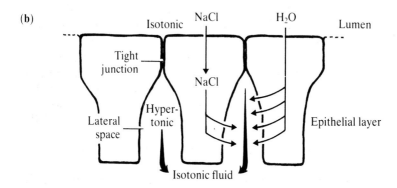

(b)

Fig. 4.17 (**a**) Diagrammatic representation of the 'standing gradient' model of isotonic water movement. This system consists of a long narrow channel closed at one end. Solute (NaCl) is actively transported into the channel across its walls, making the channel fluid hypertonic. As solute diffuses down its concentration gradient toward the open mouth, more and more water enters the channel across its walls due to the osmotic gradient. In the steady state a standing osmotic gradient will be maintained in the channel by active solute transport, with the osmolarity decreasing from the closed to the open end. A fluid of fixed osmolarity will issue from the mouth. (**b**) In the gall-bladder a standing gradient system may be achieved by NaCl being transported into the lateral spaces, closed at one end by the tight junctions but open and leading to the circulation at the other (From Diamond, J.M. (1971). *Federation Proceedings* **30**, 6–13.)

or debris during interdigestive periods and thus reduce the risk of cholesterol precipitation.

　Food provides a stimulus for gall-bladder emptying before it is released into the small intestine. This has been demonstrated in man using a sham feeding procedure. Fasting volunteers were presented with a meal of sirloin steak, french fried potatoes and water which they chewed and then spit out. Nasogastric suction was applied to some subjects to eliminate the possible effects of duodenal acidification. Their gall-bladders emptied by more than 40% within 1-2 hours. This response was eliminated by cholinergic blockade with atropine and could not be elicited in patients with vagotomies. These studies indicated that intact vagus nerves and cholinergic pathways are required for the cephalic phase of the gall-bladder emptying response.

Distension of the antral region of the stomach also produces gall-bladder contractions. A vago-vagal pylorocholecystic reflex provides bile for the emulsification of the first chyme reaching the duodenum.

The major factor controlling postprandial gall-bladder contractions in man is CCK. It is released when fat or essential amino acids are introduced into the duodenum. The resulting contractions increase the pressure of the fluid in the bile ducts. As the pressure rises the resistance offered by the sphincter of Oddi is overcome and bile is forced into the duodenum. CCK can cause contractions in two ways. It can act directly on receptors on smooth muscle membranes. In addition, however, it activates intramural neurons which release acetylcholine. Extrinsic parasympathetic nerves also have a role to play. They facilitate the gall-bladder response to CCK (NB. the vagus furthermore contributes to the maintenance of muscle tone).

In earlier sections (see page 80) it was proposed that the pancreatic enzymes released by CCK were capable of inhibiting further secretion of the hormone. In other words a negative feedback system existed to conserve enzymes. A similar self-regulating feedback loop has been established in man for gall-bladder emptying. It has been shown that bile acids inhibit the release of CCK stimulated by lipid.

Another hormone with actions on the gall-bladder is pancreatic polypeptide (PP) released from pancreatic islet PP cells. This biologically active peptide was discovered as a major contaminant during the purification of insulin. It is released by chewing food and by signals originating in the stomach and small intestine. Gastric distension is one of these. Perhaps the most potent stimuli for human PP secretion are produced by dietary proteins (e.g. those found in ground beef and steamed cod). Vago-vagal reflexes account for at least some of the PP released. PP causes relaxation of the gall-bladder. In addition it inhibits pancreatic enzyme release. These actions at first sight may seem surprising. Such effects clearly do not aid digestion. Furthermore they are directly opposite those of CCK which is also released by the products of protein digestion. A clue to the possible value of PP is provided by the finding that plasma PP levels remain elevated for at least 6 hours postprandially, long after other gastrointestinal hormones have returned to their basal levels. Thus PP may play a useful role by promoting the storage of bile and the conservation of pancreatic enzymes.

The flow of bile to the duodenum or its diversion to the gall-bladder depends on the resistance offered by the sphincter of Oddi. The basal tone of this sphincter provides a small resistance in man. However, prominent phasic contractions (2–6/min) producing much greater pressures (100–150 mm Hg) are also recorded. Bile flows passively between these phasic events. Several factors influence the sphincter contractions. One of these is CCK which decreases baseline pressure and phasic activity. The sphincter is thus more relaxed and the passive flow of bile is more easily facilitated. This effect of CCK is mediated by non-adrenergic, non-cholinergic nerves, the activity of which mask the direct excitatory effects of the hormone. Whether other regions than the gall-bladder and the sphincter of Oddi contribute to the flow of bile remains a controversial topic. What is interesting, however, is the recent observation that the canalicular contents are 'pumped' towards the bile ducts. This phenomenom has been observed in isolated hepatocytes in primary culture using time-lapse cinephotomicrography. The frequency with which canaliculi contract is increased by taurocholate. How do canaliculi contract? The answer is not known although contractile elements such as actin are recognized in a variety of non-muscle cells and are especially numerous near bile canaliculi in hepatocytes.

The flow of bile into the duodenum depends on numerous processes. These include the secretory processes of the liver and bile ducts as well as the contractions of the gall-bladder and the sphincter of Oddi. A glance at Fig. 4.18 shows how complex an event it is.

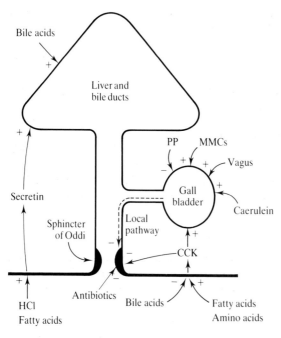

Fig. 4.18 Some events contributing to the control of bile flow into the duodenum. One must consider: (**a**) the secretion of bile by the liver; (**b**) contractions of the gall-bladder; and (**c**) the relaxation of the sphincter of Oddi. In the liver bile acids and secretin are major factors which increase bile secretion. The gall-bladder contracts in response to CCK and caerulein. The latter is a decapeptide isolated from frog (*Hyla caerulea*) skin. It has been used clinically as a secretagogue as it can cause greater contractions than CCK. The vagus also causes contractions. It does so during the cephalic phase of digestion and when the stomach is distended. Even during the interdigestive period the gall-bladder occasionally contracts. These contractions are correlated to migrating myoelectric comlexes. Gall-bladder relaxation can be produced by pancreatic polypeptide. The sphincter of Oddi is dilated by CCK and perhaps following the activation of a local reflex from the gall-bladder. Antibiotics reduce the tone of the sphincter. PP = Pancreatic polypeptide; MMC = the migrating myoelectric (and motor) complex

Bibliography

Adelson, J.W. and Miller, P.E. (1989). Heterogeneity of the exocrine pancreas. *American Journal of Physiology* **256**, G817–G825.

Beaudoin, A.R., St.-Jean, P. and Grondin, G. (1989). Pancreatic juice composition: New views about the cellular mechanisms that control the concentration of digestive and nondigestive proteins. *Digestive Diseases* **7**, 210–20.

Berridge, M.J. (1987). Inositol triphosphate and diacylglycerol: two interacting second messengers. *Annual Review of Biochemistry* **56**, 159–93.

Boyer, J.L., Gautam, A. and Graf, J. (1988). Mechanisms of bile secretion: insights from the isolated rat hepatocyte couplet. *Seminars in Liver Disease* **8**, 309–17.

Case, R.M. (1989). Physiology and biochemistry of pancreatic exocrine secretion. *Current Opinion in Gastroenterology* **5**, 665–81.

Fahrenkrug, J. and Emson, P.C. (1982). Vasoactive intestinal polypeptide: functional aspects. *British Medical Bulletin* **38**, 265–70.

Farges, O., Corbic, M., Dumont, M., Maurice, M. and Erlinger, S. (1989). Permeability of rat biliary tree to ursodeoxycholic acid. *American Journal of Physiology* **256**, G653–G660.

Fisher, R.S., Rock, E. and Malmud, L.S. (1986). Gallbladder emptying response to sham feeding in humans. *Gastroenterology* **90**, 1854–57.

Frimmer, M. and Ziegler, K. (1988). The transport of bile acids in liver cells. *Biochimica Biophysica Acta* **947**, 75–99.

Grace, P.A., Poston, G.J. and Williamson, R.C.N. (1990). Biliary motility. *Gut* **31**, 571–82.

Haddad, P. and Graf, J. (1989). Volume-regulatory K^+ fluxes in the isolated rat liver: characterization by ion transport inhibitors. *American Journal of Physiology* **257**, G357–G363.

Hall, R., Kok, E. and Javitt, N.B. (1988). Bile acid synthesis: down regulation by monohydroxy bile acids. *The FASEB Journal* **2**, 152–6.

Hofmann, A.F. (1978). Lipase, colipase amphipathic dietary proteins and bile acids: new interactions at an old interface. *Gastroenterology* **75**, 530–2.

Hofmann, A.F. (1989). Current concepts of biliary secretion. *Digestive Diseases and Sciences* **34 (12 Supplement)**, 16S–20S.

Izzo, R.S., Pellecchia, C. and Praissman, M. (1988). Internalization and cellular processing of cholecystokinin in rat pancreatic acinar cells. *American Journal of Physiology* **255**, G738–G744.

Jacyna, M.R. (1990). Interactions between gall bladder bile and mucosa: relevance to gall stone formation. *Gut* **31**, 568–70.

Knutson, L. and Flemström, G. (1989). Duodenal mucosal bicarbonate secretion in man. Stimulation by acid and inhibition by an alpha$_2$-adrenoceptor agonist clonidine. *Gut* **30**, 1708–15.

Konturek, J.W., Konturek, S.J., Kurek, A., Bogdal, J., Olesky, J. and Rovati, L. (1989). CCK receptor antagonism by loxiglumide and gall bladder contractions in response to cholecystokinin, sham feeding and ordinary feeding in man. *Gut* **30**, 1136–42.

Liebow, C. and Rothman, S.S. (1975). Enteropancreatic circulation of digestive enzymes. *Science* **189**, 472–4.

Liener, I.E., Goodale, R.L., Deshmukh, A., *et al.* (1988). Effect of a trypsin inhibitor from soybeans (Bowman–Birk) on the secretory activity of the human pancreas. *Gastroenterology* **94**, 419–27.

Lowe, P.J., Miyai, K., Steinbach, J.H. and Hardison, W.G.M. (1988). Hormonal regulation of hepatocyte tight junction permeability. *American Journal of Physiology* **255**, G454–G461.

Malfertheiner, P., Glasbrenner, B. and Büchler, M. (1988). Role of nutrients in pancreatic adaptation with implication of cholecystokinin release. *Scandinavian Journal of Gastroenterology* **23 (Supplement 151),** 108–13.

Miyasaka, K., Guan, D., Liddle, R.A. and Green, G.M. (1989). Feedback regulation by trypsin: evidence for intraluminal CCK-releasing peptide. *American Journal of Physiology* **257**, G175–G181.

Muallem, S., Schoeffield, M.S., Fimmel, C.J. and Pandol, S.J. (1988). Agonist-sensitive calcium pool in the pancreatic acinar cell. II. Characterization of reloading. *American Journal of Physiology* **255**, G229–G235.

Niederau, C., van Dyke, RW., Scharschmidt, B.F. and Grendell, J.H. (1986). Rat pancreatic zymogen granules. An actively acidified compartment. *Gastroenterology* **91**, 1433–42.

Owyang, C., May, D. and Louie, D.S. (1986). Trypsin suppression of pancreatic secretion. Differential effect on cholecystokinin release and the enteropancreatic reflex. *Gastroenterology* **91**, 637–43.

Rinderknecht, H. (1986). Activation of pancreatic enzymes. Normal activation, premature intrapancreatic activation, protective mechanisms against inappropriate activation. *Digestive Diseases and Sciences* **31**, 314–21.

Rinderknecht, H., Adham, N.F., Renner, I.G. and Carmack, C. (1988). A possible zymogen self-destruct mechanism preventing pancreatic autodigestion. *International Journal of Pancreatology* **3**, 33–44.

Rothman, SS. (1980). Passage of proteins through membranes – old assumptions and new perspectives. *American Journal of Physiology* **238**, G391–G402.

Singer, M.V. (1987) Pancreatic secretory response to intestinal stimulants: a review. *Scandinavian Journal of Gastroenterology* **22 (Supplement 139)**, 1–13.

Solomon, T.E. (1984). Regulation of pancreatic secretion. *Clinics in Gastroenterology* **13**, 657–78.

Stocker, R., Yamamoto, Y., McDonagh, A.F., Glazer, A.N. and Ames, B.N. (1989). Bilirubin is an antioxidant of possible physiological importance. *Science* **235**, 1043–46.

Thiruvengadam, R. and DiMagno, E.P. (1988). Inactivation of human lipase by proteases. *American Journal of Physiology* **255**, G476–G481.

Traber, P.G., Chianale, J. and Gumucio, J.J. (1988). Physiologic significance and regulation of hepatocellular heterogeneity. *Gastroenterology* **95**, 1130–43.

Vidon, N., Chaussade, S., Merite, F., Hutchet, B., Franchisseur, C., and Bernier, J.-J. (1989). Inhibitory effect of high caloric load of carbohydrates or lipids on human pancreatic secretions: a jejunal brake. *American Journal of Clinical Nutrition* **50**, 231–36.

5

The small intestine

The small intestine is a region in which many absorptive and secretory processes occur. In addition, it performs several complex movements. Before describing these processes, let us consider the structure and blood supply of the small bowel.

Structure of the small intestine

This convoluted tube is about 5 m long and even longer post mortem when smooth muscle tone is absent. The duodenum, jejunum and ileum are the three regions of the small intestine. The first (25 cm), beginning at the pylorus, is a curved tube devoid of mesentery. The wall of the duodenum contains mucus-secreting Brunner's glands and ducts pass through it so that pancreatic and hepatic secretions can reach the intestinal lumen. The remainder of the small intestine is a coiled tube attached to the posterior abdominal wall by mesentery. The cephalad two-fifths are recognized as jejunum and the rest as the ileum. However, this is an arbitrary division as there are no distinguishing characteristics on either side of the boundary between jejunum and ileum. Rather, a gradual change in structure occurs as the intestine is traversed. Thus the jejunum is thicker walled, more vascular and has larger and more numerous villi than the ileum. The valves of Kerkring (circular folds or valvulae conniventes) are large and thickly set in the jejunum but rare in the distal ileum. These folds retard the passage of food and provide an increased surface area for absorption. In contrast, the aggregated follicles (Peyer's patches) of the ileum are larger and more numerous than those of the jejunum.

The intestinal wall has several layers:

1. The serosal layer composed of visceral peritoneum merging with connective tissue.
2. The muscularis externa comprising a thin outer layer of longitudinal muscle and a thicker inner region of circular muscle.
3. A submucosal layer consisting of connective tissue, blood vessels and lymphatics.

4. The mucosal layer with its numerous types of cells. This can be divided into three regions:

(a) Inside the submucosa is a thin muscle layer which extends into the circular folds.

(b) A connective tissue layer, the lamina propria, in which lymphocytes, eosinophils, macrophages and mast cells are encountered.

(c) A basement membrane supporting absorptive columnar epithelial cells interspersed with mucus-secreting goblet cells.

The intestinal villi give the luminal surface a velvet-like appearance. Their structure changes along the length of the intestine. Thus broad, ridge-like villi of the duodenum give way to tall leaf-like structures in the jejunum and these are slowly modified to the shorter, finger-like processes of the distal jejunum and ileum. Each villus (Fig. 5.1) is comprised of a layer of columnar epithelial cells on their basement membrane, a lymph vessel, blood vessels, some smooth muscle fibres and connective tissue. The lymph vessel, or lacteal, originates close to the tip of the villus and drains into the plexus of vessels in the lamina propria. These vessels have an important role in the removal of chylomicrons (see pages 141 and 189). The normal villus height is up to 1 mm and the villi vary in density from 10 to 40mm³. They contribute significantly to the huge mucosal surface area that is available for absorption. T.H. Wilson calculated that the surface area was some 600 times greater than would be expected from a simple tube with the same diameter. The greatest contribution, however, appears to be made by the epithelial cells lining the villus. At their free surface are minute, parallel cylindrical microvilli, each approximately 1 μm long and 0.1 μm in diameter. These structures constitute the brush border.

Between the villi are simple tubular glands, the crypts of Lieberkuhn. A number of cells are present in these crypts, including undifferentiated cells, mucus-secreting goblet cells, Paneth cells and endocrine– paracrine cells (Fig. 5.2). Undifferentiated cells are the most numerous. These cells proliferate to provide replacements for those epithelial cells lining the villus. In contrast to some organs, e.g. brain, where cell populations are almost permanent, the small intestine has an extremely fast cell turnover. In several mammalian species the whole epithelial cell population is replaced in 1–3 days (in humans this takes about 6 days). Cells produced in the crypt stream out and up the villi. Subsequently they are lost from extrusion zones at the tips of villi and desquamate into the lumen. The rapid replacement is undoubtedly important as the epithelial cells are extremely sensitive to anoxia and other noxious stimuli.

Surprisingly, the cells lining the alimentary tract have considerable capacity of their own to recover from insults to their plasma membranes. McNeil and Ito (1989) have reported that mechanically injured and even normal experimentally undisturbed gut epithelial cells periodically develop apical membrane wounds. These wounds are sufficiently large for macromolecules to diffuse from the intestinal lumen and into the cytoplasm. Remarkably the affected cells reseal and survive. Perhaps these findings should have been anticipated. Physiologists working with microelectrodes routinely impale plasma membranes with glass pipettes, producing wounds which spontaneously reseal, before making intracellular recordings. The processes involved in wound healing remain to studied.

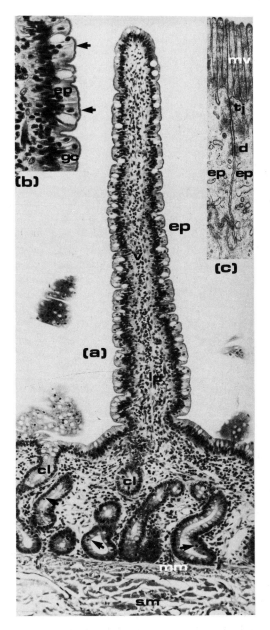

Fig. 5.1 The intestinal villus (cat). (**a**) A light micrograph of the mucosa and submucosa (sm). A single villus (v) is shown, with its absorptive epithelium (ep) and goblet cells covering a richly cellular lamina propria (lp). Several crypts of Lieberkühn (cl) are present containing dividing mucosal replacement cells (↑). Separating the lamina propria and submucosa are the muscularis mucosa (mm). (**b**) The absorptive tall, columnar epithelial cells (ep) with a brush border (←). Interspersed between the columnar cells are several mucus-secreting goblet cells (gc). (**c**) The apices of two adjoining columnar epithelial cells (ep). Their brush borders consist of microvilli (mv). Also shown is a tight junction (tj) and a desmosome (**d**). The latter is concerned with maintaining cell shape (Kindly presented by Mr R.P. Gould, The Middlesex Hospital Medical School, London.)

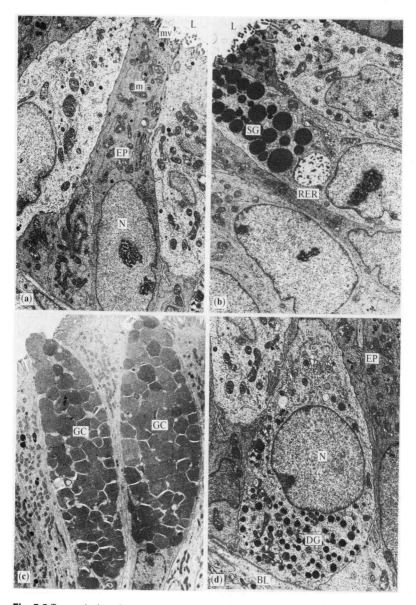

Fig. 5.2 Transmission electron micrographs of human jejunum.
(a) An immature, undifferentiated, columnar epithelial cell (EP) from a crypt. The cell lacks the well-developed microvilli which characterize the absorbing villous cell. N = nucleus, m = mitochondria, mv = microvilli and L = lumen. (b) A Paneth cell found exclusively in the crypt. It is characterized by electron-dense secretory granules (SG), a source of lysozyme, and a well-developed rough endoplasmic reticulum (RER). (c) Goblet cells (GC), packed with large homogeneous granules rich in mucus. (d) An endocrine-like cell, of which there are several different types in the crypt. Numerous dense core granules (DG) are evident at the basal pole of the cell from where they can be released into the interstitial fluid. BL = Basal lamina; EP = immature columnar epithelial cell; N = nucleus (Kindly presented by Dr K. Kyriacou, College of Medicine, King Saud University, Riyadh, Saudi Arabia.)

One factor is likely to be the self-healing properties of phospholipid bilayers.

In addition to the effects of mechanical stimuli the epithelial cells are continuously exposed to digestive enzymes and potentially harmful dietary components. Among the latter are the lectins. These can be found in numerous vegetables, cereals, fruits, nuts and spices commonly used. A single challenge to rats with raw red kidney beans (300 mg by orogastric lavage) has resulted in lectin-induced damage of jejunal absorptive epithelial cells. As early as 2 hours after the challenge dramatic structural alterations were seen. Microvilli of villous epithelia were irregular in shape. Some were short and wide, others long and thin. Even branched microvilli were found. Many vesicles could be observed in close association with the microvilli (vesiculation is thought to be the cause of microvillous shortening). Damage was largely confined to the brush border. Other organelles such as the rough endoplasmic reticulum, Golgi and mitochondria appeared unaffected. By 20 hours after challenge the microvilli had regained a more normal appearance. However, cell migration was not accelerated, suggesting that damaged cells had repaired themselves.

Paneth cells complete their life cycles at the base of the crypts. Their functions are poorly understood. Some regard them as phagocytes. The finding of spiral bacteria and the intestinal parasite *Hexamita muris* within phagosomes of Paneth cells in various stages of degeneration supports this view. Others have speculated that because Paneth cells produce a substantial secretion they may provide nutrients needed by the crypt cell population.

The number of endocrine–paracrine cells that have been identified in the small intestine has now reached double figures. Most of them produce active peptides. For example, the D, S and N cells elaborate somatostatin, secretin and neurotensin respectively. Some cells (EC cells) synthesize 5-hydroxytryptamine (5HT). The major product of a few, which include the VL cell, remain unidentified. The precise physiological roles of several of the cells also has yet to be established.

Epithelial cell proliferation and differentiation

A small number of cells in the crypts are regarded as functional stem cells. They do not migrate but give rise to columnar epithelial, mucus-secreting, endocrine–paracrine and Paneth cells. The rate at which cells proliferate can change dramatically. Thus there is atrophy during starvation and even when an animal is fed intravenously. In contrast, increased proliferative rates are recorded in regions of the intestines exposed to specific nutrients to which they are not accustomed, e.g. after intestinal resection or bypass.

There may be many factors in the control of cell proliferation. These include:

1. Local negative feedback mechanisms between functioning cells on the villi and dividing cells in the crypts.
2. Humoral factors such as enteroglucagon and EGF.
3. Luminal dietary components. In the colon, at least, short chain fatty acids may accelerate proliferation. Introducing dietary fibre, from which colonic

bacteria can release short chain fatty acids, into the food of rats previously fed fibre-free diets, increases epithelial cell proliferation.

Recently attention has been focused on a possible role of extracellular matrix factors for epithelial growth, organization and maturation. Cells derived from normal rat small intestine and resembling immature crypt cells (the IEC-6 cell line) were grown *in vitro* on basement membrane extracts harvested from Engelbreth–Holm–Swarm sarcoma cells. Mitoses were arrested and sucrase, apolipoprotein B and Na^+-dependent glucose transport were induced. Such changes are consistent with maturation. Furthermore, these cells were rapidly organized into multicellular complex structures. In marked contrast cells grown on plastic or glass remained relatively immature and proliferated rapidly.

The intestinal circulation

The blood vessels in the jejunum and ileum are derived from the superior mesenteric artery. Numerous branches are given off which supply the muscular coat and form intrinsic plexuses in the submucosal layer. From these networks tiny vessels travel to the villi and the glands of the mucosa. In man approximately 10% of the cardiac output at rest flows to the intestine. Three-quarters of this is distributed to the mucosa and submucosa, the remainder to the muscularis. This reflects the greater metabolic demands of the transporting epithelium as compared with those of the smooth muscle layer.

Measurement of blood flow

A variety of procedures have been used to measure intestinal blood flow. One of these involved an intra-arterial injection of radioactive microspheres (about 15 μm diameter and labelled with ^{85}Sr, ^{51}Cr, ^{41}Co or radionuclides with longer half-lives). Because of their size the microspheres do not appear in the veins but are trapped in precapillary vessels. The relative proportions of microspheres detected in such vessels depends on the distribution of blood to the different regions.

More recently the technique of laser Doppler velocimetry (LDV) has been developed which can be successfully applied to humans. Shepherd and Riedel (1982) built a laser Doppler flowmeter which included a helium–neon laser and a pair of fibre-optic light guides that conduct laser light to the tissue under investigation and carry back scattered light to a detector. This monochromatic light scattered by moving erythrocytes experiences a shift in its frequency which is proportional to the red blood cells' velocities. By determining mean Doppler frequencies an estimate of blood flow can be made. LDV can provide a continuous measurement of blood flow changes at tissue surfaces. As the fibre-optic probe can be passed endoscopically to the intestine changes in human mucosal blood flow can be monitored. During surgery blood flow to the muscle layers can also be investigated.

Autoregulatory escape

Nerves, hormones and local factors all contribute to the control of the intestinal circulation. The small intestine is richly supplied with sympathetic vasocon-strictor fibres which affect both pre- and postcapillary vessels. A marked increase in the resistance of precapillary resistance vessels is elicited with sustained sympathetic stimulation. Within 1 or 2 minutes, however, it rapidly declines. A new steady state is reached at which the resistance is only moderately greater than that originally recorded. Not all vessels respond. Thus there is some redis-tribution of blood. The vessels supplying the villi dilate while vasoconstriction is maintained in the more deeply situated mucosal regions (crypts). How might this phenomenon of autoregulatory escape be explained? One mechanism that has been proposed depends on adrenergic receptors adapting to continued nerve stimulation. This possibility has been regarded as unlikely because the infusion of noradrenaline during the escape phase of sympathetic nerve stimulation results in further vasoconstriction followed by a second escape. An alternative proposal has been that vasoactive metabolites accumulate during the initial vasoconstrictor response which dilate arterioles and consequently restore blood flow towards normal. Certainly the gut contains or can produce a variety of vasodilator substances. These include histamine (found in large amounts in the mesenteric vascular endothelium), prostaglandins, dopamine and adenine nucleotides.

Although histamine may mediate arteriolar responses following a meal (postprandial hyperaemia, see page 121) it is not thought to contribute to autoregulatory escape. H–1-receptor blockade with chlorpheniramine, at doses which prevent vasodilator responses to exogenously administered histamine, does not affect either vasoconstrictor or escape responses to noradrenaline infu-sions in piglets. Adenosine, on the other hand, is responsible for at least part of the escape. Vasodilator responses to adenosine can be inhibited with adenosine deaminase which converts adenosine to inosine and, therefore, prevents its accumulation. When this enzyme is administered vasoconstrictor responses to noradrenaline are increased. In contrast, steady state escape responses are reduced.

Vasoconstriction of the postcapillary capacitance vessels is usually well sustained and powerful. As a result substantial volumes of blood can be expelled from the splanchnic circulation and contribute to the maintenance of blood pressure. To appreciate these responses one has to remember that a function of the sympathetic nervous system is to adjust to the requirements of the body as a whole, often in competition with local mechanisms attempting to satisfy the needs of the immediate environment.

Vasodilator nerves

Vasodilator nerves to intestinal submucosal arterioles have been described. Some are cholinergic and project from the submucosal plexus. The acetylcholine released activates muscarinic receptors of the M_3-subtype, found on vascular smooth muscle. Thus arterioles may be dilated directly by nerves as well as indirectly following the release of EDRF from endothelial cells. We do not know the physiological role of these nerves and of other fibres to submucosal arterioles containing known vasodilators e.g. VIP, substance P and calcitonin gene related peptide? However, it is interesting to speculate. Over the past decade it has been established that submucosal cholinergic neurons promote water and electrolyte secretion. A complementary vasodilatory role of submucosal neurons might provide a simultaneous increase in blood flow to the mucosa as well as a direct excitation of secretory epithelial cells.

Local factors controlling blood flow

Blood flow can be maintained relatively constant in the face of fluctuations of arterial pressure. However, it is constantly adjusted to meet the demands of the tissue. Such control is achieved as a result of myogenic activity and of changes elicited by locally available chemical factors (autoregulation). Vascular smooth muscle has basal myogenic tone and shortens when passively stretched. It follows, therefore, that an increase in transmural pressure accompanying a rise in blood pressure will result in arterial vasoconstriction but maintained capillary perfusion. Numerous chemical agents released from the intestine have vasodilator properties. Adenosine and histamine have already been mentioned, the former thought to have a role in autoregulatory escape. However, one should look beyond these and other established vasodilators of the general circulation, e.g. K^+ and H^+. The intestinal blood vessels are exposed to substances absorbed from the lumen and present in greater concentrations than detected elsewhere in the body.

The splanchnic blood flow increases 50-300% following the intake of food with little increase in the cardiac output or blood pressure. Part of this response may be dependent on a local vasodilator reflex which is activated by light mechanical stimulation of the intestinal mucosa. 5HT, found in abundance in the argentaffin cells of the mucosa and in the myenteric plexus, has been implicated in this reflex. It may act as a neurotransmitter and/or a stimulus of nerve endings in the mucosa. A nerve reflex is thought to exist since tetrodotoxin – which blocks nerve conductivity – completely abolishes the vasodilator response to mechanical stimulation. An involvement of 5HT can also be inferred from the finding that bromo-LSD, a 5HT blocking agent, prevents the hyperaemia.

Simple mechanical stimulation is not the only stimulus for postprandial hyperaemia. Changes in bloodflow also depend on the chemical nature of the food eaten and the secretions with which it is mixed. However, these stimuli are unlikely to be of the same importance in different regions of the small intestine. Even if the composition of the luminal contents remained unaltered those factors altering blood flow would not be able to exert identical effects. They would not be carried to their sites of actions in similar concentrations because different regions have different capacities for absorption. It is well established, for example, that glucose absorption is greater in the proximal small intestine than in the distal ileum. In contrast, specific mechanisms for bile acids and vitamin B_{12} absorption are localized in the distal ileum. However, the composition of the luminal contents is not constant. Thus carbohydrate digestion and absorption are considered to be completed by the time the intestinal contents have been propelled one-third of the way along its length.

What are the luminal factors which can alter the intestinal blood flow? The hydrolytic products of carbohydrate and lipids are thought to be particularly responsible for postprandial hyperaemia in the upper small intestine. Vasodilatation is confined to those intestinal segments exposed and may be the result of endogenous histamine released after a meal. Histamine appears to act on H–1 receptors. Antagonists to such receptors e.g. tripelennamine, attenuate food-induced increases in blood flow.

Bile acids have little effect on jejunal blood flow. In contrast they appear to be important in initiating hyperaemia in more distal regions. It has been proposed that they may exert their effects in two ways. One involves a direct effect of bile acids on vascular smooth muscle. The other is the result of increased production of vasoactive metabolites (e.g. H^+ or prostaglandins) by absorbing epithelial cells and their accumulation within the interstitial fluid.

Hormones and blood flow

A number of hormones increase blood flow. These include CCK, secretin and glucagon (a polypeptide with structural similarity to secretin). Glucagon is unlikely to have a physiological role in postprandial hyperaemia. The release of this hormone depends mainly on a reduction in blood glucose concentrations and not on such increases as are likely to be observed following a meal. In contrast, CCK is regarded as a most likely candidate for increasing blood flow postprandially. Furthermore, intravenous secretin, in doses which are smaller (approximately one third) than those used to stimulate a maximal pancreatic secretion, significantly increase superior mesenteric artery blood flow in man. Thus these two hormones may work together (following their release in response to fat and the products of protein digestion or acid chyme in the duodenum) to increase blood flow as well as stimulating pancreatic exocrine secretions. The responses to these hormones are less localized than the distension effect described above.

The intestinal countercurrent system

An interesting phenomenon has been described in the villi where blood vessels are arranged in complex hairpin loops. In the cat intestine a single arterial vessel emerges from the submucosal vascular network. It lacks a muscular coat in the upper two-thirds of the villus. This vessel runs in the central core, the lamina propria, without branching. Close to the villous tip it branches into a dense subepithelial capillary network that collects into veins at the base (Fig. 5.3). The vascular arrangement in the human villus is similar.

Lundgren and his colleagues have suggested that these vessels constitute a countercurrent exchanger. Anatomically, at least, the prerequisites for such a system exist. However:

1. Blood must remain in the villus long enough,
2. The descending and ascending vessels must be close enough,

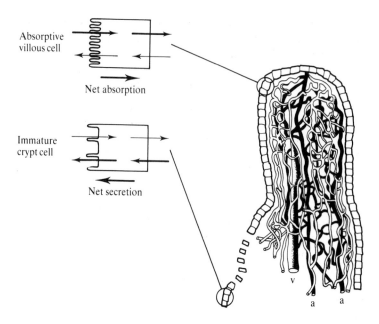

Fig. 5.3 Vasculature of the human villus. The arterial vessels (a) divide to provide an extensive capillary network. Capillaries converge on a vein (v). Columnar epithelial cells lining the villus may absorb or secrete. Usually the net result of their activities is absorption. In contrast, the cells that eventually replace them, i.e. the immature crypt cells, produce net secretory responses

3. The blood vessel walls must be sufficiently permeable, if physiologically significant exchanges are to occur.

The mean transit time for plasma is approximately 1 second even with intense vasodilatation (at rest values of about 5 seconds have been recorded). The intervascular distances in the fingerlike feline villi are 20–30 μm. As most solutes with molecular weights under 1000 achieve 75 per cent concentration equilibrium in 0.1 seconds it follows that considerable intervascular diffusion may occur, providing vascular permeability to a particular solute is high.

The intestinal blood vessels are highly permeable to lipid-soluble molecules. Such substances easily penetrate the lipid membranes of lining endothelial cells. Water movement through pores also readily occurs. Indeed the permeability of intestinal capillaries to water approaches that of lipid-soluble substances. However, the question remains as to what pores exist in intestinal blood vessels. The capillaries are fenestrated and thought to provide pores which are well suited for the transcapillary transport of small water-soluble molecules. However, these always face epithelial cells and, while valuable for the removal of absorbed substances, may be less able to contribute to exchange between blood vessels. The non-fenestrated walls of intestinal capillaries probably have permeability characteristics which result in much slower movement of hydrophilic substances (particularly if they are ionized) than lipid-soluble components.

What might be the physiological significance of the countercurrent exchanger?

Perhaps its most important function is to be a part of a countercurrent multiplier system which provides a hyperosmotic tissue compartment at the villous tip (Fig. 5.4). The existence of such a compartment is necessary to explain water absorption from the intestine in the absence of, or against, a lumen-to-plasma osmotic pressure gradient. Hyperosmolality can be established in two ways:

1. Na^+ pumping by the enterocytes produces a greater $[Na^+]$ in the subepithelial extracellular fluid and capillary network than in the artery. As blood flows along the descending limb, Na^+ diffuses from the capillary to the artery with the result that a high $[Na^+]$ is returned to the villous tip.
2. The same result can be achieved if the increased capillary $[Na^+]$ produces an osmotic flow of water from the central arterial vessel to the capillaries.

Using cryoscopic techniques a tissue osmolality at the villous tip of 1000–1200 mosmol/kg has been detected in cat small intestine (Fig. 5.5). In contrast the osmolality at the villous base was found to be approximately isotonic with plasma. The concept of water movement from the ascending vessel to the descending capillaries and, therefore, diluting their contents, is an important one. With such a system the plasma osmolality of the blood leaving the villus can be maintained close to isotonicity in spite of the absorption of fluids of very different concentrations.

If a concentration difference exists between the two limbs in which ascending exceeds descending then net diffusion should occur from the ascending limb. Such a situation exists for oxygen where concentrations are lowered in capillaries as it is utilized by absorbing epithelial cells. The result is that oxygen tensions at the tips of the villi are lower than at the bases. It has been suggested that the relatively hypoxic conditions resulting from the functioning of the countercurrent system may be one reason for the rapid turnover of epithelial cells at the villous tip.

Conversely, however, as oxygen is utilized more carbon dioxide is produced and trapped within the exchanger which lowers the affinity of haemoglobin for oxygen (Bohr effect). Thus oxygen delivery is improved at low oxygen tensions. A serious problem could develop, nevertheless, during arterial hypotension. Under such conditions there would be more time for exchange because of both a reduced perfusion pressure and the relaxation of precapillary smooth muscle. Not surprisingly ulceration of human intestine can develop within hours during hypovolaemic shock.

Several other consequences of the presence of a countercurrent multiplier have been proposed. By contributing to the development of interstitial fluid hyperosmolality it could lead to the hyperaemia associated with absorbing epithelial cells. Hyperosmolality relaxes vascular smooth muscle. Another possible consequence is that when interstitial fluid osmolality attracts water from the central arterial vessel the plasma oncotic pressure at the villous tip is increased as is the interstitial fluid hydrostatic pressure. Such alterations in the Starling forces would favour movement to the capillaries (absorption) and promote intestinal lymph flow (see below)

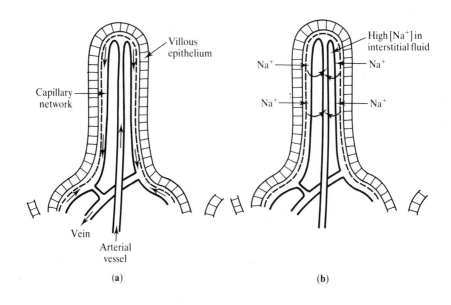

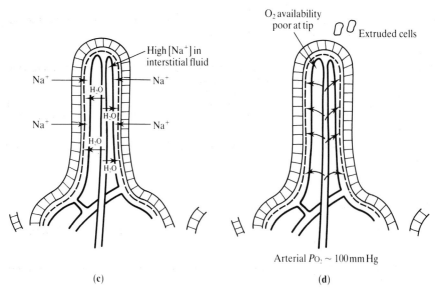

Fig. 5.4 Diagrammatic representation of the villous vasculature. The capillary vessels provide a dense network below the intestinal epithelium. The ascending arterial vessel and the descending capillary network form a hairpin vascular loop. In (**a**) the different vessels and the direction of blood flow are shown. Subsequently, in (**b**) and (**c**), exchanges are illustrated between the arterial vessel and the capillary network which may contribute to an impairment of absorption or the maintenance of hypertonicity of the interstitial fluid. The final diagram (**d**) indicates why relatively hypoxic conditions may exist at the villous tip (From Lundgren, O. (1967). *Acta Physiologica Scandinavica (Supplement)* **303**, 1–42.)

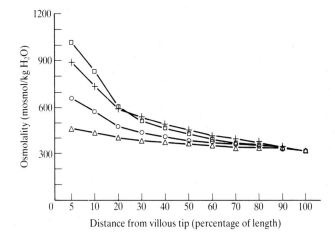

Fig. 5.5 Tissue osmolality in villi of cat jejunum. Segments of intestine were exposed to:
(a) A Krebs-glucose solution in which [Na+] = 147mmol/l and [glucose] = 30mmol/l (□–□).
(b) A Krebs–mannitol solution, which had the same composition as solution **(a)** except that glucose was replaced by equimolar mannitol (not absorbed) (+–+).
(c) A choline–glucose solution, which had the same composition as solution **(a)** except that Na+ was replaced by equimolar choline (○–○).
(d) A choline–mannitol solution, which had the same composition as solution **(c)** except that glucose was replaced by equimolar mannitol (△–△).

Note:

(1) When the intestine was exposed to solution **(a)** the tissue osmolality recorded cryoscopically at the villous tip was comparable with those recorded in the renal medulla .
(2) Glucose makes a small contribution, perhaps by stimulating Na+ absorption.
(3) In the absence of Na+ and glucose the tissue osmolality at the villous tip exceeded that of plasma. Presumably some Na+ is available from the villous interstitial fluid and from the secreting crypt epithelia.

(Data from Hallbäck, D-A., Jodal, M. and Lundgren, O. (1979). *Acta Physiologica Scandinavica* **107**, 89–96.)

Intestinal transcapillary movement

The forces involved in transcapillary fluid movement were recognized almost a century ago (Starling, 1896). They are :

1. The hydrostatic pressure exerted across the wall of the capillary which favours filtration, and
2. The effective osmotic pressure of plasma which favours the absorption of interstitial fluid.

Filtration and absorption of fluid (and water-soluble molecules) occur through pores. A number of pores with different diameters have been described. These include small perforations (0.8–2.0 nm diameter) in the endothelial cell lipid membrane which allow the transit of water and small non-polar solutes. Other pathways are through open or diaphragmed fenestrae. Such structures increase in number from the arterial to the venous ends of capillaries. The open fenestrae

(40–60 nm diameter) offer minimal resistance even to the transcapillary movement of macromolecules. The porosity of those with diaphragms is not known. Some fluid may also cross capillary walls through intercellular junctions or in pinocytotic vesicles. The latter are regarded as providing an important pathway for the transport of macromolecules particularly across continuous as distinct from fenestrated capillaries.

The rate of capillary filtration or absorption $(J_{v,c})$ is described by the equation:

$$J_{v,c} = K_{f,c} [(P_c - P_t) - \sigma_d (\pi_p - \pi_c)]$$

where

$K_{f,c}$ = the capillary filtration coefficient,
P_c = the capillary hydrostatic pressure,
P_t = the interstitial hydrostatic pressure,
σ_d = the osmotic reflection coefficient,
π_p = the plasma oncotic pressure,
π_t = the interstitial fluid oncotic pressure.

Capillary hydrostatic pressures of approximately 10 mm Hg and transcapillary oncotic pressures of 13 mm Hg have been reported. A negative interstitial fluid hydrostatic pressure (about -2 mm Hg) provides a greater than expected hydrostatic gradient driving filtration. Under conditions favouring minimal epithelial fluid transport a positive lymph flow has been reported which probably represents net capillary filtration. (NB. When describing capillary filtration/absorption it should be remembered that small venules and metarterioles make contributions.)

The capillary filtration coefficient is a measure of the hydraulic conductance of a capillary bed and is dependent on the number of capillaries perfused and the size and number of pores in each capillary. Several factors alter the $K_{f,c}$. Some of these are listed in Table 5.1. Usually situations resulting in vasodilatation are associated with an increase in $K_{f,c}$, e.g. during glucose absorption following a meal. In contrast a reduction in $K_{f,c}$ has been reported under conditions where vasoconstriction occurs, e.g. with sympathetic nerve stimulation. The osmotic reflection coefficient (σ_d) gives an indication of the leakiness of capillaries to proteins. If $\sigma_d = 1.0$ the capillary walls are impermeable to plasma proteins, and these colloids exert all their osmotic forces. In contrast freely permeable proteins do not exert an effective osmotic pressure and $\sigma_d = 0$. A value of 0.92 has been determined for cat intestinal capillaries, suggesting their relative impermeability. However, σ_d is not constant. It is reduced during fat absorption and ischaemia, and by histamine, bradykinin and *Escherichia coli* endotoxin (Table 5.1).

Bacteria may increase capillary permeability, in part, by attracting neutrophils which along with macrophages and eosinophils provide a large resident population of phagocytic leucocytes. *Escherichia coli*, for example, produces formyl-methionyl-leucyl-phenylalanine (FMLP). This peptide is regarded as a major chemotactic factor and reduces the σ_d of the rat intestinal microvasculature. However, the vascular responses to FMLP are significantly attenuated when rats are treated with antineutrophil serum. How the neutrophils exert their effects are unknown although they can release a variety of oxidative and non-oxidative agents that damage capillaries. Among them is superoxide. Superoxide-derived radicals increase vascular permeability.

Increasing the permeability of capillaries to proteins provides conditions favouring filtration. As a result greater volumes of fluid may accumulate in the interstitial spaces. This fluid may be secreted by the intestinal epithelia or contribute to an enhanced lymph flow. Certainly intestinal lymph flow is increased after a fat meal. The concentrations of plasma proteins found in lymph, however, do not fall. It has been suggested that a transient change in the capillary permeability results in an increased interstitial fluid volume and hydrostatic pressure and a means of removing recently absorbed chylomicrons (see page 141). For patients with inadequate lymph vessels (intestinal lymphangiectasia) it has been recognized that a reduced fat intake can diminish the loss of plasma proteins via the intestine.

Models can easily be constructed to illustrate how changes in the Starling forces, the degree of contraction of vascular smooth muscle and the characteristics of capillary membranes can contribute either to the supply of fluid for epithelial cell secretion (Fig. 5.6) or the removal of fluid after its absorption. Thus some of the relationships between transporting epithelial cells and their blood supply can readily be appreciated.

The fates of several substances handled by the small intestine

Had I written a text on the functions of the small intestine 40 years ago, it would have been conveniently divided into three sections. In one a description would

---

Table 5.1   Conditions that alter the filtration coefficient ($K_{f,c}$) or the osmotic reflection coefficient (σ_d) of intestinal capillaries

Factors increasing $K_{f,c}$	Factors reducing $K_{f,c}$	Factors affecting σ_d	
		Stimulus	*Value*
Glucose absorption	Luminal distension	None – control	0.92
Arterial hypotension	Portal hypertension	Bradykinin	0.65
Haemorrhagic shock	Adenosine	Fat absorption	0.70
Bradykinin	Angiotensin II	*Escherichia coli*	
Histamine	Sympathetic nerve	endotoxin	0.78
Secretin	stimulation	Ischaemia	0.59
Acetylcholine		Histamine	0.56
Cholera toxin		Histamine + cimetidine	0.90
		Histamine + benadryl	0.56

Note:
   Histamine appears to act on H-2 receptors, as its effects can be blocked by cimetidine, but not by the H-1 antagonist benadryl.
   The lack of effect of secretin and cholecystokinin on σ_d. These hormones are released by fatty acids in the small intestine. How, therefore, are lipids exerting their effects?

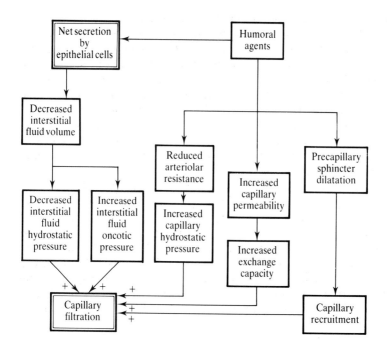

Fig. 5.6 Relationships between secreting epithelial cells and the intestinal microcirculation (Modified from Granger, D.N. and Barrowman, J.A. (1983). *Gastroenterology* **84**, 846–68.)

have been given of the juices secreted into the lumen from the liver, the exocrine pancreas and the intestinal crypts (the succus entericus). The last two would have been designated as enzyme-rich fluids continuing and completing digestion initiated in the mouth and stomach. It would have been stressed that, although bile has no enzymes, the bile acids secreted are extremely important in the solubilization of the products of fat hydrolysis. In a second section I would have dealt with the absorption of those small molecules resulting from intraluminal hydrolysis. Some comment would have been necessary on the anabolic processes (e.g. triglyceride synthesis) occurring as substances are transferred across the epithelial cells. A final section would have been devoted to intestinal motility with descriptions of mechanisms whereby the luminal content is mixed with secretions or propelled towards the colon.

Such a scheme still may be used today. However, digestion is not completed within the intestinal lumen. Many chemical bonds of ingested foodstuffs are broken down either at the mucosal surface of epithelial cells or even intracellularly. It follows, therefore, that mechanisms must exist whereby some nutrients, either whole or partially digested, can actually penetrate the epithelial cells before being hydrolysed.

What are the origins of those enzymes associated with the mucosal surface? Two possible sources are the pancreatic juice and the intestinal epithelia. The first may surprise some readers. Luminal hydrolysis undoubtedly makes an important contribution to digestion as pancreatic juice is mixed with the chyme.

However, not all pancreatic enzymes exist freely within the lumen. Some are found adsorbed to the glycocalyx or fuzzy coat, a glycoprotein layer secreted by the lining epithelial cells. These enzymes, e.g. pancreatic amylase, are involved in what has been called membrane or contact digestion (on or within the glycocalyx). Membrane digestion has an advantage over intraluminal hydrolysis in that the products are concentrated within a relatively small region close to the epithelial cells and are more available for the subsequent attack by cellular enzymes. Such products are also in closer proximity to transfer mechanisms than those derived from intraluminal hydrolysis. Furthermore, they can be carried towards these mechanisms in water flowing to and subsequently absorbed by the villous epithelium (Fig. 5.7).

Only a minor proportion of the disaccharides and small peptides resulting from the activities of pancreatic juice are hydrolysed intraluminally by intestinal enzymes. Such enzymes are not actively secreted but derived from aged cells extruded from villous tips. Much of the small peptide and disaccharide hydrolysis takes place at the luminal surface of the epithelial cells. At this site hydrolytic enzymes concerned with the final stages of breakdown of protein and carbohydrate are detected. Some peptides are not readily hydrolysed at the brush border and enter the epithelial cells before being hydrolysed by cytoplasmic enzymes. However, whether peptides are hydrolysed intraluminally, at

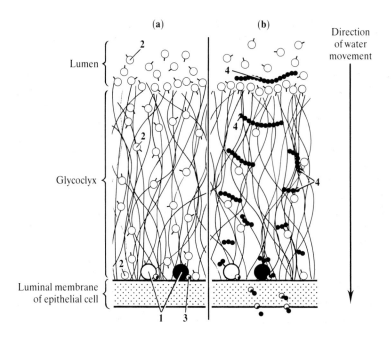

Fig. 5.7 The concept of membrane or contact digestion. (**a**) Distribution of enzymes. (**b**) Relationship of enzymes, carriers and substrates. 1 = Enteric enzymes; 2 = adsorbed enzymes, e.g. pancreatic amylase; 3 = carriers; 4 = substrates (From Ugolev, A.M. (1972). *Gut* **13**, 735–47.)

or within the brush border membrane or intracellularly, amino acids are usually the products to appear in the bloodstream.

A clear distinction no longer exists between digestion and absorption. Therefore, I propose to consider the fate of several dietary components from the time they enter the small intestine to when they or their products appear in the bloodstream. Before doing so, however, let us consider the mechanisms by which substances can be transferred and also some of the methods by which intestinal transfer processes have been studied.

Transfer of substances across the small intestine

Movement across the small intestine may be defined as the passage of substances through the epithelial barrier between the intestinal lumen and the blood or lymph vessels. It is important to remember that the small intestine transfers substances in two directions:

(a) from the lumen towards the bloodstream, i.e. absorption,
(b) from the bloodstream towards the lumen, i.e. secretion.

In other words, the transfer of a particular substance represents a balance between what is absorbed and what is secreted. If transepithelial transport is to occur, at least two membranes must be traversed. These are the luminal (or mucosal) and the basolateral (or serosal) membranes. The properties of these are not identical. For example, the characteristics of the systems transporting sugars are different at the two sites (see page 156). Furthermore, if a transfer mechanism can be demonstrated in one region it does not follow that the same mechanism exists throughout the small intestine. Thus vitamin B_{12} is absorbed by a specific process in the ileum and not readily absorbed from the jejunum.

The question remains as to whether all epithelial cells in a particular region have the same activities. In an attempt to answer it, the assumption was made that intestinal epithelial cells can be divided into two types, the immature crypt cells and the mature villous cells. Then one or the other cell type was selectively damaged and investigations carried out to determine which functions had been altered. It was found that villous cells are susceptible to osmotic shock induced by making the luminal contents grossly hypertonic e.g. by introducing 2M Na_2SO_4 for half an hour. The crypts appeared to be undamaged by such a procedure. In contrast, crypt cell functions were preferentially impaired by administering the antibiotic cycloheximide intravenously. This substance inhibits protein synthesis by the crypt cells and as a result reduces their proliferation. When these procedures were applied it was found that the secretory responses of the small intestine to cholera toxin were prevented by cycloheximide but not by Na_2SO_4 treatment. On the other hand hexose absorption was unaffected by cycloheximide but reduced following exposure to hypertonic Na_2SO_4. It appears, therefore that absorptive and secretory functions can be partially separated, the former being a function of the villi and the latter primarily of the crypts.

This view has further experimental support. In autoradiographic studies the accumulation of [14]C- and ^{3}H-labelled sugars and amino acids can be demonstrated near the brush borders of villous cells. However, uptake is poor into cells between the villi.

Several mechanisms have been postulated to transfer substances across the intestinal barrier. These include:

(a) simple diffusion,
(b) facilitated diffusion where the same equilibrium is achieved as in simple diffusion but at a more rapid rate,
(c) active transport (including pinocytosis) where an energy input is required.

Simple diffusion requires no expenditure of cellular energy. It depends on the physical forces available and occurs in the same direction as the electrochemical gradient. Diffusion across a cell membrane may involve three stages. The substance:

(a) leaves an aqueous medium and enters the hydrophobic lipid region of the membrane,
(b) crosses the lipid layer,
(c) leaves the lipid layer and returns to an aqueous medium.

Clearly, an important factor in determining whether a substance can diffuse across a membrane is its lipid solubility. In fact, correlations have been established between the rates of absorption of many substances (e.g. barbiturates) and their lipid solubilities; the greater the lipid solubility the more rapid the absorption. However, lipid solubility is not the only factor determining absorption rates by diffusion. Small molecules, e.g. urea, are absorbed much more rapidly than would be expected from a consideration of their oil:water partition coefficients. Furthermore, there is an inverse relationship between molecular size and the rate of penetration of small, lipid-insoluble molecules. The concept has been developed, therefore, that water-filled channels extend through the membranes and that small lipid-insoluble molecules diffuse through these hydrophilic regions.

Finally one must recognize that a transcellular pathway is not the only means by which small molecules can diffuse across an epithelial barrier. When I was a student a tight junction was thought to be well named and not a zone across which diffusion could take place. Today, however, many small molecules are known to use a paracellular (around the cell) route during absorption (Fig. 5.8).

Most substances are transferred across the intestinal epithelia by processes other than simple diffusion. When substances are transferred by mechanisms which are independent of cellular energy, the term facilitated diffusion is used to describe the process. The characteristics of facilitated diffusion are as follows:

1. As with simple diffusion, the movement of a substance takes place down its electrochemical gradient.
2. Saturation phenomena. The rate of transfer of a substance is initially proportional to the concentration gradient, but this decreases at concentrations that saturate the mechanism.
3. The substance transferred is released from the membrane in its original

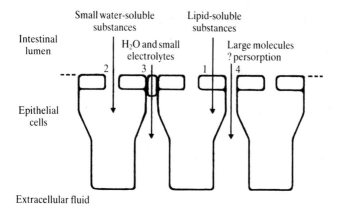

Fig. 5.8 Possible sites for diffusion from the intestinal lumen. 1 = Lipid membrane of epithelial cell; 2 = Small water-filled channels; 3 = 'Not so tight' junctions; 4 = Spaces left by extruded cells. Two processes are transcellular, the others are intercellular

form. For a non-electrolyte, the concentrations achieved on either side of the membrane should be equal.

4. The transfer system functions equally well in either direction.

5. There may be competition between structurally related substances. Thus the rate of transfer of a substance is reduced in the presence of another substance which can be transferred by the same process. The strongest inhibitory effect is exerted by the substance with the highest affinity for the transfer process.

6. Evidence that strongly supports the view that transfer is via facilitated diffusion is the demonstration of countertransport. In countertransport the movement of a substance down its electrochemical gradient is linked with the movement of a structurally analogous molecule in the opposite direction against its electrochemical gradient.

What mechanisms are involved in facilitated diffusion? They are thought to be minor components of the membrane and, because the substance being transferred is not modified, any interaction between the system and the transferred molecule involves only hydrogen, hydrophobic and/or electrostatic bonds. The transfer process may not be rigidly fixed in the membrane (although see page 156) but may move within it (Fig. 5.9). For such systems the term carrier was introduced and may well involve proteins because:

1. Proteins are the only molecules with properties of controlled selectivity and specificity necessary to impart the specificity characteristics of transfer systems.

2. The kinetics of carrier-mediated transfer are similar to the kinetics of enzyme–substrate interactions.

3. Transfer processes can be inhibited by agents that react with proteins.

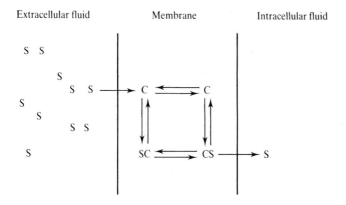

Fig. 5.9 Facilitated diffusion. The substance S binds to a receptor site on the carrier at one surface of the membrane. The complex diffuses through the membrane and dissociates at the other surface releasing S. In this figure the mechanism transfers S from the extracellular to the intracellular fluid. The reverse process can also occur. The net result is that S moves down its electrochemical gradient

An alternative proposal is that facilitated diffusion may occur via protein channels or pores inserted in the membrane. Only a part of the protein, and this includes the region to which the transferable substance binds, has mobility. Movement of this region would allow a substance bound on one side of the membrane to appear at the opposite surface. It is assumed that the binding sites can be exposed on both sides of the membrane, but not simultaneously (see page 156).

The characteristics of active transport are the same as for facilitated diffusion, except that the former requires the expenditure of energy to drive the mechanism against an electrochemical gradient. Probably ATP is the source of energy. Most writers include pinocytosis in any list of mechanisms. It is an active transport process since a requirement for energy and a degree of specificity can often be demonstrated. Pinocytosis, or the engulfing of particles or dissolved materials by vesiculation, is regarded as the most primitive mechanism of food digestion, largely lost during the process of evolution. Some examples still remain. In the newborn calf soluble protein can be absorbed for a short time after birth.

However, mechanisms other than pinocytosis may account for the absorption of particles. When students (common laboratory animals!) were given 200 g potato starch suspended in water, starch granules were detected subsequently in blood. The granules appeared 4 minutes after ingestion, and in maximum concentrations after 10 minutes. From similar studies with rats it was concluded that large particles can be kneaded through the epithelial cell layer, passing between cells preferentially in the areas of desquamation at the villous tips. The term persorption was used to describe this process (see Fig. 5.8).

Methods of studying intestinal transport processes

Many techniques have been developed to study intestinal absorption. None of them can be described as ideal and results obtained using a combination of different procedures are the most desirable for together they will yield more information concerning intestinal function under physiological conditions than any taken singly. The methods available can be divided into two groups (a) *in vivo*, (b) *in vitro*. The advantage of the former is that absorption can be measured where the circulation and the extrinsic nerves are intact. However, with such methods it is difficult to study in detail all the aspects of absorption. For example, the collection of absorption products in blood or lymph is not easy. In contrast, repetitive sampling of fluids bathing the serosal surfaces of *in vitro* preparations is often a straightforward procedure.

In vivo methods

In several methods the disappearance of a substance from the intestinal lumen is measured. Often a known amount is given by mouth. Subsequently, the faeces are analysed for the substance. The difference between the amount given and the amount recovered is assumed to be the amount absorbed (a balance experiment). One means of conducting such a study is to keep the subject on a diet free of the test substance for some time. A single dose of the test substance is then given. The faeces are collected until there is reason to believe that none of the substance remains in the GI tract and the faecal output is determined.

In a human study of cyanocobalamin absorption faeces were collected until two successive samples contained less than 1% of the dose given. This required 4–13 days. Marker substances were used in another type of balance study. Chromium sesquioxide is fed along with the substance to be tested and the ratio of the marker and test substance is determined in the diet and the faeces. If these ratios are X and Y, the percentage absorption is given by the equation $100 \times (X - Y) / X$.

Several intestinal absorption studies have been undertaken by means of swallowed tubes. Abbott and Miller advocated the use of the triple lumen tube. Inflating balloons via two of these lumina isolated a segment of intestine leaving the third available for taking samples. However, to occlude the intestinal lumen the balloons had to be inflated to pressures of 25–40 cm H_2O. This results in changes in motility and blood flow. Furthermore, the possibility of leakages past the balloons and discomfort for the subject has to be considered. To overcome these problemss, it was proposed that a fine tube should be swallowed and allowed to pass all the way to the anus. With this technique there is no obstruction to the movement of the luminal content and subjects can tolerate the tube's presence for several days. Sampling the luminal residue has provided valuable information as to the sites of absorption of several dietary components.

When interpreting data derived from balance studies, one must remember that the substance investigated may have been:

1. Utilized by intestinal bacteria and not absorbed.

2. Produced by intestinal bacteria, e.g. vitamins.
3. Involved in the enterohepatic circulation, e.g. cholesterol.

Furthermore, some animals, e.g. rats, practices coprophagy. A grid through which the faeces can fall does not prevent coprophagy as they may be eaten as they are excreted. A different approach, applicable to the unanaesthetized animal, is to measure absorption from surgically prepared loops of intestine. The Thiry-Vella loop is the loop prepared when a segment of intestine is separated from the remaining intestine and is brought to the surface of the abdomen. An objection to these procedures is that there is an absence of daily intestinal contact with chyme, which may result in abnormal digestive functions. In addition, the small intestine is exposed to bacteria not normally encountered.

In vitro methods

Of the many procedures devised to study intestinal absorption, probably none has been used as frequently as the everted sac technique developed by Wilson and Wiseman in 1954 (Fig. 5.10). Many earlier techniques involving the use of tied segments had given erratic results because of inadequate oxygenation of the mucosal epithelial cells. Wilson and Wiseman turned the intestine inside out so that the epithelial layer was on the outer surface. The sacs produced after tying both ends of the segment could be placed in large volumes of incubation medium and readily oxygenated. This technique offers other advantages:

1. Fluid absorption can be estimated gravimetrically.
2. The volume of fluid bathing the mucosal surface can be large so that as transport occurs there are no large changes in concentrations of the substances in the incubation medium. This is useful in kinetic studies where one measures transport rates at different concentrations.
3. Substances absorbed can be detected either in the gut wall or in the small volumes of the fluid bathing the serosal surface. Because the volumes of these two compartments are small, there is an excellent opportunity for determining whether substances are transferred against their concentration gradients.

A further method frequently used to assess intestinal transport mechanisms was originally introduced to study the properties of frog skin. Small segments of intestine are carefully opened along their mesenteric border to produce sheets which can be clamped between two Perspex compartments (the Ussing chamber, Fig. 5.11). With such a preparation fluid transport (absorption or secretion) can be determined by measuring the dilution of an inert non-transported marker introduced into the mucosal fluid, e.g. mannitol or inulin. By using radioisotopes the movement of solutes can also be monitored. Furthermore, the resistance of intestinal tissue and the electrical changes associated with transport processes can be monitored if measurements are made of potential differences and short circuit currents.

The volumes of fluid on either side of the sheets are small. As a result it has been necessary to use only small amounts of expensive chemicals (e.g. hormones) to produce effective concentrations. In addition hormones can be

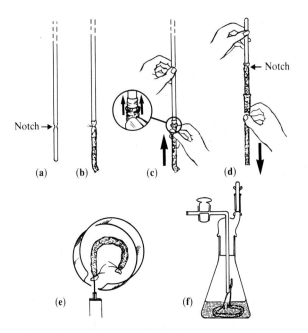

Fig. 5.10 The everted sac technique. Some of the stages are illustrated above. Eversion of the intestine is shown from (**a**) to (**e**). A glass rod is used with a groove for a ligature (**a**). This is inserted into the intestine which is then tied close to the end (**b**). The eversion is started by pushing the gut upwards over the place where it is tied (**c**). The eversion is completed by inverting the rod and pulling the intestine downwards (**d**). In the lower part of the figure the process of filling the sac is shown. The sac lies on a modified Petri dish which is used for weighing the gut (**e**). Finally, the sac is lowered into an incubation flask which can be gassed so as to provide aerobic conditions for the tissues (**f**). (From Smyth, D.H. (1963). In *Recent Advances in Physiology*, 8th edn. Ed. by R. Creese, J. and A. Churchill, London. pp 36–68.

added directly to the serosal side of the tissue, the side from which they normally exert their effects. This option is not readily available with everted sac preparations.

A major problem when studying intestinal absorption *in vitro* is that the gut wall is composed of many different cell types. In addition to absorbing epithelial cells there are muscle, connective tissue and mucus-secreting cells. Thus with everted sacs the concentrations of substances measured within the intestinal wall does not reflect the concentrating ability of the epithelium. For those using intestinal sheets the problem can be partially resolved if they are skilful enough and can carefully remove the muscle layers.

It was hardly surprising, therefore, that techniques were developed to separate and collect viable epithelial cells. Subsequently, sealed vesicles have been prepared of both brush border and basolateral membranes. As a result detailed analyses can be made of transport processes albeit in non-physiological conditions. These processes may be studied in isolation, unaffected by intracellular metabolic events.

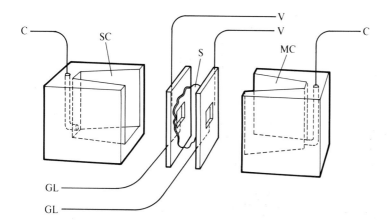

Fig.5.11 The Ussing chamber for measuring electrolyte transport across the intestine and electrical parameters (current, resistance and voltage). Sheets of intestine (S) are clamped between two Perspex, saline-filled compartments. The mucosal compartment (MC) contains fluid which bathes the transporting epithelial cells. Fluid in the serosal compartment (SC) can readily be sampled or added to during experiments. Gas lines (GL) ensure adequate oxygenation of the tissue. Agar : KCl bridges (V) lead to voltage measuring equipment. Current can be passed using Ag/AgCl electrodes. Such electrodes are not introduced directly into the fluids bathing the intestine because of the toxic effects of Ag+ ions. To overcome this problem wide bore salt-bridges (C) are used

One method of isolating brush border membranes has been to homogenize thoroughly intestinal cells or mucosal scrapings. Non-brush-border particulate matter can then be precipitated with 10 mmol/l Ca^{++} or Mg^{++}. The brush borders, because of their greater density of negative surface charges, are not precipitated and remain in the supernatant fluid. Centrifugation of this fluid provides a pellet of membrane vesicles, 95% of which have the same membrane orientation as in the intact epithelial cell (i.e. they are 'the right side out').

To study basolateral membranes it is necessary to have a source of isolated epithelial cells. Basolateral membranes have similar properties to other non-epithelial cell membranes and cannot readily be separated from them. They can be made available by differential centrifugation followed by separation on a density gradient or free flow electrophoresis.

The fate of fat

In Western Europe, 60–100 g lipid is the daily dietary intake. This is mainly in the form of triglyceride, although cholesterol, phospholipid and fat-soluble vitamins are also nutritionally important. Fat digestion takes place mainly in the small intestine. Enzymes active against triglycerides with short chain (gastric lipase) and long chain (lingual lipase) fatty acids may cause some lipid hydrolysis in the stomach. However, the major contribution of the stomach to fat absorption appears to be its ability to deliver fat into the duodenum at a rate which can be handled by the small intestine. Furthermore, the stomach may not release lipids until the aqueous gastric contents have been emptied. As fats are warmed to body temperature they form droplets which are likely to float to the surface and not be available to be propelled through the pyloric sphincter. Fat digestion can conveniently be divided into the following four stages.

Emulsification and hydrolysis of fat

Dietary fats are insoluble in water, yet are acted upon by enzymes secreted in an aqueous medium. At body temperatures, many fats exist as oils so that pancreatic lipase exerts its effects at an oil:water interface. Thus the larger the surface area of this interface the greater the probability that fat-hydrolysing enzymes will exert their effects. By mechanical mixing in the stomach and the upper small intestine, triglyceride droplets can be broken down to minute particles. However, these would reunite to larger droplets were it not for emulsifying agents present within the luminal contents. These include fatty acids, monoglycerides, cholesterol, lecithin and its derivative lysolecithin, protein and bile salts. The bile salts alone are poor agents but in combination with polar lipids such as monoglycerides or lecithin form powerful emulsifying mixtures. Stable particles of 0.5–1.0 μm diameter are produced.

Conjugated bile acids have a further effect in that they alter the pH optimum of pancreatic lipase from 8.9 to 6.7. This should ensure greater activity of the enzyme in the small intestine into which the acidic contents of the stomach have been emptied. The products of pancreatic lipase are 2-monoglycerides and free fatty acids. The 2-monoglycerides can be hydrolysed but only very slowly. However, fatty acids can migrate spontaneously from one alcohol group to another. As a result 2-monoglycerides can be converted to 1-monoglycerides which are then rapidly broken down to the more water-soluble glycerol with the release of a further fatty acid. Only about 30% of the triglycerides are completely hydrolysed the major products being monoglyceride and free fatty acid. NB: pancreatic lipase can act on the 1-fatty acid of lecithin with the formation of lysolecithin.

The formation of micelles

Free fatty acids and monoglycerides are not readily soluble in water and, were there no means of solubilizing them following their release from triglyceride, they would be absorbed very slowly from the luminal aqueous environment. Further, such a mixture would produce a balance between hydrolysis and re-esterification and so effectively inhibit triglyceride breakdown.

More rapid digestion and more complete absorption are brought about through the formation of very small highly stable units called micelles (Fig. 5.12). These units, 4–5 nm diameter, are capable of incorporating and maintaining the products of fat digestion in a water soluble form. The micelles are formed from bile acids. At low concentrations bile acids exist as monomers. However, when they are present in the intestinal lumen above their critical micellar concentrations they form polymolecular aggregates. The structure of these units is such that hydrophilic groups face the aqueous medium while

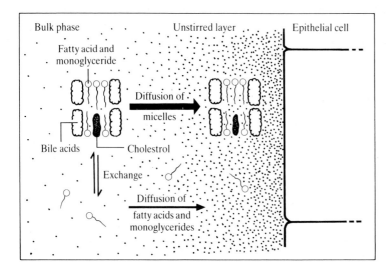

Fig. 5.12 The role of micelles in fat absorption. 1. They incorporate and maintain the products of fat digestion in a dissolved form in the luminal aqueous contents. 2. They cause more rapid movement of fatty acids and monoglycerides through the unstirred layer (After Davenport, H.W. (1977). *Physiology of the Digestive Tract,* 4th edn. Year Book Medical Publishers, Chicago.)

hydrophobic groups face one another to form a core. In this core monoglycerides (but not di- and triglycerides), free fatty acids and fat-soluble vitamins (A, D and K) can be carried in a soluble form. The critical micellar concentrations of bile acids are lower when aggregates with fatty acids, monoglycerides and lecithins are formed. Such units are mixed micelles.

Usually the concentrations of conjugated bile acids encountered in the jejunal contents exceed the critical micellar concentrations and the products of fat digestion are maintained in a soluble form. However, some bile acid molecules are deconjugated by bacteria as they pass along the intestine. The bile acids produced have similar critical micellar concentrations as the conjugated forms but are more lipid soluble. As a result they are more readily absorbed across the lipid membranes of absorbing epithelial cells and more likely to be precipitated producing lower bile acid concentrations within the lumen. The micelles form complexes with colipase at the oil/water interface. This binding brings the micelles close to the site of hydrolysis facilitating the removal of end products and preventing feedback inhibition of lipid digestion. A further important function of micelles is that they carry fatty acids and monoglycerides to the absorptive surface. They do so at rates faster than can be accounted for by the diffusion of individual molecules. This seems unlikely as large molecular aggregates diffuse more slowly than individual molecules. Indeed, it has been calculated that the diffusion coefficient of a micelle is only one-seventh that of a fatty acid molecule. However, at the luminal face is an unstirred water layer, 0.05–2 mm thick, across which substances must diffuse if they are to be absorbed. This layer acts as a barrier to the movement of relatively water-insoluble molecules whilst the micelles containing relatively large concentrations of fatty acids and monoglycerides readily diffuse to the luminal membrane.

The unstirred water layer differs from the aqueous intestinal contents in that it is more acidic. It has a uniquely low pH estimated to be between 5.1 and 6.3. This acid microclimate is thought to be due to hydrogen ion secretion (see page 162) and the presence of mucus which prevents the otherwise rapid diffusion of hydrogen ions away from the site of their release. As many pharmacological agents are weak acids or weak bases, e.g. acetylsalicylic acid and morphine, their degree of ionization and, therefore, absorption may be different from that anticipated from bulk pH measurements. Those substances absorbed by simple diffusion through lipid membranes are transferred more rapidly if they are present as the undissociated lipid-soluble form than when they exist in the more water-soluble ionized state.

The absorption of the products of fat digestion

Free fatty acids and monoglycerides are absorbed mainly in the duodenum and proximal jejunum having been released from micelles. At the brush border fatty acid monomers, for example, are in equilibrium with micellar aggregate forms. As the monomers are absorbed this equilibrium is disturbed and more fatty acid is released from the micelle. The low pH encountered in the unstirred water layer may also contribute to fatty acid absorption by reducing the solubility of fatty acids in micelles.

It has been suggested that more fatty acids would be released from micelles in a protonated, highly soluble form. Because of their lipophilic character it has usually been assumed that the major products of fat hydrolysis are absorbed by simple diffusion through the phospholipid bilayer of the luminal membrane. This may not be the complete story. A membrane fatty acid binding protein (MFABP), molecular weight 40 000, has been identified in jejunal microvillous membranes and evidence presented to show that fatty acid uptake can be mediated by this protein. Using rat isolated jejunal cells a saturable (K_m = 93 nmol/l) and temperature sensitive (optimum = 37°C) oleate uptake system was demonstrated. Pretreatment of the cells with a monospecific antibody of MFABP inhibited the uptake of several long chain fatty acids and even of the monoglyceride monopalmitin. The presence of this protein with such high specificity for fatty acids does not exclude simple diffusion as an important means of absorption but indicates that uptake may be more complex than previously thought.

Lysolecithin appears to be transported into the mucosal epithelial cells without alteration. Once inside the enterocyte, a phosphodiesterase system removes the base while the fatty acid is removed due to phosphatidase activity. Finally, non-specific phosphatases bring about the production of glycerol and phosphate.

Triglyceride resynthesis and its delivery to lacteals

The absorbed products of fat digestion are incorporated into triglycerides. A cytoplasmic fatty acid binding protein appears to play a role in the transport of the fatty acids from the brush border to the smooth endoplasmic reticulum where re-esterification takes place. Two pathways are involved (Fig. 5.13). The major system is the monoglyceride pathway. Longchain fatty acids are activated with coenzyme A in the presence of ATP to form fatty acyl-coenzyme A. This is condensed with mono- and diglycerides respectively. The minor process is the α-glycerophosphate pathway in which α-glycerophosphate, derived from the glycolytic pathway or absorbed glycerol, reacts with two molecules of fatty acyl-coenzyme A. The phosphate group is then removed and a third fatty acid group added.

When the carbon chain length of the fatty acid falls below twelve there is less ready incorporation of fatty acid into triglyceride. These fatty acids are not bound to the cytoplasmic fatty acid binding protein which has been regarded as a crucial step for re-esterification and may help to explain why such fatty acids pass unaltered to the portal blood. Triglyceride droplets, once formed are transferred through the endoplasmic reticulum to the Golgi apparatus in the supranuclear region of the cell. Here they are enveloped in a hydrophobic coating and enclosed within vesicles. The coat is made up of protein, phospholipid and cholesterol. The particles produced, the chylomicrons, have diameters which range from 76 to 600 nm. Phospholipids can be synthesized by epithelial cells but appear to be derived from luminal sources e.g. the lecithin of bile. In contrast a number of specific proteins are synthesized within the mucosa e.g. apolipoprotein B (see page 184). The vesicles migrate to the basolateral membranes where they fuse and release their contents. by exocytosis (reverse pinocytosis).

The movement of chylomicrons across the subepithelial basement membrane may depend on the thixotropic properties of this structure i.e. its capacity to undergo gel–sol transformations. It has been suggested that instead of being a rigid structure acting as a barrier it may be continuously deformed and reformed allowing the movement of chylomicrons or migrating cells of the immune system, e.g. lymphocytes and macrophages.

Chylomicrons, because of their size, rarely pass into the mucosal capillaries. Even the open fenestrae of these vessels are only 40–60 nm in diameter. However, chylomicrons can reach the central lacteals probably aided by the bulk flow of water during absorption (Fig. 5.14). Subsequently they enter these lymphatic channels through interendothelial cell gaps and so pass to the systemic circulation.

The fate of protein

When considering what happens to protein, several questions must be asked:

1. Where are the products of the gastric and pancreatic phase of digestion hydrolysed within the small intestine?
2. What are the products of this hydrolysis?

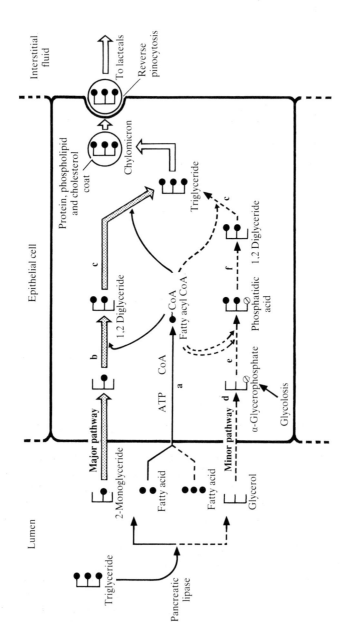

Fig. 5.13 The fate of triglyceride in the small intestine. A number of enzymes are necessary for these steps. A knowledge of them is, perhaps, beyond the requirements of this book. For those biochemically minded, however: a = Fatty acid CoA ligase; b = monoglyceride acyltransferase; c = diglyceride acyltransferase; d = glycerokinase; e = glycerophosphate acyltransferase; f = phosphatidate phosphohydrolase (Modified from Gangl, A. and Ockner, R.K. (1975). *Gastroenterology* **68**, 167–86.)

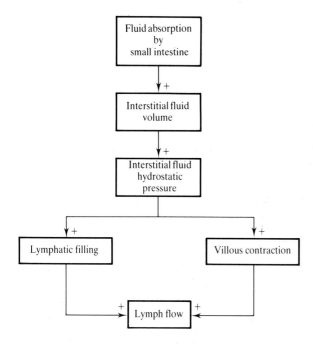

Fig. 5.14 The influence of intestinal fluid absorption on the flow of lymph

3. Which substances can be transferred from the lumen towards the bloodstream?

4. What is known of the mechanisms involved in the transfer of these substances?

The finding that only the component amino acids of proteins appeared in the bloodstream has led to many supporting the classical but erroneous view that proteins are completely hydrolysed within the lumen. Few listened to R.B. Fisher when he pointed out in 1950 that 200 hours would be required for the liberation of 90 per cent of the amino acids from proteins subjected to the successive actions of the known proteolytic enzymes. Such a sequence of events would be much too slow to account for the rapid disappearance of protein from the intestinal lumen. A number of possibilities remain. One is that enzymes concerned with the final stages of digestion are active at sites other than the lumen. Another is that products other than amino acids are absorbed.

Consider, first of all, the problem of the site of peptide hydrolysis (Fig. 5.15). After the proteolytic enzymes of gastric and pancreatic juice have exerted their effects, a mixture remains of free amino acids and small peptides. Two distinct groups of intestinal enzymes are thought to be involved in peptide hydrolysis. One is associated with the brush border membrane, while the other is located in the cytoplasm. It is believed that any peptidases present within the luminal contents are derived from sloughed epithelial cells.

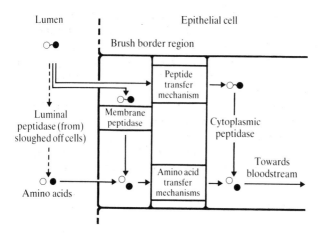

Fig. 5.15 The three different sites for the hydrolysis of peptides. 1. Some peptides are absorbed from the lumen and hydrolysed by cytoplasmic peptidases. 2. Some peptides are hydrolysed by brush border enzymes and their component amino acids transferred by specific mechanisms. 3. Some peptides are hydrolysed intraluminally as a result of peptidase activity from cells sloughed off at the villous tip. Very little peptide appears in the bloodstream

The question must be asked as to which peptides are hydrolysed by cytoplasmic enzymes and which by those associated with the brush border. The di- and tripeptides containing proline appear to hydrolysed almost exclusively by cytoplasmic enzymes. Peptidases in the brush border have virtually no activity against them. Peptides containing glycine, aspartic and glutamic acid may also be hydrolysed in the cytoplasm. In contrast, peptides containing arginine, lysine, methionine and leucine appear to be hydrolysed in the brush border region.

This leaves us with the question as to which digestive products are absorbed and what processes are involved. Let us consider the intestinal handling of amino acids.

Absorption of amino acids

Prior to 1950, the absorption of amino acids was considered to be a passive event, the driving force for it being the difference in luminal to plasma amino acid concentration. This view was supported by the finding that uptake was reciprocally related to the molal volume. However, even at that time some sort of 'accelerating mechanism' was being considered, because amino acid movement was more rapid than that of other substances of similar size. More evidence favouring this concept was the finding that, if one measured the absorption of amino acids from racemic mixtures, then the movement of the L-form was the most rapid (Table 5.2). Subsequently, transport of some amino acids against a concentration gradient has been demonstrated. From autoradiography studies, the amino acids being transferred across the intestinal wall were found to be concentrated in the microvilli, with much smaller accumulations at the basolateral membranes. This suggests that the brush border membrane is the site at which amino acids are actively transported, the result being the development of high concentrations intracellularly. Clearly, the subsequent diffusion of amino acids from a high to a low concentration might account for their appearance in the bloodstream.

Our understanding of the processes by which amino acids can be transferred across intestinal epithelial cell membranes has been greatly increased in the last 20 years. The advent of isolated membrane vesicle preparations has provided a valuable tool for the systematic study of both brush border and basolateral membranes. The brush border has several unique transport pathways not found in non-epithelial membranes. These include:

1. The NBB (Neutral Brush Border) system, which can transport most neutral amino acids.
2. The IMINO system, which exclusively transports proline and hydroxy-proline.
3. The PHE system, which has phenylalanine and methionine as typical substrates.

Two more processes have been described. One involves a carrier which transfers the basic amino acids (e.g. lysine, and including cystine). The other is concerned with the transport of dicarboxylic acids such as glutamic acid.

Passive diffusion makes some contribution to the movement of amino acids across basolateral membranes. These membranes are more leaky than those of the brush borders. In addition, however, there are several systems for the removal of amino acids with characteristics similar to those in plasma membranes of non-epithelial cells. The L system appears to provide the major route and has broad specificity for neutral amino acids. A further mechanism

Table 5.2 Absorption of L- and D-amino acids from D L mixtures introduced into the lower ileum of anaesthetized rats (From Gibson, Q. H. and Wiseman, G. (1951). *Biochemical Journal* **48**, 426–9.)

D L amino acid	Amount introduced (μmol)	L-form (μmol)	D-form (μmol)	L : D
Histidine	232	84	14	6.0
Phenylalanine	156	54	10	5.4
Glutamic acid	192	49	10	4.9
Lysine	168	38	10	3.9
Valine	222	69	22	3.1
Aspartic acid	206	46	17	2.7
Leucine	200	48	21	2.3
Alanine	256	48	22	2.2
Isoleucine	184	54	25	2.2
Methionine	272	104	64	1.6

is available whereby basic amino acids can exit. It appears to be of limited capacity.

The systems referred to above transfer the L-amino acids. What happens to the D-isomers? Several of the amino acid carriers are capable of transferring them. However, the affinities of the D-amino acids are low and little transport of the D-form occurs because of the competition with the L-forms derived either from food or endogenous sources.

A requirement of many of the brush border amino acid transfer mechanisms is for the presence of Na$^+$. Without it amino acid transfer is inhibited. Indeed a reduced transfer in the absence of Na$^+$ cannot be limited to amino acids. A number of other substances, listed in Table 5.3 are also affected.

Table 5.3   Sodium-dependent mechanisms in the intestine for the transfer of water-soluble organic substances. The substances have all been shown to be transferred by mechanisms that are sensitive to sodium. It does not follow that all these mechanisms depend on sodium in the same way. Furthermore, even when the sodium dependency of the system is established in one species, it would be extremely dangerous to assume that the process in another species was similarly dependent.

1. Amino acids:
    (a) Acidic, e.g. glumatic and aspartic.
    (b) IMINO, e.g. proline.
    (c) NBB, e.g. most neutral amino acids.
    (d) PHE, e.g. phenylalanine.
2. Bile salts, e.g. taurocholate.
3. Monosaccharides, e.g. glucose and galactose.
4. Phosphate.
5. Vitamins:
    (a) Ascorbic acid.
    (b) Biotin.
    (c) Folic acid.
    (d) Inositol.
    (e) Thiamine.

How might Na$^+$ alter the ability of the small intestine to absorb amino acids? Several possibilities have been considered:

1. The Na$^+$ could influence amino acid transport indirectly, perhaps modifying membrane structure so that the transport sites are more readily accessible.
2. The Na$^+$ could be involved in the coupling of metabolic energy to the transport systems, e.g. through Na$^+$-sensitive ATP-ases.
3. The Na$^+$ could affect the reactions involved in metabolism and so alter the availability of energy.
4. A more direct relationship can be imagined in which the movements of Na$^+$ and amino acids are coupled.

Many have investigated the relationships between Na$^+$ and amino acid transfer. As a result the following model is available to explain transepithelial amino acid movement (Fig. 5.16). It is proposed that amino acids and Na$^+$ combine with a membrane carrier to form a ternary complex. This complex is capable of traversing the membrane. The amino acid and Na$^+$ are released into the cell.

These movements of Na$^+$ and amino acids result in the amino acids accumulating within the epithelial cells and being unable to be transferred back towards the lumen readily by the same mechanism because Na$^+$ is less available in the intracellular fluid as compared with the extracellular fluid. Less Na$^+$ is present intracellularly as the result of the activity of an active transport process, located in the basolateral membranes, removing Na$^+$ from the epithelial cells. When one accepts this model, it can be argued that, while amino acid transfer can occur against a concentration gradient, no energy need be fed into the amino acid transport system. Rather, it can be seen that active transport of Na$^+$ creates an asymmetric distribution of Na$^+$ across the luminal membrane, and this Na$^+$ asymmetry provides energy for amino acid transport. This concept is known as the Na$^+$-gradient hypothesis and was proposed by R.K. Crane.

The movement of amino acids out of the epithelial cells across the basolateral membranes is primarily by Na$^+$-independent mechanisms. However, Na$^+$-dependent processes (A and ASC) have been recognized which may accelerate amino acid uptake from the interstitial fluid under conditions where amino acid availability in the lumen is limited.

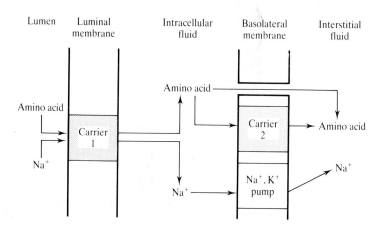

Fig. 5.16 Amino acid transport from the lumen to the interstitial fluid. Na$^+$ is required for amino-acid entry into the cell (via carrier 1). This process is one of facilitated diffusion. Na$^+$ is pumped out of the cell at the basolateral membrane. Thus amino acids accumulate intracellularly and diffuse out of the cell down their concentration gradients (Crane's Na$^+$-gradient hypothesis). Both simple and facilitated (carrier 2) diffusion are thought to contribute to the removal of amino acids from the cell at the basolateral membranes

Can peptides be absorbed?

At the beginning of the present century, the view was held that proteins did not have to be completely hydrolysed to their component amino acids before absorption from the intestinal lumen took place. Today we support that concept although peptides with four or more amino acids appear to be unsuitable for absorption. Favouring the concept that some peptide absorption occurs has been the finding that a few peptides are transferred to the bloodstream, e.g. peptides of proline and hydroxyproline have been detected after gelatin ingestion, while carnosine (β-alanylhistidine) and anserine (β-alanylmethylhistidine) appear after a meal including chicken breast. Such peptides are difficult to hydrolyse.

What do we know of the mechanisms involved in peptide absorption? Our knowledge is, as yet, incomplete. Only a few peptides have been studied and there are many possible amino acid combinations to provide dipeptides (400) or tripeptides (8000). In man, one system of extremely broad specificity has been detected. In some animals, e.g. rabbit, two mechanisms have been described. Competition between different peptides has been demonstrated. Peptide movement is thought to occur by an active transport process against an electrochemical gradient with di- and tripeptides sharing the same system. Such movement is inhibited by anoxia and metabolic inhibitors. Initially peptides were described as being absorbed by yet further Na^+-dependent systems from the lumen. However, the relationship between Na^+ and peptides may be less direct than that described for amino acids. A Na^+-proton exchange process is thought to provide an inwardly directed proton gradient at the brush border. These protons stimulate a proton-dependent but Na^+-independent peptide movement. The overall result of course is that Na^+ and peptides are transferred (Fig. 5.17). Nevertheless, in the absence of Na^+ a reduced uptake of peptides would be expected.

More evidence in favour of peptide transport has been obtained from studies of patients with amino acid transport defects. Two such abnormalities are cystinuria and Hartnup disease. These conditions are relatively rare, and were originally described as renal tubular transport disorders. Subsequently, it was appreciated that transport across the small intestine could also be deranged. In cystinuria the basic amino acids lysine, ornithine and arginine, and the sulphur-containing amino acid cystine are poorly transferred. In Hartnup disease several neutral amino acids, e.g. tryptophan, are not absorbed at normal rates. However, if amino acids are introduced in the form of small peptides these can be absorbed and the needs of the body satisfied.

In some less specific malabsorption states, e.g. coeliac disease, amino acid absorption is markedly reduced while peptide absorption seems to be less severely affected. Diets with di- and tripeptides rather than free amino acids for such patients have several advantages. As well as providing a source of amino acids, peptides are less osmotically active than free amino acids. Hypertonicity is poorly tolerated. In addition, diets containing peptides are more palatable.

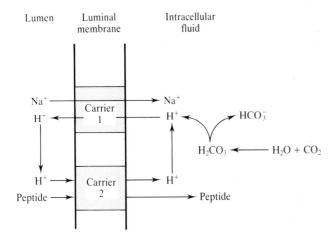

Fig. 5.17 The absorption of peptides from the intestinal lumen. Carrier 1 exchanges Na+ for H+. The latter is cotransported with peptide by carrier 2.

Protein absorption

In the adult mammal, intact dietary protein does not reach the mucosal epithelial cells in appreciable amounts. Nevertheless, small amounts may escape complete digestion, reach subepithelial sites and induce the elaboration of antibodies against them. Such protein movement may occur in one of several ways:

1. By diffusing through the extrusion zones at the tips of villi.
2. Via the remnants of mechanisms described in the fetus and newborn.
3. As the result of specific transport processes whereby macromolecules can be 'sampled'.

In contrast to the situation encountered in the adult, the small intestine of the fetus and the neonate display a transient but pronounced permeability to some macromolecules. As a result passive immunity can be transmitted from mother to offspring. In primates transmission occurs entirely before birth. However, the intestine would not appear to be a major route for antibody transfer. Only small amounts of such proteins as IgG reach the amniotic fluid, from which they could be swallowed by the fetus and, subsequently, absorbed. The primary route for immunoglobulin transfer from mother to fetus is across the chorio-allantoic placenta. In many mammalian species, maternal antibodies are transferred mainly after birth. These proteins are available as the newborn ingests colostrum and milk. The permeability of the intestine to antibodies is rapidly lost, e.g. after 18 days in rats.

The fetuses of several animals (including man) have an additional means of removing macromolecules from the intestinal contents. From the fourteenth gestational week to shortly before birth, the human fetus is capable of pinocytosing radio-opaque markers into ileal vacuoles. These macromolecules do not pass through the cells into the lamina propria as such, but are thought to be degraded by lysosomal enzymes intracellularly before being released. It has been suggested that this form of digestion may play a role in the nutrition of the immature animal before the establishment of efficient luminal digestion.

The question remains as to whether macromolecules are specifically sampled from the intestinal lumen. It would appear that they are. Thin membranous (M) cells have been identified as part of the epithelial covering of intestinal lymph nodes (Fig. 5.18). They have the unique capacity to transport antigens and macromolecules in vacuoles and present them to the underlying Peyer's patches. The M cells may be derived from absorptive epithelial cells as the result of interactions with closely associated lymphoid tissue. They differ in appearance from normal epithelial cells in that:

(a) their luminal membranes possess far fewer, shorter and often wider brush borders,
(b) the glycocalyx is poorly developed,
(c) there are no lysosomes.

Such features might be expected in cells which had adapted for the transport of macromolecules. In addition, fewer mitochondria are observed.

What happens when antigens are released into the subepithelial space? It must be remembered that the gut provides a major subdivision of the body's immune system, and when antigens are presented to the Peyer's patches lymphocytes are stimulated. Some proliferate and are committed to specific immunoglobulin A (IgA) production (plasma cells) in the lamina propria of the intestine. Other activated cells migrate via the mesenteric lymph nodes and the thoracic duct to the blood in which they 'home in' on specific sites e.g. salivary gland, breast, lacrymal gland and the urinogenital tract.

IgA is the principal secretory immunoglobulin found at the mucosal surface. It provides protection, not because of any limited capacity to cause bacteriolysis or opsonization, but because it can prevent adherence and penetration of bacteria, viruses and other antigens, e.g. *Streptococcus* and *Escherichia coli*. The IgA released from plasma cells is in the dimeric form. Within the cells monomers are connected by a glycoprotein (molecular weight about 150 000) called the J or junctional piece. To reach the intestinal lumen the dimer is complexed with yet another glycoprotein, the secretory component (molecular weight about 70 000). Secretory component is a constituent of the basolateral membranes of epithelial cells transporting IgA to the lumen. When IgA binds to secretory component, endocytosis occurs and vesicles containing IgA are transferred to the luminal membrane. At this site the IgA dimer–secretory component complex is released (Fig. 5.19). The secretory component renders the IgA more resistant to proteolytic enzymes such as trypsin and chymotrypsin.

A rich source of IgA in the intestinal lumen is bile. Up to 90% of the newly synthesized specific IgA antibodies may reach the lumen via hepatic secretions. As in the intestine the secretory component appears to be the hepatocyte's receptor for IgA. Once bound, vesicles are produced which transfer IgA from the sinusoidal membrane to the bile canaliculus. The concept of antigens within the food swallowed activating the intestine and resulting in the release of specific IgA proximally is an important one. Furthermore, the capacity of the lactating mother to release IgA into her milk in response to antigen challenge would be useful particularly as the intestinal barrier of the neonate has been regarded as immature.

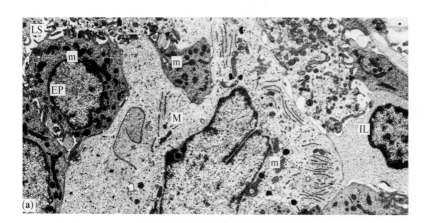

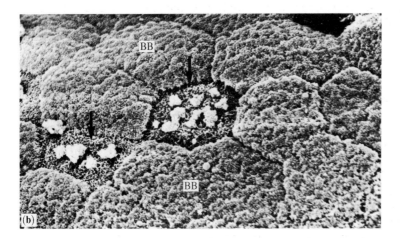

Fig. 5.18 (**a**) Transmission electron micrograph of baboon duodenum showing a longitudinal section through a villus. Note the M cell (M) in intimate contact with an intraepithelial lymphocyte (IL). The M cell has abundant cytoplasm but few mitochondria (m). This contrasts with the numerous mitochondria encountered in the surrounding absorbing epithelial cells (EP). The lateral spaces (LS) separating these columnar cells, important for fluid transport, can readily be discerned. (**b**) Scanning electron micrograph of baboon duodenum showing the luminal surface of villous epithelial cells. The characteristic brush border (BB) of the normal absorbing cells is replaced on the M cells by numerous microfolds (↓) (Kindly presented by Dr K. Kyriacou, College of Medicine, King Saud University, Riyadh, Saudi Arabia.)

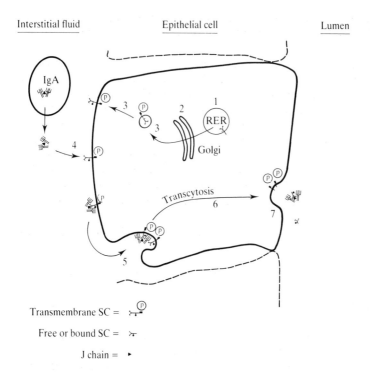

Interstitial fluid   Epithelial cell   Lumen

Transmembrane SC =

Free or bound SC =

J chain =

Fig. 5.19 A model for the transport of IgA from the interstitial fluid to the intestinal lumen. 1. Secretory component (SC) is synthesized in the rough endoplasmic reticulum (RER). 2. SC undergoes glycosylation (●) in the Golgi complex. 3. Subsequently, SC is phosphorylated (P) and incorporated into the basolateral membranes. 4. SC binds with the dimeric form of IgA. 5. Endocytosis of IgA : SC complex (and excess SC). 6. Transcytosis of vesicles. 7. Release of a part of SC, either free, or bound to IgA. During exocytosis stabilizing disulphide bridges are formed between SC and IgA (Simplified from Brandtzaeg, P., Sollid, L.M., Thrane, P.S. et al. (1988). *Gut* **29**, 1116–30.

The fate of carbohydrate

Whereas the small intestine is capable of absorbing small peptides or amino acids derived from the hydrolysis of protein, it appears unable to transfer, in appreciable amounts, products of carbohydrate digestion other than mono-saccharides. Thus extremely small amounts of the non-digestible disaccharide lactulose (4-O-β-D galactopyranosyl D-fructose) are absorbed. The breakdown of polysaccharides, started by salivary amylase and continued by the pancreatic hydrolase, results in the formation of maltose, maltotriose and α-dextrins. These and other carbohydrates (e.g. the disaccharides, sucrose and lactose) are further hydrolysed by oligosaccharidases distributed throughout the small intestine, but with greatest activity in the jejunum. Where do these enzymes exert their effects? Doubtless, salivary and pancreatic amylase act within the lumen of the stomach and small intestine respectively. However, Ugolev has suggested that pancreatic amylase is adsorbed to the jejunal surface and that at this site 'membrane' or 'contact' digestion may be an important mechanism in carbohydrate breakdown (see Fig. 5.7).

Oligosaccharidases concerned with the final stages of carbohydrate digestion are elaborated by mucosal epithelial cells. These enzymes can be detected in brush border preparations of villous but not crypt cells. They appear to be globular structures attached to the external surface of the luminal membranes by anchoring systems. Two means of attachment have been described. One is characterized by a hydrophobic sequence of about 20 amino acids which spans the membrane. Enzymes anchored by this peptide (e.g. sucrase) may be separated from the membrane by the plant proteolytic enzyme papain. The other system involves a covalent linkage between the C-terminal amino acid of the enzyme and the diacylglycerol part of a membrane phosphatidylinositol (phospholipid).

Several brush border enzymes contribute to the production of monosaccharides. These include:

1. Glucoamylase (or maltase) which can release glucose from small oligosaccharides with $\alpha 1, 4$ linkages.
2. Isomaltase which is essential for the hydrolysis of $\alpha 1,6$ linkages in tri- and tetrasachharides.
3. α-limit dextrinase which more readily hydrolyses the $\alpha 1,6$ linkages of penta- and hexaoligosaccharides than isomaltase.
4. Sucrase (or invertase) which as its name suggests releases glucose and fructose from sucrose. This enzyme also has maltase activity. Different active sites are required for the two hydrolytic events. Sucrase and isomaltase exist together as a complex.
5. Lactase, a β-galactosidase which hydrolyses lactose to glucose and galactose. The disaccharide is normally ingested only in milk and milk products. Usually, lactase activity declines during childhood to low adult levels. However, some people in Northern Europe and the Hamitic people of Africa do not follow this pattern and lactase levels remain high.

As the result of the activities of the first four enzymes the glucose polymers and sucrose are broken down to monosaccharides. Under normal circumstances these enzymes are not rate limiting for carbohydrate digestion and absorption, i.e. they can release monosaccharides more rapidly than the hexose transport process can remove them.

It has been recognized that if these enzymes were to be specifically and reversibly inhibited, then a means would be available to reduce the rates at which monosaccharides are absorbed. Normally, carbohydrate digestion and absorption is completed in the first third of the small intestine. By carefully inhibiting monosaccharide production more distal intestinal sites would, perhaps, be utilized for absorption. It would, however, take longer for absorption to occur. Absorption could still take place because the small intestine has considerable reserve capacity for monosaccharide transport, and sugars need not pass to the colon where they would be fermented by bacteria. By delaying absorption postprandial rises in blood glucose concentration might be minimized and the longer term complications of diabetes mellitus reduced.

Recently, a reversible inhibitor (BAY m1099, a derivative of 1-deoxy-nojirimycin) has been synthesized in microbial culture. Studies in man indicate it is tolerated well and in appropriate doses can regulate postprandial glycaemia without causing malabsorption.

One is left with the problem of monosaccharide transport. Evidence to suggest a special mechanism started to accumulate more than half a century ago:

1. Glucose and galactose are absorbed from the intestine at similar rates, which are very much faster than those recorded for mannose, xylose and arabinose. Fructose disappears at a rate intermediate to these two extremes. Thus molecular configuration and not size determines the rate of absorption of sugars.

2. Glucose and galactose can move across the epithelial cell against their chemical potential.

3. The rates of absorption of some sugars are not proportional to their luminal concentrations.

4. Several sugars, e.g. glucose and galactose, compete with each other for the absorption mechanism, if present together in the intestinal lumen.

5. Absorption of glucose is inhibited by a number of substances. The most striking of these is phlorrhizin (phloretin $2'\beta$-D glucoside). This substance specifically and reversibly blocks the entry of glucose and galactose into the epithelial cell from the lumen. With such an inhibitor it has been possible to study the specificity of the glucose carrier mechanism. It is suggested that phlorrhizin acts by attachment of the glucosyl unit to the glucose sites on the carrier and that the phloretin group makes the affinity of the glucosyl unit for the sites greater than that of glucose.

Substances that interfere with the provision of energy for cellular functions, e.g. 2,4-dinitrophenol, also interfere with glucose transport. Hence, unless one argues that such inhibitors generally disrupt cellular activity, one must conclude that glucose transport is an energy-requiring process.

Obviously, some monosaccharides are transferred across the gut by a 'special mechanism'. Several theories were put forward to explain glucose transfer. One was the phosphorylation theory in which it was postulated that glucose was trapped within the epithelial cell following its phosphorylation at the luminal border. The hexose was thought to be transferred across the cell in this form and subsequently dephosphorylated with the release of free glucose which diffuses out of the cell into the subepithelial space. No real evidence for this theory was ever produced. It was suggested as a reasonable explanation of the inhibition of glucose absorption by substances which interfered with phosphorylation, e.g. iodoacetate. Evidence against the theory has accumulated. For example, the two phosphate esters of glucose that can be detected are glucose-1-phosphate and glucose-6-phosphate. However, hexose derivatives are available which can utilize the glucose transfer mechanism but are unable to be phosphorylated at carbon 1 or 6.

Rather than hexose phosphorylation occurring at the luminal membrane, dephosphorylation should be recognized. Phosphorylated sugars cannot be absorbed and their hydrolysis may be an important function of the brush border alkaline phosphatase. This enzyme has broad substrate specificity, and many biologically important esters other than glucose 1- and 6-phosphate can easily be hydrolysed, e.g. phosphoserine, -glycerophophate and nucleotides. The enzyme increases inorganic phosphate (P_i) availability. Furthermore, alkaline phosphatase has considerable affinity for P_i at physiological pH. Thus, after the hydrolysis of esters it may transiently sequester the P_i and donate it to the brush border Na^+-dependent phosphate carrier.

What is known about monosaccharide absorption? As regards glucose and galactose (the important aldohexoses in the diet) transport a similar picture has emerged to that previously described for amino acids. Thus at the brush border membrane a Na^+-dependent mechanism is available for hexose entry from the lumen. Na^+ may be available from:

1. Dietary sources and saliva,bile and pancreatic secretions
2. Secretions of the small intestine (see page 164)
3. Paracellular movement of Na^+ from the subepithelial extracellular fluid.

The countercurrent multiplier (see page 123) may contribute to an increased availability of Na^+, particularly towards the villous tip where absorption primarily occurs. Na^+ and hexose are transferred together (i.e. cotransported). The removal of Na^+ by the energy requiring Na^+,K^+-pump in the basolateral membranes may prevent hexoses returning to the lumen and maintains Na^+ and K^+ electrochemical gradients.

This cotransport system does not require a direct input of energy. Nevertheless, sugars have been shown to accumulate intracellularly at concentrations 70 times greater than outside the cell. Energy is, however, utilized to maintain the Na^+ and K^+ gradients and is vital for hexose accumulation. The term secondary active transport has been coined to describe such processes using energy indirectly.

Several questions have been asked about the brush border system. For example:

1. Is there only one Na^+-dependent mechanism?
2. Which binds first, Na^+ or hexose?
3. What is the stoichiometry between Na^+ and glucose?
4. What sort of carrier is involved?

Some answers are slowly appearing. Initially data collected were compatible with the existence of a single specific mechanism and a contribution from simple diffusion. Even then, however, a more complex situation was suspected. Recent studies with bovine brush border membrane vesicles provide support for the presence of two systems. The major one is a high-capacity, low-affinity system with a 1:1 stoichiometry of Na^+:glucose. A low-capacity, high-affinity mechanism involving a 3:1 relationship between Na^+ and glucose provides a minor route. An ordered sequence of binding to the cotransporter has been proposed with Na^+ binding first and increasing the affinity of the hexose binding site. Considerable progress has been made in our understanding of the carrier in the last decade. It has stable structural and functional asymmetry. Thus the structure it exposes at the two sides of the membrane react differently with SH-reagents or proteases. Furthermore, influx and efflux rates of glucose across brush border membrane vesicles are by no means identical under equivalent but mirrored conditions. Such evidence is against a carrier rotating in or diffusing across the membrane but favours the existence of a 'pore' or 'channel'.

This does not mean that the carrier has no movement. Indeed, models have been presented in which part of the protein, including the Na^+ and hexose binding sites has mobility. In one of these (Fig. 5.20) a negatively charged gate and a sugar binding site are visualized within a channel. These sites can be exposed on both sides, although not simultaneously. They preferentially face the intracellular compartment. However, a membrane potential (negative inside) results in the gate and glucose binding site moving towards the extracellular surface and becoming accessible to luminal Na^+ and glucose. Na^+ binds to the gate. This produces an increase in the affinity of the sugar binding site for glucose. The neutralization of the gate allows the mobile part of the carrier to 'snap back' to its preferred orientation exposing it and the glucose-laden site to the intracellular fluid. Following the release of Na^+ (and glucose) the gate again becomes negatively charged and the process repeated.

The structure and biochemical characteristics of the cotransport system is the subject of exciting investigations by Ernest Wright and his colleagues in Los Angeles. The transporter has been identified as a protein with molecular weight about 75 000. It has significant homology with the *Escherichia coli* Na^+, proline cotransporter suggesting an evolutionary link between bacterial and mammalian (human) Na^+-cotransport systems. Recently the protein has been cloned from rabbit intestinal brush borders and expressed in Xenopus oocytes. Its characteristics there are similar to those determined in intestinal brush borders, e.g. the substrate specificity in both preparations is D-glucose > D-galactose >> D-mannose = L-glucose. A method is, therefore, available with which a more detailed examination can be made of the specific properties of the cotransporter.

At the basolateral membrane an Na^+-independent facilitated diffusion process and simple diffusion account for the removal of hexoses from the epithelial cells. The facilitated process is similar to that described for non-epithelial cells. Its capacity to transfer glucose can be varied. Two distinct changes have been reported as a result of hyperglycaemia. One occurs within 2 hours at which time carriers already inserted in the membrane can transfer more hexose. Subsequently, even greater sugar transport occurs because of the recruitment of new carriers. The system is said to be 'upregulated'. The question remains as to its functional significance. The changes might represent an increased capacity for the transport of an important energy-rich nutrient from the lumen. Alternatively, if glucose is more readily transferred from the interstitial fluid (or bloodstream) energy would be available for either:

(a) the absorption of slowly absorbed substances normally present within the diet, or

(b) the greater absorption of water and electrolytes observed when the sympathetic nervous system is stimulated (see page 166).

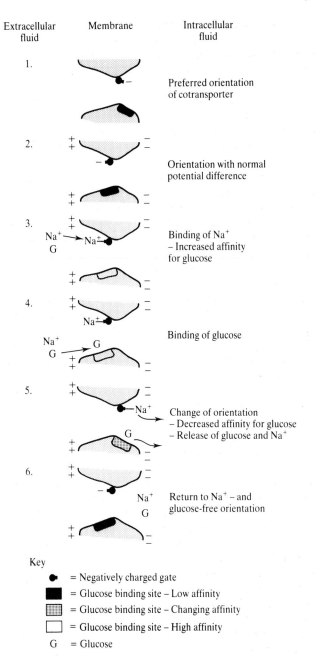

Extracellular fluid	Membrane	Intracellular fluid

1. Preferred orientation of cotransporter

2. Orientation with normal potential difference

3. Binding of Na$^+$
   – Increased affinity for glucose

4. Binding of glucose

5. Change of orientation
   – Decreased affinity for glucose
   – Release of glucose and Na$^+$

6. Return to Na$^+$ – and glucose-free orientation

Key

● = Negatively charged gate

■ = Glucose binding site – Low affinity

▨ = Glucose binding site – Changing affinity

☐ = Glucose binding site – High affinity

G = Glucose

Fig. 5.20 Model for glucose transport across the luminal membrane of absorbing epithelial cells (Modified from Kessler, M. and Semenza, G. (1983). *Journal of Membrane Biology* **76**, 27–56.)

Energy requirements for transport

From the preceding paragraphs it is clear that energy is not fed directly into hexose and amino acid transport systems. Rather, the energy requirement is for Na^+ extrusion from the mucosal cells. The question arises as to the source of energy. Is glucose metabolism, for example, the major source of energy? One might have anticipated that this would be an easy question to answer, particularly as the intestinal mucosa is regarded as one of the most actively respiring tissues in the body. In contrast, metabolism in the other layers is slow, e.g. muscle contributes under 10% of the total lactic acid production of the intestinal wall. However, several different metabolic pathways are involved and these are affected markedly by such factors as age, stress and diet. Thus the following questions need to asked, although not all of them can be answered:

1. Are the substrates and/or metabolic pathways providing energy during absorption identical with those used in the postabsorptive state? (During absorption there is an increased energy requirement).
2. Are the substrates metabolized the same in different regions of the small intestine?
3. What additional substrates are present within the gut wall which may be utilized to provide energy for transport?

To illustrate the complexity of the problem, consider the situation in rat small intestine. The major respiratory substrates in the jejunum after fasting are glucose, glutamine and ketone bodies. Although plasma glucose and glutamine concentrations in 48-hour fasted rats were 7.5 mmol/l and 1.5 mmol/l respectively, more glutamine is metabolized than glucose. In contrast, in the fed animal, glutamine utilization was less than half the rate of glucose metabolism.

Glucose is undoubtedly a major energy source, although glutamine can also be utilized. However, under certain conditions, e.g. starvation, the intestine may utilize non-carbohydrate substrates so as to preserve plasma glucose levels. As a result the energy needs of those tissues that are more carbohydrate dependent, e.g. brain, might be satisfied for longer periods of time. During starvation the rat intestine appears to adapt in another way with the ileum, perhaps, becoming a more important region for glucose absorption. To support this view it has been found that glucose metabolism is reduced in both the jejunum and the ileum in the fasted animal. However, the ileum is less dependent on glucose metabolism than the jejunum. Hence, ileal absorption processes may be less susceptible to changes in glucose metabolism. In fact, the ileal capacity to absorb glucose is increased during starvation and substances introduced into the stomach reach the ileum more rapidly. Both these findings:

(a) increased glucose transport capacity, and
(b) reduced transit time,

may indicate a greater importance of the terminal ileum during starvation (Fig. 5.21).

Usually the transfers of sugars and amino acids are markedly reduced if intestinal tissue is incubated anaerobically. Some exceptions, however, have been reported. For example, the small intestine of the rabbit fetus, subject to more hypoxic conditions than adult tissues, is able to support transport processes in the absence of oxygen. In the adult animal there is evidence that the limited energy available from anaerobic metabolism can be used preferentially by certain transport processes. Thus glucose can double the anaerobic transport of methionine *in vitro*. This effect partially overcomes the inhibition that oxygen deficiency produces of the uptake of this essential amino acid. In contrast, glucose does not alter alanine transport under anaerobic conditions.

Fructose absorption

This ketohexose is absorbed at a slower rate than glucose and galactose but at a more rapid rate than several hexoses, such as mannose, which have the same molecular weight. Probably fructose is absorbed from the lumen by a Na^+-independent facilitated diffusion process and cannot be transported against a concentration gradient.

Evidence for a specific transfer mechanism has been obtained from measurements of sugar absorption across the luminal membrane of rabbit ileum in the presence of phlorrhizin. When phlorrhizin occupies the carrier sites for galactose, the residual transfer of this hexose should represent simple diffusion.

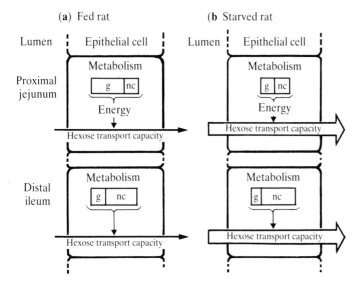

Fig. 5.21 The effect of starvation on hexose transport by rat small intestine. (**a**) Fed rat, (**b**) starved rat. The hexose transport capacity for both proximal jejunum and distal ileum is increased following starvation for 3 days. Energy needed for transport is derived from both glucose (g) and non-carbohydrate (nc) sources, and the energy available from glucose is reduced in fasting. In the distal ileum more energy comes from non-carbohydrate and this maintains the increased hexose transport induced by fasting. The proximal jejunum is more dependent on glucose metabolism, and hexose transport cannot be increased because of decreased availability of energy. The above does not take into consideration possible alterations in non-carbohydrate metabolism (From Sanford, P.A. and Smyth, D.H. (1974). *Journal of Physiology* **239**, 285–99.)

Fructose, a sugar of similar chemical and physical properties, would be expected to diffuse across the luminal border at a comparable rate if only absorbed by simple diffusion. However, fructose penetrated at six times the rate observed for galactose. These results have been explained by postulating the existence of a fructose carrier with no affinity for glucose, galactose or phlorrhizin (Fig. 5.22). The fructose mechanism may be specific for sugars that exist in the furanose form.

Hydrolase-related transfer of sugars

It is generally thought the intestine is unable to absorb molecules larger than monosaccharides in appreciable amounts. At one time, however, it was suspected that some disaccharidases were able to act as vectorial enzymes and transfer their products directly across the brush border membranes independently of the systems described for monosaccharides. Black lipid membranes were prepared which were normally impermeable to sucrose, glucose and fructose. Subsequently, purified sucrase–isomaltase complexes were incorporated into these membranes. As a result the permeability of the membrane to glucose and fructose derived from sucrose, but not to free glucose and fructose was increased. While support for disaccharide absorption is lacking fructose absorption from sucrose has been shown to be more rapid than from fructose itself. This may reflect the greater concentrations of fructose produced intraluminally as a result of glucose-stimulated water absorption.

The fate of water and ions (Na^+, K^+, Cl^-, and HCO_3^-)

Bidirectional movement

The view that epithelial cells represent a barrier which is traversed by the movement of substances through the cells has had to be modified. A major component

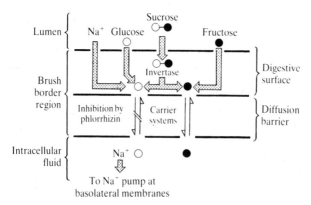

Fig. 5.22 The digestive surface of the epithelial cell. The digestion of sucrose and the absorption of glucose and fructose (From Crane, R.K. (1977). *International Review of Physiology* **12**, 325–65, University Press, Baltimore.)

of salt and water transfer is by way of the 'not so tight' junctions. These are zones at which epithelial cells are somewhat loosely attached. Transfer through tight junctions is said to occur via the paracellular pathway.

With such a pathway, water movement will depend on either osmotic gradients between the luminal and interstitial fluids or hydrostatic pressures. Because the lateral spaces are open to the interstitial fluid at one end but closed by tight junctions at the other, one might predict that alterations of the hydrostatic pressure in the lumen would have little effect on fluid movement,* whereas changing interstitial fluid pressure would have a marked effect. Some evidence to support this prediction is available. If the plasma volume is rapidly expanded by saline administered intravenously, then absorption is depressed. However, fluid absorption can be enhanced on reducing plasma volume by haemorrhage (but see page 123).

Fluid will also move along the paracellular pathway in response to osmotic gradients. If the intraluminal fluid is hypotonic with respect to the interstitial fluid, an absorption of fluid is expected. In contrast, if the luminal fluid is hypertonic, then fluid secretion results. In either case the luminal contents tend to become isotonic.

Electrolyte movement via the paracellular pathway occurs through water-filled pores, assumed to be located in the tight junctions. How large are these pores? One approach used to determine the approximate dimensions has been to measure the reflection coefficients of solutes which have diameters of the same order as those gaps in the tight junctions. The reflection coefficient (σ) is the ratio of the osmotic pressure a penetrating solute exerts across a membrane to that exerted by a molecule which is unable to be transferred. (NB. The reflection coefficient has already been introduced while considering the leakiness of intestinal capillaries to plasma proteins.) The human jejunum is impermeable to mannitol. The sugar alcohol, therefore, has a reflection coefficient of 1.0. However, Na^+ and K^+ penetrate this intestinal barrier. Values of 0.4 and 0.5, respectively, have been calculated. Using the data derived from such measurements, it has been suggested that the diameter of human jejunal pores is approximately 0.8 nm, while ileal pores are only half that size. The contribution of the paracellular pathway to electrolyte transfer in the ileum, therefore, is thought to be smaller.

The water-filled pores of the tight junction are not unselective. Both jejunal and ileal pores are more permeable to cations than to anions, suggesting that the pores are lined with negative charges.

Following a meal, a number of different substances are present in the lumen. Many of these are absorbed by processes coupled to transcellular active Na^+ transport. An accompanying anion (e.g. Cl^-) helps to maintain electrical neutrality. It might be expected, therefore, that osmotic gradients would be developed between the luminal fluid and the interstitial fluid and that water would be osmotically attracted into the lateral spaces via the paracellular

---

*Michael Hobsley reminded me, however, that if the rise in intraluminal pressure causes the veins to collapse, then absorption is grossly impaired, e.g. during intestinal obstruction.

pathway. Such fluid movement takes along with it electrolytes small enough to penetrate the water-filled pores. This phenomenon of water pulling electrolytes is known as solvent drag. Clearly, Na^+ movement can be either transcellular or intercellular, the contribution of the different pathways depending on the environmental conditions.

Transcellular absorption

A number of mechanisms have been proposed by which electrolytes may be transferred from the lumen to the interstitial fluid across the brush border and basolateral membranes. None of them, except the Na^+, K^+-pump located in the basolateral membrane is directly linked to an energy input. At the brush border a potential difference of about 35 mV has been measured (inside negative). Thus Na^+ entry is down an electrochemical gradient. The coupled transfer of Na^+ with non-electrolytes has already been discussed (see page 146). In addition electroneutral transfer occurs and is regarded as the major step for NaCl absorption in the absence of sugars and amino acids (Fig. 5.23). Two systems have been suggested. In one Na^+ and Cl^- are transferred together on a single carrier. In the other two separate, but coupled carriers, are proposed, one exchanging Na^+ for H^+, the other Cl^- for HCO_3^- (or OH^-). Both systems may exist, the latter contributing to the maintenance of intracellular pH and/or the provision of an acidic microclimate at the external surface of the brush border.

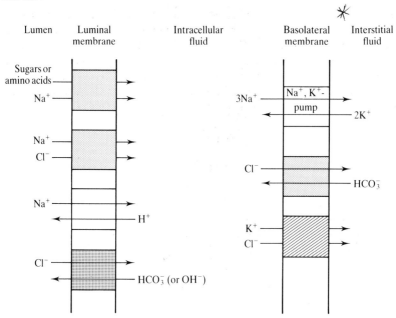

Fig. 5.23 Mechanisms proposed for the transport of Na^+ and Cl^- across the luminal and basolateral membranes of absorbing epithelial cells

The removal of Na^+ from the cell can be explained by the basolateral Na^+,K^+-pump which exchanges three Na^+ for two K^+. Na^+ is transported against both an electrical (about 36-41 mV, inside negative) and chemical gradient. The electrochemical gradient for Cl^- is such that this anion might be transferred by simple diffusion. This possibility, however, is thought unlikely, and carriers transferring K^+ and Cl^- or exchanging Cl^- and HCO_3^- have been suggested.

A model for HCO_3^- transport is presented in Fig 5.24. In it HCO_3^- as such is not transferred across brush border membranes. However, as a result of $Na^+:H^+$ exchange carbonic acid is formed which dissociates to CO_2. The lipid-soluble gas diffuses into the epithelial cell where the acid is reformed. Carbonic acid provides a source of H^+ for further $Na^+:H^+$ exchange and HCO_3^- which accompanies Na^+ to the interstitial fluid to provide electrical neutrality.

K^+ appears to be absorbed passively in response to electrochemical gradients. Indeed both the basolateral and brush border membranes have high K^+ permeability and cellular K^+ is continually lost. However, the Na^+,K^+-pump restores and maintains intracellular $[K^+]$. There is some evidence for a reciprocal relationship between the activity of the pump and the permeability of the basolateral membrane to K^+.

Intestinal secretion

In addition to its absorptive functions, the small intestine is able to secrete large volumes of fluid. Luminal hyperosmolarity may be one cause of secretion. However, secretion occurs in the absence of osmotic gradients, so other stimuli must be considered. Hydrostatic pressure and active transport are two possible driving forces. The former exerts a considerable effect on fluid movement but provides an insufficient force to explain the massive water and electrolyte losses observed in non-inflammatory diarrhoeas, e.g. cholera. Thus some secretion

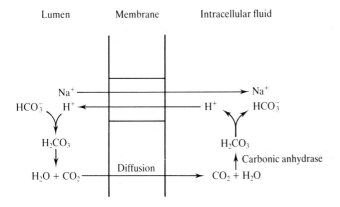

Fig. 5.24 A model for bicarbonate transport across the luminal membrane

may be dependent on transcellular electrolyte movement. Two questions must be asked:

1. Are the cells that are capable of secreting the same as those with absorptive functions?
2. Which ions are secreted?

The available evidence suggests that the immature cells of the crypts of Lieberkühn are primarily involved in secretion, while those cells lining the villi, although capable of secreting, are more concerned with absorption (see page 132).

To identify the ions secreted by the small intestine has been difficult, particularly as secretion and absorption occur simultaneously. Normally the result is net absorption. However, the data support the view that both the major anions Cl^- and HCO_3^2 are actively secreted. More is known about the first mentioned.

A model for Cl^- transport has been presented (Fig. 5.25). Cl^- enters secreting epithelial cells via a frusemide-sensitive, electrically neutral process along with Na^+ and K^+. A low intracellular $[Na^+]$ is maintained by the basolateral Na^+,K^+-pump. The stoichiometry for $Na^+:K^+:Cl^-$ is probably 1:1:2. This is an attractive feature because such a mechanism is likely to be less energy-requiring than one which transfers Na^+ and Cl^- in equal proportions. Other features of the model include K^+ channels in the basolateral membranes and Cl^- channels in the luminal membranes. The basolateral channels allow K^+ entering the cell by the Na^+,K^+-pump or the Cl^- entry process to diffuse to the extracellular fluid. This provides a 'safety valve', preventing the cells from swelling and eventually rupturing.

Loss of K^+ increases the intracellular negativity and contributes to the driving force for Cl^- transfer across the luminal membrane. The Cl^- channels are opened by cAMP (and probably a number of other intracellular mediators also contribute). This opening is probably the major means by which secretion can be stimulated. The cation accompanying Cl^- to the luminal fluid is mainly Na^+. It is transferred by the paracellular route which is cation selective. NB. In the colon K^+ channels are found predominantly sited in the luminal rather than the basolateral membranes. As a result a K^+-enriched secretion is produced. The question remains as to what stimulates the intestine to secrete. A wide range of potential secretory agents are recognized. These include neurotransmitters, hormones, local metabolites, components of gastrointestinal secretions and factors released from luminal bacteria.

Neurological mechanisms

A role for the autonomic nervous system has been suspected for a long time. When loops of mammalian intestine were sympathectomized, a spontaneous secretion was observed. The finding that this secretion was inhibited by atropine pointed to an involvement of parasympathetic extrinsic nerves or local nerve networks. *In vitro* studies have demonstrated that adrenaline and noradrenaline enhance Na^+ and Cl^- absorption, whereas Cl^- secretion is stimulated by acetylcholine. These observations have led to the attractive possibility that cholinergic nerves are concerned with the control of secretion , adrenergic nerves with absorption.

A complete picture of the neural control of intestinal transport has yet to emerge. Nevertheless, there is strong support for the view that local enteric neurons are activated spontaneously by firing pacemaker cells in the myenteric plexus (see page 190) to provide a stimulus for electrolyte secretion. Such a mechanism would ensure a continuous source of fluid and electrolytes, e.g. Na$^+$. A supply of Na$^+$ may be of considerable value. It has been calculated that the demand for Na$^+$ in the absorption of sugars and amino acids is greater than that provided by the diet and other gastrointestinal secretions.

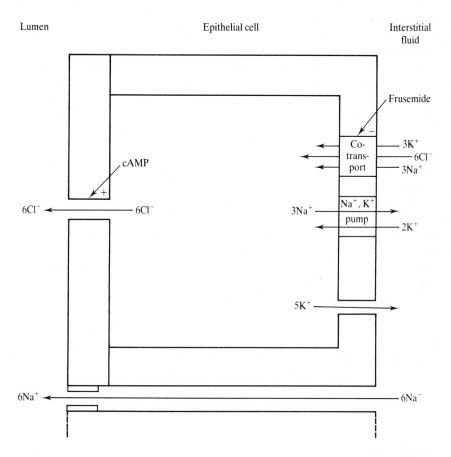

Fig. 5.25 A model for chloride secretion by crypt epithelial cells of small intestine. Several carriers and channels are involved. These include the Na$^+$,K$^+$-pump and an electrically neutral Na$^+$,K$^+$,2Cl$^-$-cotransporter in the basolateral membrane. A K$^+$ channel in the basolateral membrane prevents cell swelling. Cl$^-$ reaches the intestinal lumen via a cAMP-activated channel. Na$^+$ maintains electrical neutrality, reaching the lumen from the interstitial fluid by a paracellular route. + and − refer to stimulation and inhibition respectively.

A spontaneous secretion may be of importance but the major neurally activated secretion is the result of a reflex originating in the mucosa. It has been proposed that luminal secretagogues activate one of the various endocrine-like cells of the mucosa to release their products (peptides and/or amines) into the interstitial fluid. There, they activate adjacent nerve endings and this stimulates an intramural secretory reflex (ISR). What might be released from endocrine-like cells? Two possibilities are 5-HT and neurotensin, elaborated in EC and N cells respectively. Both induce a secretion which can be abolished by nerve blocking agents and both can be released by cholera toxin. Two nerve pathways have been proposed to the secreting epithelial cells. One releases acetylcholine at the effector cells and is probably stimulated by the heat-stable enterotoxin of *Escherichia coli*. The other may release VIP and be stimulated by cholera toxin, the deconjugated secondary bile acid deoxycholate and mechanical stimulation. The nicotinic antagonist, hexamethonium, blocks the neurally mediated response to both bile acid and *Escherichia coli* enterotoxin. Thus it is likely that cholinergic synapses are involved in both reflex pathways. The question remains as to whether there is any overlap between the two pathways. Are acetylcholine and VIP released from the same nerve endings (see page 35)?

A role for extrinsic nerves has already been referred to. Sympathetic denervation of intestinal segments resulted in brisk secretions. These responses have been attributed to the removal of extrinsic antisecretory sympathetic adrenergic nerves. Because the antisecretory effects of noradrenaline could be inhibited by TTX (e.g. in guinea-pig ileum) it has been suggested that sympathetic nerves may modulate the ISR at a ganglion level. However, a more direct effect on crypt cells has also been proposed with noradrenaline, released from nearby sympathetic varicosities, binding to specific receptors detected on basolateral membranes (Fig. 5.26).

It has been reported that all adrenergic nerves found in the small intestine are extrinsic in origin. They can be detected in both the crypts and the villi, although they are rarer in the latter. The increased water and electrolyte absorption measured when sympathetic nerves to the cat jejunum are stimulated could reflect, therefore, either increased absorption by the villous epithelium, decreased secretion by the crypts or both these events. The major effect of sympathetic nerves appears to be to modulate the secretory event with little or no effect on the absorbing cells. The significance of the greater net absorption in response to increased adrenergic activity is that the small intestine may contribute to the control of body fluid volume. To test this possibility studies have been carried out, with cats and rats, in which the sympathetic nervous system was reflexly stimulated by:

(a) carotid baroreceptor unloading accomplished by carotid occlusion, or
(b) cardiopulmonary receptor unloading produced by positive pressure ventilation.

Greater fluid absorption was observed with both these procedures. This suggests that when the extracellular fluid volume is depleted, e.g. as the result of a haemorrhage, the intramural pathways involved in digestion are inhibited and

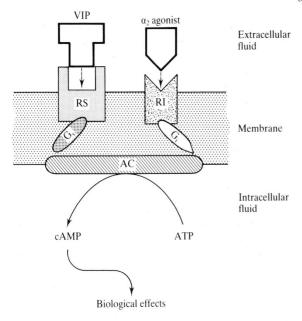

Fig. 5.26 The control of intestinal secretion. Agents stimulating secretion (e.g. VIP) bind to their specific receptors (RS). As a result adenylate cyclase (AC) is activated via the stimulatory G proteins (G$_s$). The cAMP produced increases intestinal secretion. In contrast, noradrenaline binds to its specific site (RI) and alters the orientation of inhibitory G protein (G$_i$). This change prevents the production of the intracellular messenger and so reduces intestinal secretion

fluid needed by the hypovolaemic patient is available to prevent circulatory collapse (Fig. 5.27).

A significant increase in net fluid and NaCl absorption also occurs in man when circulating blood volumes are reduced. A reduction was achieved by changing the lower extremities from an elevated (30° above horizontal) to a downward position. At the same time tourniquets were applied to the thighs (50 mm Hg) to produce stasis. By doing this it is assumed that blood pools in the lower extremities. It has been calculated that fluid absorption by the small intestine may be increased by 600–900 ml per hour by this procedure.

The importance of extrinsic nerves in the growth and biochemical development of epithelia has already been stressed (see page 36). Clearly such nerves also influence epithelial transport in the small intestine. These facts must be recognized by those considering the possibility of transplantation for patients with intestinal failure. (NB. The vagus as well as the sympathetic nerves has been shown to modify intestinal secretion. The physiological significance of the increased secretion induced by the vagus has yet to be established.) Renewed interest in transplantation has recently been generated by the finding that long term survival of transplants in animals can be achieved by immunosuppression with cyclosporin A. Histological examinations showed little damage to the villi. Carbohydrate and amino acid absorption were not significantly impaired.

However, it was recognized that the absence of extrinsic sympathetic nerves may result in diarrhoea and electrolyte losses, and be a major limiting factor in intestinal transplantation.

Hormones and locally produced factors

A number of circulating hormones modify intestinal electrolyte transport. Among these are the glucocorticoids and atrial natriuretic factor (ANF). Glucocorticoids enhance Na^+,Cl^- coupled absorption and inhibit secretion. To achieve the latter they induce the production of lipomodulin, a protein which

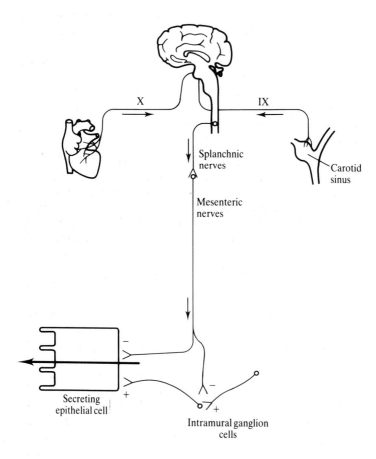

Fig. 5.27 A model for the cardiovascular reflex control of jejunal fluid secretion. When there is a loss of body fluid volume, the discharges of carotid sinus and cardiopulmonary mechanoreceptors are altered. Fewer impulses from these receptors travel to the brain in the IXth and Xth cranial nerves respectively. As a result the sympathetic nervous system is activated. Efferent fibres in the splanchnic nerve supply the intestine and inhibit fluid secretion. They may act directly on the epithelial cells or indirectly at the ganglion level, blocking mechanisms which promote fluid secretion. Net absorption is, therefore, increased

inhibits phospholipase A2. By doing so the release of arachidonic acid from plasma membranes and the production of prostaglandins, causing secretion, is reduced (see below). An inhibition of water and Na^+ absorption by ANF might have been anticipated. This newly discovered peptide is present in atrial muscle cells, particularly on the right side. It is thought to be released by atrial stretch. By increasing renal Na^+ excretion, and concomitantly water loss, the extracellular fluid volume is reduced. ANF may act in several ways to reduce renal Na^+ reabsorption e.g.:

(a) by reducing renin secretion from the juxtaglomerular apparatus, and
(b) by directly inhibiting aldosterone release from the adrenal cortex.

The inhibition of intestinal salt and water absorption by ANF presumably leads to the renal effects of the peptide being less compromised. Interestingly ANF is found not only in the heart. ANF-immunoreactive cell bodies have been detected throughout the brain. One proposal is that ANF acts on the central nervous system to reduce water intake and salt appetite. Thus, smaller volumes of fluid and electrolytes may be presented to the intestine for absorption.

Several substances affecting intestinal transport are released close to the secreting epithelial cells during inflammatory responses induced by bacteria, viruses, radiation and chemically noxious agents. They include:

1. The secretagogues histamine and 5-hydroxytryptamine (5HT). Both can be derived from mast cells. Histamine is thought to exert its effects both directly on enterocytes and indirectly by activating local nerve networks. The close association of some mast cells with enteric nerves would facilitate the latter mechanism. The relationship between mast cells and nerve fibres is more complex. The finding that the H-1-blocker, pyrilamine, inhibits the secretory response to electrical field stimulation suggests that some nerves elicit their effects, partially at least, by stimulating histamine release. 5HT from mast cells (and endocrine-like cells) activates nerve reflexes to produce a secretion.

2. Prostaglandins, derived from arachidonic acid. This polyunsaturated fatty acid (see page 6) is released during the breakdown of membrane-bound phospholipids. It then follows either the cyclo-oxygenase pathway with the formation of prostaglandins or the lipoxygenase pathway in which leukotrienes are elaborated. Some prostaglandins directly stimulate intestinal secretion. One of these is PGE_2. It is effective at concentrations detected in the diarrhoeal diseases caused by Salmonella and Shigella. Prostaglandins are thought to be important for the secretions induced by mechanical stimulation. Prostaglandins have numerous effects throughout the body, although under normal circumstances they affect mainly those cells in which they are produced, and thus act as local regulators. An example of prostaglandins having effects at sites distant to where they are produced is afforded by patients with medullary carcinoma of the thyroid. Such patients commonly excrete an excess of prostaglandins from their tumours and it is thought likely that these substances play a part in the diarrhoea frequently observed.

3. Bradykinin, a peptide released from a plasma globulin. In addition to

causing vasodilatation and increasing vascular permeability it evokes a secretion. It does so mainly as a result of stimulating prostaglandin release.

From the above discussion it is clear that in response to various noxious stimuli, the small intestine produces a secretion which may dilute and wash away the 'offending' agent. At any one time a mixture of secretagogues can be released, some acting directly on the epithelial cells, others acting via local nerve networks.

Cholera – a disease producing diarrhoea without inflammatory changes

Cholera is an infectious disease in man caused by *Vibrio cholerae*. The vibrio elaborates an enterotoxin (mol. wt. = 84 000) which elicits a voluminous diarrhoea, resulting in hypovolaemic shock, metabolic acidosis and, if untreated, death. Death can occur within 4–5 hours of the onset of the symptoms. Cholera is endemic in the delta of the River Ganges and has been considered responsible for seven major pandemics during the last century and a half. It was not until the 1880s that the *Vibrio cholerae* was identified as the aetiological agent of the disease. Nevertheless, cholera had been carefully studied earlier and the involvement of contaminated water was clearly indicated. In 1857 John Snow described the outbreak of cholera in London and had pointed out that, if the handle of the communal pump in Broad Street were removed, the outbreak might be controlled. This suggestion was adopted with excellent results.

Man is the only natural host and victim of *Vibrio cholerae*. The vibrio shows remarkable susceptibility to gastric acid and even ten billion organisms will not consistently produce clinical disease in healthy adult volunteers. One might expect, therefore, that those producing less acid would be more at risk. The greater incidence of cholera in individuals with total or subtotal gastrectomy in recent outbursts in Italy and Israel support this concept.

Studies of tissue obtained by peroral biopsy provide data to show that mucosal damage is not the cause of the water and electrolyte losses. No evidence has been obtained to suggest that membrane selectivity is changed in cholera. In other words, the permeability or 'effective pore size' of the intestinal barrier is not altered.

If permeability of the mucosa is not altered, then large hydrostatic gradients would be necessary for ultrafiltration to account for fluid secretion. The continuing fluid and electrolyte losses observed clinically even when the patient is grossly hypotensive and dehydrated would be difficult to explain in terms of ultrafiltration.

From the above discussion, it seems that fluid losses in cholera are mediated by functional rather than anatomical alterations of epithelia. Several pieces of evidence favour the view that a reduction in intestinal absorption may contribute to, but by no means accounts for, the symptoms of cholera:

1. Complete cessation of intestinal absorption should not produce more than 7–8 litres fluid stool per day, the normal volume of gastrointestinal secretions. However, the average fluid output on the first day of cholera is 8.3 litres, and volumes as high as 16 litres have been described.

2. Glucose absorption is unaltered. This fact has been used as a means of decreasing the requirements of patients for intravenous replacement of fluid and electrolytes. Glucose, as it is absorbed, is accompanied by increased Na^+ movement. Both hexose and Na^+ absorption stimulate fluid absorption. The use of glucose/saline solutions in the oral treatment of patients with cholera has been of immense benefit, particularly in those parts of the world where intravenous solutions are not readily available or are very expensive.

It must be remembered that oral rehydration fluids cannot greatly exceed plasma osmolarity without the risk of increased diarrhoea and hypernatraemia. Water would quickly be drawn by luminal hypertonic fluids from the interstitial fluid through the 'leaky' intestinal barrier. To provide increased amounts of glucose the sugar must be available in a form with low osmotic activity e.g. starch. This polymer is a major product in many natural foods e.g. rice, wheat, potato, millet and plantain. Substituting starch for glucose in oral rehydration solutions has been shown to effectively replace fluids and reduce the duration and severity of diarrhoea. Starch can provide large quantities of glucose without incurring an osmotic penalty.

One means by which cholera enterotoxin could produce diarrhoea is by stimulating secretion. It does so although not all regions of the intestines are similarly affected. A definite involvement of the proximal jejunum has been described, this region being in a net secretory state during the acute phase of the disease and reverting to normal absorption 7–14 days later. Net secretion can also be demonstrated in the ileum of many, but not all, patients. By contrast, the colon absorbs normally. To appreciate the mechanism by which the enterotoxin increases secretion it is necessary to know something about its structure. It is an acid-labile protein consisting of A (dimer) and B (pentamer) subunits (Fig. 5.28). The latter binds tightly to a brush border receptor, a monosialoganglioside (GM1). Part of the A subunit (A_1) is capable of stimulating adenylate cyclase and can, therefore, elicit a cAMP-mediated secretion. However, adenylate cyclase is in the basolateral membranes. How could it be activated? One possibility is that following endocytosis the A_1 component might be released and diffuse through the cytoplasm to the enzyme. There is no convincing evidence that this occurs.

An alternative proposal involves Gs proteins (see page 000). These can be detected in brush border (and basolateral) membranes and are made up of three subunits, i.e. α, β and γ. It has been suggested that subunit α is dissociated from the membrane-bound subunits β and γ following the binding of cholera enterotoxin. The subunit is then free to cross the cell and activate the adenylate cyclase. The subunit also has GTP-ase activity and when GTP is hydrolysed intracellularly the subunit becomes reassociated with β and γ subunits and inactive. By inhibiting the GTP-ase activity of the subunit cholera enterotoxin has a further effect. It maintains the subunit in a permanently activated form. A direct stimulation of secreting epithelial cells is not the only means by which cholera enterotoxin may exert its effects. The ISR can also contribute to the diarrhoea.

Evidence pointing to a role for intramural nerve networks has been the finding that the effects of cholera enterotoxin can be reduced by tetrodotoxin, hexamethonium and the local anaesthetic lidocaine. Not all events occurring during cholera increase secretion. Recently it has been reported that the pituitary gland produces a protein, molecular weight about 60 000, with antisecretory properties. Its physiological significance has yet to be established. Might such a protein, however, increase our tolerance to the enterotoxin?

VIP and somatostatin

Two peptides with effects on water and electrolyte transport by the small intestine deserve further consideration. One is VIP which, in man under normal conditions, is a neurotransmitter, and not a hormone. Its probable importance in the neural control of intestinal secretion has already been referred to. Renewed interest, however, was generated by the finding of high circulating levels of the peptide in patients with pancreatic cholera syndrome (the Verner-Morrison syndrome) now known to be a VIP containing Fumour (VIPoma). The condition is associated with life-threatening diarrhoea. An attempt was made to reproduce the diarrhoea of this endocrine tumour with prolonged administration of VIP to healthy subjects. The volunteers received a continuous infusion of 400 pmol/g body weight/hour. Within 2 hours the plasma VIP levels had risen from 15.3 to 129 pmol/l. This is in the range reported for

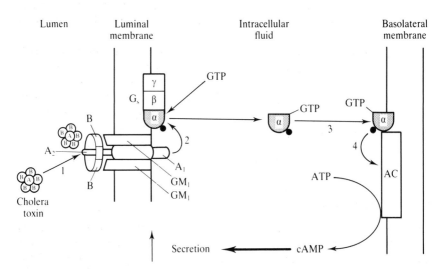

Fig. 5.28 A model for the mechanism by which cholera toxin increases intestinal secretion. 1. The toxin binds to a monosialoganglioside (GM_1) by means of its B subunits. 2. The A_1 component following endocytosis, releases the α subunit of guanylate nucleotide binding protein (G_s) from the luminal membrane. It also inhibits the GTPase activity of the subunit (●). It achieves this by catalysing a covalent linkage of adenosine diphosphate ribose to the subunit. 3. The subunit diffuses through the cytoplasm. 4. At the basolateral membrane adenylate cyclase (AC) is activated by the subunit. The cAMP produced increases the secretion of water and electrolytes. GTP hydrolysis is necessary for subunit inactivation. As GTPase activity is inhibited the subunit remains permanently activated

patients with pancreatic cholera syndrome. In every subject watery diarrhoea developed. The mean stool weight was 2441 g as compared with normal values of less than 250 g/day. The faecal $[Na^+]$, $[HCO_3^-]$ and pH increased. The large HCO_3^- excretion resulted in metabolic acidosis, a characteristic feature of the syndrome. It was suggested, therefore, that VIP is at least one of the mediators of the watery diarrhoea in pancreatic cholera syndrome.

Somatostatin is the other peptide to be discussed. It is found in both endocrine-like cells (highest concentrations in the duodenum, decreasing towards the ileum) and nerve fibres. Several reports show that somatostatin inhibits nutrient absorption. For example, glucose, glycine and oleic acid absorption from human perfused jejunum can be reduced by intravenous infusion of somatostatin. It has been suggested that somatostatin might be a physiological regulator in the homeostasis of absorbed nutrients by modulating the rates at which they are absorbed.

A reduction of intestinal absorption is only one of the inhibitory effects of somatostatin. Gastric acid, pepsin, intestinal fluid and pancreatic secretions and splanchric blood flow are other events affected. Some may be directly inhibited, others modified because somatostatin interferes with the release of many gastrointestinal hormones, e.g. gastrin and VIP. Because of its potent inhibitory effects the possibility is recognized that the peptide might be of considerable therapeutic value. However, somatostatin has a short half life, and its clinical use limited. Nevertheless, it has been an effective agent in the conservative treatment of persistent peptic ulcer bleeding where the risk of emergency surgery is too great.

Analogues of somatostatin have been synthesized in an attempt to provide potent inhibitors with longer lasting effects. One of these is the octapeptide SMS 201-995 (Sandoz). Several patients with severe diarrhoea associated with gut and pancreatic endocrine tumours (VIPoma and carcinoid syndrome) have been treated with this analogue. The results obtained were dramatic. Two daily subcutaneous injections (50 μg) were sufficient to reduce stool volumes. Liquid excretions were replaced by semi-solid or normal stools. The analogue is well tolerated and currently regarded as a valuable tool for such patients.

The fate of calcium   *facilitated diffusion*

In addition to a variable dietary intake, further sources of calcium appearing in the intestinal lumen are derived from gastrointestinal secretions and desquamated cells. Calcium absorption is not a simple function of the luminal content. A number of substances inhibit absorption. For example, fatty acids form insoluble soaps with Ca^{++}. This should not be a problem for the healthy individual but may result in less Ca^{++} being available when lipids are malabsorbed. Oxalates and phytates also complex with Ca^{++} and could inhibit absorption. Oxalates are found in some fruits and vegetables, e.g. rhubarb and spinach. These are, perhaps, infrequent dietary components for many people, and often tea is likely to provide over 50 per cent of the daily dietary oxalate intake. Many cereals, rich in phytates, also possess phytases which release Ca^{++} from the complex formed.

One cereal, the oat, contains little of the enzyme. Some who reside south of Hadrian's wall in the United Kingdom have, therefore, politely enquired as to whether the 'traditional Highlander's breakfast' might render those who live further north prone to rickets. Fortunately Scottish volunteers were able to provide evidence that they could absorb Ca^{++} effectively, perhaps because bacterial enzymes release the complexed cation. Dietary fibre (see page 215) may also bind Ca^{++}. In many tropical diets so much fibre is ingested that the binding capacity can exceed the total intake of Ca^{++}. Microbial fermentation in the colon breaks down some of this fibre so that eventually Ca^{++} becomes available for absorption.

Several agents improve Ca^{++} absorption. These include gastric acid, bile acids and lactose. In the stomach, some Ca^{++} is probably converted to the more soluble chloride. In the small intestine Ca^{++} reacting with conjugated bile acids is rarely precipitated. A less soluble product is formed with deconjugated bile acids. Enhanced Ca^{++} absorption in the presence of lactose has been recognized for more than half a century although how lactose produces its effects is puzzling. Milk is a rich source of both Ca^{++} and lactose. Thus they are presented together to the intestine, and the disaccharide's effects can be important in promoting the absorption of the available Ca^{++}. One possible mode of action of lactose is to be a source of glucose. It has been suggested that the relatively slow hydrolysis of lactose at the brush border provides glucose (and galactose) which is important for controlling the dimensions of the paracellular pathway, i.e. the sizes of the spaces between the epithelial cells. By increasing the permeability of the tight and gap junctions more paracellular transport occurs. Certainly, paracellular Ca^{++} transport is one means by which Ca^{++} is absorbed. Transport by it varies with the luminal $[Ca^{++}]$ and is independent of physiological regulation. Alternatively, Ca^{++} can be absorbed transcellularly (Fig. 5.29). There are three stages to the saturable process involved.

1. Entry at the brush border which does not require the expenditure of energy. A steep electrochemical gradient exists. The intracellular $[Ca^{++}]$ is less than 1 μM, less than 1/1000th of that in the extracellular fluid. The potential gradient across the brush border membrane is about 35 mV (inside negative). Two factors are thought to be important for Ca^{++} entry:
   (a) the lipid composition of the membrane, and
   (b) a protein with affinity for Ca^{++} which may act as a carrier.
   NB. The brush border has a high cholesterol:phospholipid ratio resulting in high viscosity and poor Ca^{++} permeability. Viscosity can be reduced and Ca^{++} permeability improved by increasing the unsaturated fatty acid content of the membrane.
2. Once inside the cell Ca^{++} is translocated to the basolateral membranes. An intracellular calcium binding protein (CaBP) preferentially binds Ca^{++} and may act as an intracellular ferry. Other cellular organelles may also play a role. These include mitochondria and the Golgi complex which have large capacities for Ca^{++} accumulation.
3. At the basolateral membrane Ca^{++} must be pumped out of the cell against a steep electrochemical gradient. Two mechanisms are available:

(a) a calcium pump utilizing ATP for energy. A Ca^{++}-ATPase stimulated by nanomolar concentrations of Ca^{++} is located in the basolateral membranes and may be a component of this pump;

(b) a Na^+:Ca^{++} exchanger driven by the Na^+,K^+-pump.

The absorption of Ca^{++} is improved in infants with rickets by administering cod liver oil. The important factor in the oil is vitamin D. Several vitamin D compounds exist, the most important being cholecalciferol (D_3). It is available in the diet or formed in the skin as a result of ultraviolet irradiation of 7-dehydrocholesterol and stored in the liver. The active form of vitamin D is 1,25-dihydroxycholecalciferol ($1,25(OH)_2D_3$) which is produced by:

1. hydroxylating cholecalciferol to 25-hydroxycholecalciferol in the liver, and

2. further modification to the 1,25-dihydroxy-derivative in the kidney.

The conversion of 25-hydroxycholecalciferol to the active form requires parathyroid hormone. $1,25(OH)_2D_3$ has a number of effects on Ca^{++} absorption (Fig. 5.29). One is to increase the permeability of the brush borders to Ca^{++}. Inhibitors of protein synthesis such as cycloheximide fail to block this response, which is thought to be due to a change in the membrane

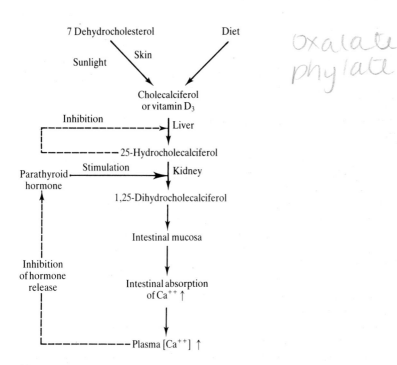

(a)

Fig. 5.29 (a) The relationship between vitamin D_3, parathyroid hormone and intestinal Ca^{++} absorption.

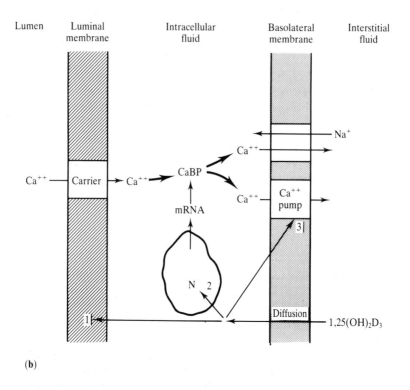

| Lumen | Luminal membrane | Intracellular fluid | Basolateral membrane | Interstitial fluid |

(b)

Fig. 5.29 (b) The mechanisms by which vitamin D_3 (1,25-dihydroxycholecalciferol; 1,25(OH)$_2$D$_3$ is the active form) may act to regulate Ca++ transport in the small intestine. The vitamin has several effects. 1. It stimulates Ca++ entry at the luminal membrane, perhaps by altering the lipid composition of the brush border and, therefore, changing the motility of the Ca++ carrier. 2. It stimulates the production of specific messenger RNA (mRNA) in the nucleus (N) and the subsequent translation into calcium binding protein (CaBP). This protein may act as an intracellular ferry for Ca++. 3. It increases Ca++ removal from the cell at the basolateral membrane by stimulating the Ca++ pump

phospholipid composition (the liponomic effect). By increasing the brush border content of polyunsaturated fatty acids membrane viscosity decreases and Ca++ permeability increases. Such a change could alter the activity of the Ca++ carrier, perhaps allowing its easier movement, or increase the size of membrane Ca++ channels. Whatever the mechanism, this effect reminds us that steroids penetrating membranes can exert their effects by means other than the stimulation of protein synthesis. 1,25(OH)$_2$D$_3$ also stimulates CaBP synthesis, Ca++-ATPase activity and Ca++ efflux at the basolateral membrane thus providing greater absorptive capacity for the Ca++ available.

The question remains as to which mechanisms are where in the small intestine. The non-saturable paracellular system exists all the way along the intestine, playing a major role in the ileum. In contrast the transcellular route is confined largely to the proximal intestine. This mechanism is influenced by age. For example, active Ca++ transport is not observed in newborn rats. It reaches peak activity, however, by 30 days and then decreases. In adult humans Ca^{++} absorption also decreases with age. In the elderly, malabsorption of Ca^{++} can occur primarily due to vitamin D deficiency. Both impaired absorption of, and decreased responsiveness to the vitamin are thought to contribute.

Although the capacity for transport may vary considerably from one region of the gut to another, this does not mean that the area with the greatest capacity absorbs the most. Passage through the duodenum is rapid and may not allow enough time for absorption. In contrast, in the ileum transit of intestinal contents is slower, and longer contact between the epithelial cells and the luminal contents can favour Ca^{++} absorption. Furthermore, a contribution of the colon cannot be ignored. Even though net Ca^{++} absorption does not occur in the colon in normal subjects, a sensitivity of the absorption process to $1,25(OH)_2D_3$ has been reported.

The fate of iron

Iron is unique in that body levels are maintained primarily through the regulation of intestinal absorption, there being only a limited capacity for excretion. Iron uptake occurs mainly in the duodenum and upper jejunum.

Absorption from the lumen

A large number of intraluminal factors modify iron movement, e.g. tea markedly reduces absorption by forming iron tannate complexes. Furthermore, oxalates, phosphates and phytates form poorly absorbed sources. This can be a problem in areas where people use under-milled cereals as a staple food. Thus in Northern India the dietary intake of iron can be 22 mg/day, far greater than in the Western diet, yet less iron is available. Ferrous salts (Fe^{++}) are more soluble than ferric (Fe^{+++}) salts at the pH of the intestinal contents. The bivalent form is, therefore, more easily absorbed. Indeed ferric salts are insoluble at pH values over 3. The HCl in the stomach is, however, useful in that it provides a medium in which Fe^{+++} is not precipitated and is available to form complexes which can subsequently be absorbed from the small intestine.

Several factors enhance absorption. Thus a soluble absorbable complex is formed with citrate. Some sugars and amino acids also bind iron and maintain it in a soluble, monomeric form. They interfere with the formation of water bridges between iron molecules and so prevent polymerization. Ascorbic acid is another dietary constituent which aids iron absorption. It maintains iron in the reduced, more soluble form, and also reacts to produce iron chelates. The value of fresh fruit and vegetables in the prevention of anaemia probably lies more in their ability to facilitate iron absorption than in their actual iron content.

Not all substances complexing with iron and maintaining it in a soluble form facilitate absorption. For example, ethylenediamine tetraacetic acid (EDTA) enhances the solubility of iron but decreases its absorption. EDTA probably acts by binding to all six coordinating bonds of iron so that receptors on mucosal epithelial cells no longer recognize it. This complexing agent is one of the most widely used chelating agents in the American diet, being added to prevent oxidative damage by free metals to foods which may not be immediately consumed.

Only a fraction of the villous epithelial cells appear to be adapted for iron absorption. These cells are randomly distributed. For uptake from the lumen several processes contribute (Fig. 5.30). At low concentrations the uptake of inorganic iron is at least partially energy dependent, although at high concentrations a non-saturable and non-energy requiring process appears to prevail. A further system transfers haeme, derived from the partial breakdown of haemoglobin (in dietary meat) by the action of duodenal secretions. Once absorbed, iron is released by xanthine oxidase.

Movement within the epithelial cell

How iron is transferred across epithelial cells is controversial. It has been found associated with the rough endoplasmic reticulum and free ribosomes. Several iron-containing compounds have also been detected. These include:

1. A low molecular weight substance, possibly an amino acid-iron chelate, which might ferry iron from the brush border to the basolateral membranes.
2. A vitamin D-dependent calcium binding protein, which might be a part of a common pathway for iron and calcium absorption (see page 174). Calcium in the diet can diminish the absorption of iron. Furthermore, when the production of this protein is stimulated, the absorptions of both iron and calcium are increased.
3. Ferritin, a protein found in all tissues, particularly the liver, spleen, bone marrow and intestinal mucosa. Its major function is to store iron. In this way it protects cells from oxidative damage due to free iron. It is also a reserve source of iron. Ferritin consists of a shell of apoferritin which has enzymic properties so that ferrous iron becomes oxidized within the shell to ferric iron and is stored as ferric oxyhydroxide. It tends to accumulate in secondary lysosomes, especially when the body has an excess of iron. When epithelial cells are sloughed off from the villous tip this iron-containing protein is also released. Thus ferritin contributes to the elimination of excess iron.

Transfer from the epithelial cell

Movement of iron across the basolateral membranes is not a simple process. It depends on the iron status of the animal, a fact illustrated by the responses of three groups of rats to ^{59}Fe-labelled ferric chloride introduced into the stomach. These animals had previously been fed either:

(a) a stock diet;
(b) an iron-deficient diet for several weeks,
(c) an iron-deficient diet for several weeks, but given a large dose of iron twenty four hours before administering the ferric chloride.

In the first group, a small quantity of ^{59}Fe was detected in the blood stream ten minutes after its administration. However, there was no further increase in the blood over the next twenty minutes, even though ^{59}Fe gradually accumulated within the epithelial cells. Blood ^{59}Fe was greater after ten minutes in animals that had been fed an iron-deficient diet. This level continued to rise during the subsequent 20 minutes, yet smaller amounts accumulated in the epithelia. The results obtained with the final group (c) followed a similar pattern to those

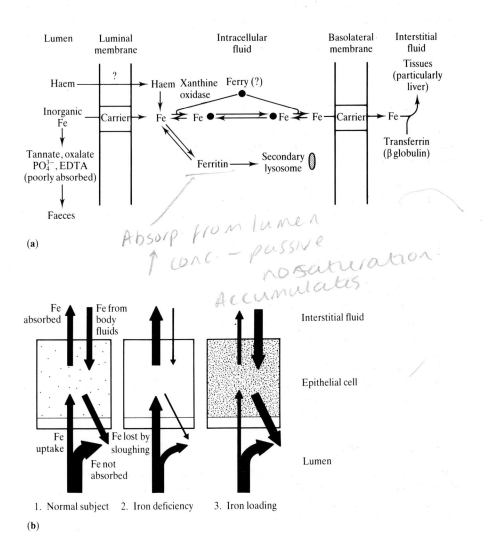

1. Normal subject   2. Iron deficiency   3. Iron loading

(b)

Fig. 5.30 (a) Absorption of iron. Iron is derived from both organic and inorganic sources. Several intracellular constituents bind iron. Some may ferry the iron across the epithelial cells. **(b)** A model for the control of iron absorption. In normal subjects intracellular iron, obtained from either the lumen or the body fluids, is bound to receptors, and contributes to the control of absorption. Thus, with iron excess, uptake from the lumen is limited. However, cellular iron is available to meet the body's requirements and can be lost when cells are sloughed from the villous tip. In contrast, in iron deficiency, more cellular receptors are free. Greater luminal uptake and transport to the interstitial fluid occurs. Iron loss from sloughed cells decreases

obtained with animals fed a stock diet. Thus decreased iron stores are associated with increased iron absorption.

Iron can enter the cells through the basolateral membranes. Hence, some have postulated that a mechanism may operate to remove excess iron from the bloodstream. A further means by which iron can be eliminated is by the infiltration of iron-laden macrophages through the mucosal barrier.

Regulation of iron absorption

Evidence is presented above to show that decreased iron stores are associated with increased iron absorption. Hypoxia and enhanced erythropoiesis would be expected, therefore, to stimulate iron absorption. What mechanisms are involved? Almost 50 years ago Hahn (1943) suggested that mucosal iron-sensitive receptors might have a role to play. The concept has been developed that such receptors facilitating intestinal iron absorption may be loaded or unloaded (the mucosal block theory). When loaded, because of either excess iron from the lumen or from the interstitial fluid, absorption is inhibited. In contrast, if iron is not bound to the receptors, then absorption occurs.

The influence of a hormone was suspected following studies with parabiotic rats. When one of the pair was subjected to hypoxia, the intestinal mucosa of the partner presented an increased ability to absorb iron. The identity of such an agent remains a mystery. Some have speculated that erythropoietin, released during hypoxia may be involved. However, there is evidence against a direct effect of erythropoietin. If the bone marrow is depressed by irradiation the hormone fails to increase iron absorption.

Water–soluble vitamin absorption

It is thought that most water-soluble vitamins are absorbed as consequences of intricate metabolic and transport phenomena. Movement of these substances into and across epithelial cells is characterized by stereospecificity and saturation kinetics, suggesting the existence of carriers. It appears that several vitamins are absorbed by Na^+-dependent mechanisms and the Na^+-gradient hypothesis formulated for sugar and amino acid transport also holds for these vitamins. Only in the case of pyridoxine has no convincing evidence been presented for carrier-mediated transport. It is assumed that simple diffusion accounts for its movement. Limitations of space permit only one vitamin to be discussed in any detail. Vitamin B_{12} has been selected.

The fate of vitamin B_{12} (cobalamin)

The concept of dietary sources of vitamin B_{12} (methyl-, deoxyadenosyl- and hydroxy-cobalamin are the major forms) binding to intrinsic factor (IF), produced in the stomach, so that it can be effectively absorbed in the ileum is an important one. The vitamin is required for DNA synthesis. Without it cells fail to mature. Pernicious anaemia is one result. Only recently, however, have we started to appreciate what happens to vitamin B_{12} . Dietary sources reaching the stomach (the liver and kidney provide the richest supply) are rapidly released from food proteins.

This release is facilitated by pepsins and HCl. The free form preferentially binds to R protein, a constituent of both saliva and gastric juice. This has surprised many, the author included, who thought that vitamin B_{12} bound immediately to IF. However, human salivary R protein binds vitamin B_{12} with affinities 50 and 3 times higher than human IF at pH 2 and 8 respectively. In the duodenum and jejunum pancreatic proteolytic enzymes break down the R protein. Again freed, the vitamin B_{12} now binds to IF, which is resistant to pancreatic digestion. Furthermore, the pancreas is an additional source of IF. Reports of vitamin B_{12} malabsorption in patients with pancreatic insufficiency may be explained in terms of the unavailability of enzymes for R protein hydrolysis. The IF-vitamin B_{12} complex reaching the ileum binds to highly specific membrane receptors located at the bottom of pits between the microvilli. The binding is Ca^{++}-dependent. Neither free IF nor free vitamin B_{12} bind to the receptor. Both components are necessary, and vitamin B_{12} bound to other proteins is not absorbed. Nor are potentially harmful vitamin B_{12} analogues which are ubiquitous in nature.

The absorption of vitamin B_{12} is said to be an astonishingly slow process, taking hours to complete. What mechanisms are used? Is vitamin B_{12} released from the complex before or after its uptake at the brush border membrane? Certainly the complex does not appear in the urine. The fate of IF continues to be debated. The favoured view is that IF is internalized with vitamin B_{12} by receptor-mediated endocytosis. The IF-vitamin B_{12} complex becomes part of an endosome (vesicle). Within the ileal epithelial cell vitamin B_{12} is released. To explain this, two hypotheses have been put forward. One involves lysosomal fusion and subsequent proteolysis. The alternative proposal is that vitamin B_{12} release is the result of the acidification of the vesicle containing the IF-vitamin B_{12} complex without lysosomal involvement. The latter, perhaps, is the most attractive. IF is very resistant to lysosomal proteolytic enzymes but releases vitamin B_{12} in an acidic medium. The concept of intracellular compartments having a pH very different to the surrounding cytoplasm, because of proton pumps, has already been introduced (see page 78).

What happens to intracellular IF? Its accumulation at the brush border membrane some time after absorption suggests that some may be recycled. It may be released at the basolateral membrane into the interstitial fluid (transcytosis) and eventually excreted in the urine. When liberated, vitamin B_{12} can be transferred to transcobalamin II (TCII) and carried in the circulation to target tissues where the complex can be internalized. More information is required about the mechanism of removal of vitamin B_{12} across the basolateral membranes and where the TCII-vitamin B_{12} complex is formed. It has been suggested that TCII, produced by ileal epithelial cells, and vitamin B_{12} may interact intracellularly within acidic vesicles. Furthermore TCII may be necessary for vitamin B_{12} transport. Patients with inherited TCII deficiency have been reported to have impaired vitamin absorption.

(Colonic bacteria can synthesize vitamin B_{12} . However, this is not available to man as it is produced distal to the region it is absorbed.)

Malabsorption

From the above discussion it is clear that for efficient absorption to occur a number of events must be closely coordinated. Digestion within the lumen of the gastrointestinal tract, or even at a cellular level results in absorbable substances being produced. Subsequently these are transported across the epithelial barrier by many different processes. Following their absorption they are removed by the bloodstream or in lymph vessels. Any one or all these steps might be altered and result in malabsorption (Fig. 5.31). Thus:

    a. A substance may fail to reach the absorbing epithelium.
    b. Substances normally absorbed are unavailable.
    c. Substances may pass rapidly through the small intestine.
    d. There may be loss of absorptive surface.
    e. Columnar epithelial cells may lack specific digestive enzymes or transport processes.
    f. The blood supply to the mucosa or lymphatic system may be inadequate.

A substance may fail to reach the absorbing epithelium

This can occur when a gastrocolic or jejunocolic fistula is formed and luminal contents bypass the small intestine. A gastrocolic fistula usually arises from carcinoma of the transverse colon penetrating both the stomach and the colon.

    Alternatively, abnormal or excessive numbers of normal bacteria within the small intestine may utilise dietary components. The proximal small intestine

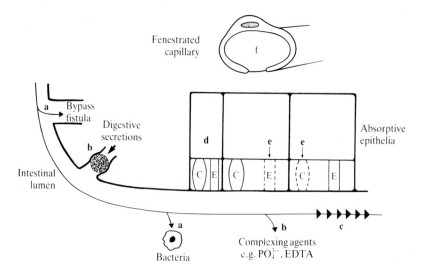

Fig. 5.31 Ways in which malabsorption can occur. **a** = Failure of substances to reach the absorbing epithelium. **b** = The substances are not available to be absorbed. **c** = Insufficient time for absorption to be completed. **d** = Loss of absorptive surface. **e** = Specific defects of epithelial cells, e.g. loss of digestive enzymes (E) or carriers (C). **f** = Inadequate drainage by blood or lymph vessels

usually has a sparse microflora. These are aerobes. This picture can change dramatically in diverticulosis or hypochlorhydria, situations associated with stagnant intestinal contents or the loss of the protective gastric acid bath. The numbers of bacteria rise and anaerobic species thrive. Aerobic forms probably lower the oxygen tension of the luminal contents to a level at which the anaerobes can survive. Some anaerobes are capable of binding to vitamin B_{12}, causing its malabsorption, and making more likely the subsequent development of pernicious anaemia.

Substances normally absorbed are unavailable

The substances normally absorbed may not be available as such either because of:

1. A failure of digestive processes, or
2. the presence of factors which maintain substances in undigestible or unabsorbable forms.

Thus in patients with chronic pancreatitis or obstructive jaundice the availability of pancreatic enzymes or bile acids is greatly reduced, resulting in incomplete digestion and losses of fat and fat-soluble vitamins. The variable absorption of both calcium and iron have already been referred to and are hardly surprising. Perhaps less expected was the report of incomplete carbohydrate absorption in healthy volunteers ingesting starch in the form of macaroni or bread made from all-purpose wheat flour. In this form starch is surrounded by a protein network. In contrast, carbohydrate absorption from rice flour, which has much less protein, was almost complete. Physical and/or chemical interactions between protein and carbohydrate, preventing digestion, were suggested to be the cause of this malabsorption.

Rapid passage through the small intestine

A substance may pass through small intestine so rapidly that the mucosa is exposed to it for an insufficient time to allow complete absorption. This may occur after gastric surgery when the pylorus is either destroyed or bypassed. Hypertonic meals are quickly 'dumped' into the duodenum where they are diluted by excessive intestinal secretions. Such luminal contents are rapidly propelled. Hypertonic glucose solutions may reach the terminal ileum within 5 minutes of their ingestion.

Loss of absorptive surface

There may be a loss of absorptive surface. However, one should remember that the intestine has considerable reserve capacity to compensate for any reductions (see page 185). In the event of the loss of jejunal mucosa the distal regions can assume the proximal region's functions. It receives secretions and products of digestion at concentrations to which it is not normally exposed. Nevertheless, malabsorption can result when massive resections have been necessary, e.g. for patients with gangrene induced by the involvement of the bowel in a volvulus and for those with widespread disease e.g. Crohn's regional enteritis. In some cases the mucosal layer is damaged and its surface area reduced. For example, in coeliac disease, where there is a unique sensitivity to dietary gluten, the villi become flattened and the brush borders of the epithelial cells are abnormal. Why the intestines of coeliac patients are so sensitive to gluten is still debated. Several theories have been proposed to account for the pathogenesis of the disease. These include:

1. The presence of surface receptors that allow gluten binding with subsequent toxic effects on epithelial cells,
2. Immunological hypersensitivity to specific protein components.

A final picture has yet to emerge although it appears that the local immune system has a major role to play.

Columnar epithelial cells lack enzymes of transport processes

Columnar epithelial cells may lack specific digestive enzymes or transport processes. The cells, otherwise, function normally. In the absorption of the products of fat digestion the proteins of the chylomicrons quantitatively form only a small proportion of the mass but are vital for triglyceride transport to the interstitial fluid. Some patients have a rare inherited defect (abetalipoproteinaemia) and are unable to form these proteins with the result that the villous epithelial cells are engorged with large triglyceride droplets even under fasting conditions. Occasionally a patient is presented with a specific transport process missing. Those with cystinuria or Hartnup disease have genetic defects in which dibasic or a neutral amino acid transport process is absent. More than 30 patients have been reported who are unable to absorb glucose and galactose effectively. A specific defect of the jejunal Na^+-dependent uptake mechanism has recently been demonstrated using brush border membrane vesicle preparations. Whether this represents fewer carrier sites or a defective carrier function remains to be determined. Defective absorption can also be specific for vitamins. Three children, of parents who are first cousins, were found to have selective vitamin B_{12} malabsorption (the Imerslund–Grasbeck syndrome). Apparently the defect in the ileal receptors for IF-vitamin B_{12} complex was not present at birth. Vitamin B_{12} deficiency was not recognised until the children were 4, 11, and 13 years old. The number or functional quality of the ileal receptors presumably declined as time passed.

Congenital lactase deficiency, described in children, is an example of an enzyme defect. Patients with it fail to thrive and frequently produce watery stools. The condition is thought to be due to autosomal recessive transmission. The congenital defect should not be confused with acquired lactase deficiency (hypolactasia) which is found in many parts of the world. A high incidence of acquired lactase deficiency is seen in certain racial groups, e.g. Negroes and Greek Cypriots. In affected populations, there is a gradual regression as maturation proceeds and this is comparable with what happens in most animal species. In fact, it could be argued that those who retain high lactase activity are abnormal.

Inadequate blood supply

The blood supply to the mucosa or the lymphatic system draining this region may be inadequate. The most widely recognized condition associated with lymphatic insufficiency is lymphangiectasia. This may be classified as a primary development defect of a group of lymphatic vessels, or secondary to a variety of conditions which result in obstruction of these vessels. As fat in the diet causes increased capillary permeability and the lymphatic vessels are inadequate for fat removal, a protein losing enteropathy is a problem. In the treatment of this condition a low fat intake is recommended.

Adaptation

Having described how malabsorption might occur, it is important to remember that the small intestine has considerable reserve capacity. Furthermore, the capacity of any one region to absorb is not constant. The small intestine can adapt to altered circumstances. Examples are the change in Ca^{++} absorption that accompanies hypocalcaemia and the increased transport of glucose that can be monitored in a number of situations, e.g. diabetes mellitus, gestation and lactation and intestinal resection. How might these increases be brought about? W.H. Karasov and J.M. Diamond reminded us that not even all the signals were known which induced the changes observed. Several plausible candidates could be put forward. For example, in diabetes mellitus, insulin deficiency, raised blood sugar levels or increased intracellular glucose concentrations in enterocytes or other cells could provide stimuli. But which of them, if any, are involved? They also reminded us that absorption could be modified by changes in:

1. The carrier density in either the brush border or basolateral membranes,
2. The type of carrier available.
3. Passive permeability.
4. The electrochemical gradient for Na^+.
5. The thickness of the unstirred water layer.
6. The cell maturation rate.
7. The number of transporting cells.

Clearly so many factors have to be considered in any adaptive response. An increase in the intestinal absorptive surface area, achieved mainly through mucosal growth, would appear to be the primary means of increasing glucose absorption in the situations mentioned above. However, in diabetes mellitus there is also a specific stimulation of the glucose transport system.

Motility of the small intestine

Several events result from the movements of the small intestine:

1. Chyme from the stomach is mixed with the secretions of the liver, pancreas and intestine.
2. The luminal contents are brought into contact with the absorbing cells,
3. The contents are propelled towards the ileocaecal junction.

   The latter may represent the movement of indigestible material towards the colon. However, this is only one possibility. Some substances are preferentially absorbed in the ileum, e.g. bile acids and vitamin B_{12}. In addition, localized distension of the intestine results in contractions whereby intestinal contents are squeezed away from that region, to be mixed in and absorbed from others less mechanically stimulated.

Gastroenterologists have talked of two types of muscle contractions:-

1. Segmenting contractions, which are dependent on circular muscle, are concerned with the mixing of luminal contents.
2. Peristaltic contractions, which are more dependent on longitudinal muscle, are concerned with propulsion over short distances (a few cm).

However, segmentations accomplish some propulsion, contractions squirting chyme both in oral and aboral directions. Furthermore, peristaltic movements result in some mixing.

Segmenting contractions

Segmenting contractions are localized, involving only small segments of bowel (1–2 cm). The lumen is constricted and the contents separated. The original description of segmentation by Cannon in 1902 was as follows:

'A string-like mass of food is seen lying quietly in one of the intestinal loops. Suddenly an undefined activity appears in the mass, and a moment later constrictions at regular intervals along its length cut it into little ovoid pieces. The solid string is thus quickly transformed by a simultaneous sectioning, into a series of uniform segments. A moment later each of these segments is divided into two particles, and immediately after the division neighbouring particles rush together, often with the rapidity of flying shuttles, and merge to form new segments. The next moment these new segments are divided and neighbouring particles unite to make a third series, and so on.'

Alvarez, in 1915, recognized that the rates of rhythmic contractions of any segment of the small intestine varied inversely with the distance from the pylorus. In man, the rate in the upper small intestine was about 11/min, while slower rates (8/min) were recorded in the terminal ileum. However, Cannon's rhythmic segmentations are now regarded as relatively rare. In 1939, Douglas and Mann studied unanaesthetized dogs. They exteriorized loops of small intestine, with nerves and blood supply intact, enclosed in bipedicled tubes of skin. From an analysis of almost a week of recordings, Cannon's rhythmic segmentations were observed during less than 3% of the time.

A more common type of rhythmic segmentation is where several segments contract from above downwards, i.e. a progressive type. These movements are unaffected by feeding, fasting or extrinsic nerves. However, vigour and amplitude of these contractions can vary greatly. Thus movement may be barely visible during fasting but pronounced after feeding.

The absence of an effect of extrinsic nerves on the rate of segmentation despite a gradient of activity along the length of the small intestine suggests a relationship between different regions either through intrinsic nerves or smooth muscle cells. That this is so has been demonstrated by transplanting jejunal segments to the lower ileum. This procedure was accompanied by a fall in the rate of the segment's rhythmic contractions.

Transecting the jejunum also reduced the rate of contractions of muscle distal to the site. The rate did not alter if the bowel was hemisectioned. One explanation of these findings is that the rhythmic activity of the jejunum is coordinated. When the intestine is transected and re-anastomosed, the union depends on non-excitable fibrous tissue and excitation cannot be transmitted. The intestine distal to the section takes up its own inherent rhythm. The ventricles do this when separated from the atria by division of the bundle of His.

How can the different rates of segmental contraction along the small intestine be explained? It appears that segmenting contractions are controlled by pacemakers within the intestinal wall. These may be either longitudinal smooth muscle cells or cells in the boundary between the longitudinal and circular smooth muscle layers, possibly the interstitial cells of Cajal. The pacemakers generate a basal electrical rhythm (or BER, Fig. 5.32), also called pacesetter potentials, slow waves or electrical control activity. Two mechanisms have been proposed by which the BER could be produced. In one the electrogenic Na^+,K^+-pump is rhythmically switched on and off. The alternative is that there might be periodic changes in membrane ion conductance, particularly to Na^+ and Cl^-. Both mechanisms may exist with the former dominant. Why

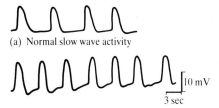

(a) Normal slow wave activity

10 mV

3 sec

(b) Slow wave activity with diastolic depolarizations

Fig. 5.32 Slow-wave activity (BER) recorded from rat jejunum *in vitro*. (a) Normal slow wave activity; (b) Slow wave activity with diastolic depolarizations. Amplitude of slow waves = 2–18 mV; duration of slow waves = 1–3msec; frequency = 10–15/min; time of peak = 400–600 ms. The resting membrane potential of the muscle cells could be separated into two groups. (1) 30–55 mV negative – perhaps longitudinal muscle. (2) 55-65mV negative - perhaps circular muscle. Usually membrane potentials between slow waves remain constant. In some cases, however, a depolarization proceeded the slow wave. Because of the similarity to the diastolic depolarization of the sinoatrial node of the heart this is termed diastolic depolarization (From Zelcer, E. (1979). *Pfügers Archiv für die gesamte Physiologie des menschen und der Tiere* **381**, 185–94.)

two systems should exist and whether there is any interaction between them is unknown. Did one of them evolve at an earlier time?

BER waves, while not initiating muscle contractions, increase and decrease the excitability of muscle cells so that a contraction to a given stimulus is more or less likely. In the duodenum, close to the entry of the bile ducts, a rhythm of a given frequency is generated which travels some distance down the small intestine. The frequency of the BER in this segment is greater than that of an adjacent segment of more distal intestine, and if the two segments are sectioned each displays different rates of contractions. The small intestine is made up of a number of segments each with a BER frequency lower than that immediately above it, and may be regarded as a series of oscillators, each having a characteristic frequency. If the coupling between adjacent oscillators is strong enough, then the oscillator with the higher frequency will drive that with the lower frequency.

However, as the small intestine is traversed, eventually a segment will be reached where the smooth muscle cells will be incapable of following the driving frequency of the duodenal oscillator. In this region the BER frequency falls and another rate is established. One can imagine several such falls along the intestine and, therefore, the gradient of segmenting contractions that have been described from duodenum to terminal ileum.

Propulsive contractions

The first detailed description of peristalsis was by Bayliss and Starling in 1899. They prepared dogs with intestine which they hoped was devoid of extrinsic nerves and described the advancing wave of contraction by which luminal contents were propelled. To produce peristalsis, a bolus of cotton wool covered in Vaseline and introduced into the lumen was the most effective stimulus. They concluded that irritation caused impulses to be transmitted both up and down the small intestine producing excitation (contraction) above and inhibition (relaxation) below the stimulated site. This response has been called 'the law of the intestine'. The myenteric plexus is concerned with the control of this response. In addition to the descending pathway causing relaxation, a descending excitatory pathway has also been proposed which has a longer latency so that the circular muscle contracts after a relaxation phase. The 'peristaltic wave' moves slowly (1–2 cm/s) and for short distances. A rare propulsive movement, sweeping rapidly along the whole length of the intestine, has been described as the peristaltic rush. The activity in the coils of the intestine has given the appearance of turning wheels, hence the alternative term 'rollbewegunen' used to describe it. Peristaltic rush is regarded as a characteristic motor activity occurring immediately *post mortem*.

However, although abnormal, peristaltic rush can be recorded in living animals, e.g. in acute enteritis due to bacterial or viral infections. Some involvement of extrinsic nerves has been established because cutting the vagi prevents the response. More recently other terms have been used to describe rapid, powerful contractions migrating considerable distances along the intestine. These include the propagating power contraction (PPC), the giant migrating contraction (GMC) and the prolonged propagated contraction (also PPC). In several other instances a confusing, overlapping terminology exists, e.g. the BER. With tongue in cheek, N.W. Read has suggested a solution. He believes that funds should be made available to send 'the opinion leaders in gastrointestinal motility' to a tropical island. Furthermore, strict instructions should be given to whoever conveys them not to return until they have agreement as to which terms should be used.

PPCs propelling the luminal contents distally do not necessarily involve the whole intestine. Indeed such events in the ileum are not uncommon even under normal circumstances. They are stimulated by the introduction of short chain fatty acids, deconjugated bile acids (products of bacterial metabolism) or a slurry of colonic contents into the ileum. The propulsive wave induced continues into the large intestine and provides a means by which refluxed colonic contents can be returned.

The picture presented so far, of segmenting and propulsive contractions, is undoubtedly a gross oversimplification. Other events have been described. One is antiperistalsis, where a wave of contraction moves in an oral direction. Many have doubted its existence even though patients have been known to vomit enemas and suppositories introduced rectally. It was thought that some intestinal contents would move orally as a result of segmenting contractions. However, retrograde propagating contractions can be recorded in the proximal intestine which propel the luminal contents into the stomach, an event frequently associated with vomiting.

Mucosal folds and movements of villi

The muscularis mucosae contract in response to gentle mechanical stimulation, e.g. touch. The result is that the mucosal surface is thrown into a complex pattern of folds. These patterns can rapidly change. Sympathetic nerve stimulation produces muscle contraction (in contrast to the inhibition of motility normally recorded in longitudenal and circular muscle). Vagal stimulation has little effect.

The intestinal villi also show movement. Piston-like contractions and relaxations were discribed more than a century ago. These contractions are thought to facilitate the removal of the products of fat digestion from the lacteals. The concept is that absorption takes place into a relaxed villus. Subsequently, the pressure in the lamina propria increases and intercellular channels between lacteal endothelial cells are opened. As a result interstitial fluid enters the lacteal. When the villus contracts the increase in intralymphatic pressure closes the lacteal and lymph is propelled into more distal segments of the lymphatic system. Valves in the submucosal lymphatic vessels prevent reflux when the villus subsequently relaxes. An increase of interstitial fluid pressure is one of the factors eliciting a myogenic contraction of muscle fibres in the lamina propria.

Villous contractions may also facilitate the rapid repair of the epithelial cell barrier after an injury. It appears that epithelial defects quickly shrink by a neurally mediated (TTX-inhibited) shortening of the villi. This reduces the surface area to be resealed. One suggestion is that a subepithelial network of myofibroblasts may be responsible for this process as well as providing a supportive tonus.

In addition to pumping movements villi can also sway. Such pendular movements could agitate the chyme and, therefore, enhance absorption. Local mechanical changes or chemical stimuli (amino acids and fatty acids, but not glucose or pH changes in the physiological range) are thought to elicit these movements.

Control of intestinal motility

The contractions of the small intestine are modified by at least four mechanisms.

1. Inherent smooth muscle cell activity.
2. Activity of intrinsic nerves.
3. Activity of extrinsic nerves.
4. Circulating or locally released chemicals.

What is the nerve supply of the intestine? Many intrinsic neurons are found in several plexuses. The most prominent, between the circular and longitudinal muscle layers, is the myenteric or Auerbach's plexus. Lying in the submucosa is Meissner's plexus. These are not completely separate anatomically and some authors refer to the two of them as the myenteric plexus. Many cell bodies in the plexus are considered cholinergic. However, not all cells release acetylcholine. In fact, the list of putative agents released by, or modifying the action of intrinsic nerves is bewildering. Roles for peptides, amines and nucleotides have been proposed. The fact that some peptides:

(a) are present in both nerves and endocrine-like cells, and
(b) may exert their effects in several ways if released from nerves or endocrine-like cells, further confuses the issue (Fig. 5.33).

Peptides modifying intestinal motility include VIP, somatostatin, substance P and opioids. Interestingly, opioids may make an important contribution to the control of gastrointestinal function. Related opium alkaloids have been used for centuries as potent antidiarrhoeal agents and analgesics. Endogenous opioids acting on distinct receptors (χ, μ and δ) are thought to inhibit reflex peristalsis, induce segmentation and increase circular muscle tone.

Cells in the myenteric plexus innervate both the longitudinal and circular muscle layers. These neurons receive signals from intestinal receptors, e.g. those responding to stretch, so that local reflexes occur without the participation of the central nervous system. In addition basic patterns of motility may be programmed in neural circuitry of intrinsic nerves.

Nerves from both branches of the autonomic nervous system reach the myenteric plexus. The parasympathetic fibres, derived from the dorsal vagal nucleus, are mainly preganglionic fibres. These enter the myenteric plexus to synapse with intrinsic nerves. The latter, therefore, are postganglionic fibres of the parasympathetic nervous system. Each preganglionic fibre innervates several thousand myenteric plexus cells. Thus vagal control of intestinal function may not be discrete. The sympathetic fibres originate in the coeliac and superior mesenteric ganglia and reach the intestine in splanchnic nerves. Axons synapse either in the myenteric plexus or directly with smooth muscle cells.

We must now enquire whether the central nervous system has any control on motility. Usually, stimulating sympathetic nerves inhibits contractions. The result may depend on a number of events:

1. When sympathetic nerves to intestinal blood vessels are stimulated, the resultant vasoconstriction and diffusion of the neurotransmitter from the blood vessels to the muscle cells may contribute to the inhibition of muscle contraction.

2. Sympathetic fibres may act within the myenteric plexus inhibiting those nerve fibres that produce muscle contractions when stimulated. The extrinsic nerves modify presynaptic nerve terminals, preventing the release of neural transmitters at the synapse.

3. Following general sympathetic stimulation, both adrenaline and nor-adrenaline are released from the adrenal medulla. These substances diffuse to the intestinal smooth muscle and exert their effects.

An example of the involvement of sympathetic nerves in modifying intestinal motility is afforded by the intestino-intestinal reflex. This is a mechanism to prevent powerful contractions completely obliterating the lumen. If an intestinal segment is distended, contractions in the remainder of the small bowel are inhibited. The receptors sensitive to stretch are found in the longitudinal muscle layer. Both the afferent and efferent limbs of this reflex reside in the sympathetic nerves, although the transection of the cervical spinal cord does not abolish the reflex (see page 232).

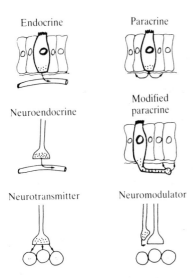

Fig. 5.33 The different mechanisms by which peptides may influence gastrointestinal function (After Weinbeck, M. and Erckenbrecht, J. (1982). *Clinics in Gastroenterology* **11**, 523–43.)

Trauma of other abdominal organs, e.g. kidney and gonads, also leads to inhibition of intestinal motility. The atonic bowel (paralytic ileus) is regarded as a manifestation of this physiological principle. In many animal experiments, no intestinal movements are observed until the splanchnic nerves have been cut, as tonic inhibitory impulses are conveyed in this nerve.

What about the role of the parasympathetic nervous system? Stimulating the vagus can induce contractions of intestinal muscle. However, sectioning the vagus has little effect on motility. A picture is emerging to show that, while the extrinsic nerves may exert a general control over the small intestine, local events, by releasing chemical agents or stimulating local nerve pathways, are the cause of much of the smooth muscle activity.

Extrinsic nerves are assumed, however, to be important in the ileogastric reflex. When the ileum is distended, gastric motility is inhibited. Such a response would slow down the passage of chyme from the stomach and not further embarrass the already distended bowel. This reflex is only one of many examples where activity in one part of the alimentary tract modifies the functions of another region and vice versa. Thus, associated with gastric secretion and emptying is an increased ileal motility, clearing the intestine of residual content and preparing it to receive more recently ingested food. This relationship is called the gastroileal reflex. The contribution of the nervous system to the gastroileal reflex, however, is debatable. Gastrin may be a major factor in eliciting the response. This hormone, in physiological amounts, increases segmentation in the terminal ileum (a similar mechanism may explain the greater colonic motility observed after taking a meal - the gastrocolic reflex, see page 233).

If extrinsic nerves modify motility, what parts of the central nervous system are involved? Roles for the cerebellum and the pituitary have been suggested. Unco-ordinated motor activity in the duodenum is recorded after hypophysectomy. When the nucleus fastigius is stimulated, ileal tone* is increased. However, the jejunum responds inconsistently, sometimes with an increase, at other times with a decrease in tone. The mechanism of this effect may be an inhibition of the tonic activity of sympathetic nerves.

One might ask why the jejunum and ileum act differently or why stimulation of the cerebellum produces variable changes in the jejunum. These questions are not easily answered, but it is worth remembering that nerves are not uniformly distributed along the small intestine, e.g. the sympathetic supply is absent from the proximal jejunum and irregularly distributed to the distal ileum in dogs and rabbits.

I wish I did not have to comment on the influence of peptides (released from endocrine-like cells and neurons) on motility. I question whether any subject has snowballed in the last 20 years to the same extent as gastrointestinal peptides. How many of the proposed effects elicited by these substances are pharmocological rather than physiological? Doubtless, however, they have

---

*One property of gastrointestinal smooth muscle that I have not examined in detail is its tone (or resistance to stretch). Tone, however, is important as it provides the background for other muscle activity. If tone is low, and there is little resistance, then mixing will be weak and intestinal transit slow.

important roles to play. Both gastrin and CCK disrupt the fasting pattern of motor activity (see page 195). This has led to the view that after a meal endogenous gastrin and CCK induce postprandial motor patterns. This may be part of the story in the stomach and duodenum. These peptides appear to be relatively less effective in more distal regions.

Four other peptides should be mentioned. One is VIP, a strong candidate to be the neurotransmitter producing relaxation when distension results in propulsive movements (Fig. 5.34). The peptide has been demonstrated in axons which originate in the myenteric plexus and project anlwards to innervate the circular smooth muscle layer. Enteroglucagon and neurotensin are two others to note. The former is released from ileal and colonic mucosal L cells. It is detected in the plasma in large concentrations when foodstuffs pass unduly rapidly to the distal small intestine, e.g. in patients with dumping syndrome or who have had jejuno-ileal bypass operations (Fig. 5.35) . Hyperosmolar glucose solutions and triglyceride emulsions are stimuli for enteroglucagon release. Two functions have been proposed:

1. To increase mucosal growth – The peptide stimulates DNA synthesis in cultures of jejunal mucosa. Furthermore, a patient with a benign renal tumour producing high concentrations of enteroglucagon was found to have gross mucosal hypertrophy. A more normal mucosa could be seen when the tumour was resected. Thus the intestine may adapt to a loss of absorptive area by promoting growth of the epithelial surface area available.

2. To slow intestinal transit – By doing so more time would be allocated for the complete digestion and absorption of fat and carbohydrate.

Neurotensin is produced by endocrine-like N cells found mainly on the villi, and with increasing frequency towards the distal ileum. Nutrients, particularly fats, release it. This peptide also inhibits propulsive movements. After a meal the rate

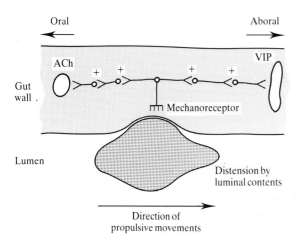

Fig. 5.34 The concept of elongation of smooth muscle fibres by VIP and their contraction by acetylcholine. Distension by luminal contents stimulates mechanoreceptors and activates local nerve networks

of propagation of the BER is reduced, probably as a result of the uncoupling of intestinal muscle cells. Some have speculated that neurotensin could be one of the factors contributing to this uncoupling. Neurotensin has a further effect. It causes vasodilatation. By doing so it could steepen the mucosa to serosa gradient for absorption across the epithelia and, therefore, enhance absorption.

Enteroglucagon and/or neurotensin might contribute to the inhibition of jejunal motility and delayed transit that follows the infusion of partial digests of fat, long chain or medium chain fatty acids into the ileum. This inhibitory effect of ileal lipid is known as the 'ileal brake'. However, although both peptides are released by ileal infusions correlations between the rises in plasma peptide levels and the reductions in jejunal motor activity were poor. A better correlation was achieved with yet another peptide released by lipid. This recently discovered hormone has been given the name peptide YY or PYY. It is elaborated by mucosal cells of both the ileum and the colon. PYY can also inhibit gastric emptying when administered to human volunteers in doses that produce similar rises to those seen after ileal lipid infusions.

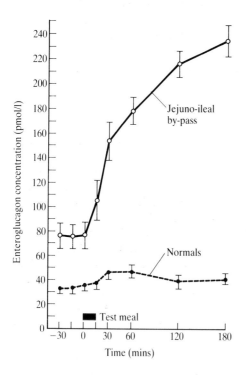

Fig. 5.35 Plasma enteroglucagon concentrations following a 530 calorie test breakfast in patients (n = 19) after jejuno-ileal bypass (o——o) and in a matched group (for sex and age) of normal subjects (n = 16) used as controls (●——●). The vertical bars represent standard error (SE) of each mean value (From Bloom, S.R. and Polak, J.M. (1982). *Scandinavian Journal of Gastroenterology Supplement* **74**, 93–103.)

The migrating myoelectric (and motor) complex – the MMC

If one measures simultaneously the electrical activity of muscle at several points along the stomach and intestine of fasting, conscious dogs, a recurring band of intense action potential activity is observed (Fig. 5.36). This is detected in the stomach and duodenum before it sweeps aborally along the intestine. As one front reaches the terminal ileum, the subsequent complex starts in the duodenum. These cycles occur in dogs at approximately the same time each day and are propagated at a faster rate (5.7–11.7 cm/min) in the proximal than in the distal intestine (0.9–2.5 cm/min). The complex takes 105–135 minutes to reach the terminal ileum from the duodenum.

The myoelectric complex can be modified by introducing into the stomach:

(a) 400 ml milk;
(b) 400 ml air to distend an intragastric balloon.

However, each stimulus produces a different response. Milk interrupts the complex already present and eliminates the next expected cycle. Air distension was found to interrupt the complex in the duodenum and stomach but had less effect than milk in the lower two-thirds of the intestine. These results have been interpreted as showing that both (1) gastric distension and (2) the passage of liquids into the small intestine affect the interdigestive myoelectric activity.

The questions remain as to:

(a) the type of muscle contractions to which these electrical events are related;
(b) the functions of these contractions,
(c) the activation and control of this activity.

In fasting dogs the myoelectrical activity correlates with segmenting contractions. It has been suggested that the complex has the role of an 'interdigestive housekeeper', maintaining the muscle in condition and cleaning the digestive tract. Powerful persistent contractions, aided by coordinated gastric and pancreatic secretory activity, remove residual undigested food particles, secretions, cell debris and even bacteria from the villi and propel them distally.

While complexes can be recorded experimentally using chronically implanted sensors, in man other procedures must be considered. David Wingate and his colleagues (Valori *et al.*, 1986) have induced young adults to swallow pressure-sensitive radio pills. They tethered a thread attached to the pill to the teeth or cheek after allowing the device to pass beyond the duodenum. Motor complexes were detected as episodes of contraction. These occurred at the rate of 9–11/min and between seven and seventeen were recorded daily, i.e. more variable than in animal studies.

The initiation and migration of the complex appears to depend on enteric neural mechanisms. A basic oscillator may reside in the enteric nervous system. The mechanism may be modified by both extrinsic and intrinsic neural input and by hormonal factors. Thus, truncal vagotomy, splanchnectomy, coeliac and superior mesenteric ganglionectomy or combinations of these do not prevent MMCs, suggesting that MMCs are initiated by local events. Mental stress inhibits MMC cycling.

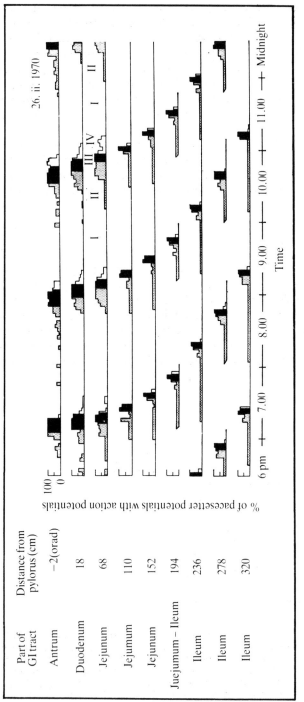

Part of GI tract	Distance from pylorus (cm)
Antrum	−2(orad)
Duodenum	18
Jejunum	68
Jejunum	110
Jejunum	152
Juejunum – Ileum	194
Ileum	236
Ileum	278
Ileum	320

Fig. 5.36 Three interdigestive myoelectric complexes starting in the stomach and duodenum and migrating to the terminal ileum during a 6-hour recording session made 30–36 hours after the onset of fasting in a dog. As one complex ends in the ileum another starts in the stomach and duodenum. The electrical activity was measured using electrodes placed at various sites in the stomach and small intestine. Four phases of myoelectrical activity have been recognized.

Phase 1: Relative absence of action potentials.
Phase 2: Persistent, but random, action potentials.
Phase 3: Bursts of continuous action potentials with every slow wave.
Phase 4: A rapid decrease in incidence and intensity of action potentials.

(From Code, C.F. and Marlett, J.A. (1975). *Journal of Physiology* **246**, 289–309.)

Numerous peptides have effects on gastrointestinal motility. One of them is motilin, a major source of which is the mucosa of the duodenum and proximal jejunum. Initially this hormone was regarded as a possible initiator of MMCs. The plasma motilin concentrations showed cyclical changes which were correlated with the MMCs. Maximum peptide levels were recorded when bursts of continuous action potentials (phase III, Fig. 5.36) started to be produced in the upper small intestine. No doubt motilin has an important role to play. However, rather than initiating MMCs it is thought more likely that motilin is released as a result of the MMC. Once released motilin may help to coordinate motor (and secretory) events.

Interestingly in man MMCs reach the ileocaecal sphincter only occasionally. Most 'fade out', merging with unique patterns of contraction that develop in the distal ileum (e.g. see page 189). Only now are some of the contractile mechanisms regulating ileal emptying and minimizing bacterial contamination being investigated.

The ileocaecal sphincter

Only the terminal part of the ileum, separating the rest of the small intestine from the colon, remains to be discussed. Many specific transfer processes are not encountered in the colon. In contrast, the colon has a bacterial population that is not normally associated with the small intestine. This suggests that the ileocaecal junction may have a role in controlling the backward movement of bacteria and the movement of substances useful to the body beyond the absorbing areas. Many believe that the terminal ileum is of little importance

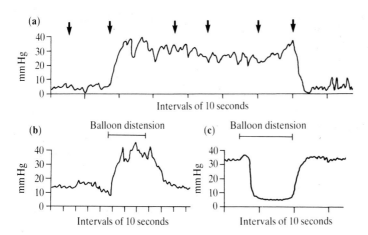

Fig. 5.37 The elevated pressure zone of the ileo-caecal region in man. (**a**) The pressure profile of the region; each arrow represents a 1 cm movement of the recording device from the colon through the region and into the ileum. (**b**) The effect of distending a balloon in the colon. There is a prompt, sustained increase in the pressure of the junctional zone. (**c**) The effect of distending a balloon in the ileum. In this case the pressure in the ileo-caecal region fell to a value only slightly above the mean colonic pressure (From Cohen, S., Harris, L.D. and Levitan, R. (1968). *Gastroenterology* **54**, 72–5.)

in the absorption of substances other than those specifically absorbed in that region, e.g. bile acids and vitamin B_{12}. This view is understandable as the terminal ileum constitutes only a small proportion of the total intestine, and absorption occurs rapidly as chyme traverses the jejunum and proximal ileum. However, if in some way the ileocaecal sphincter restricted the movement of the luminal contents to the colon, then these contents would be able to be digested and absorbed for a longer time. The ileum may take on a more important role.

This region in man is a zone about 4 cm long with a resting pressure approximately 20 mm Hg greater than that measured in the colon. This pressure changes when either the ileum or the colon is distended (Fig. 5.37). Inflating a balloon in the ileum results in a pressure drop in the ileocaecal region. The reverse occurs on distending the colon. One would expect, therefore, that retrograde movements of the luminal contents from the colon would be prevented but transit of ileal contents would be facilitated.

Some may question the adequacy of the sphincter in preventing retrograde movement, as barium reflux into the ileum can be observed during the course of a barium enema. However, colonic pressures exceeding 90 cm H_2O may occur with this procedure. These may be sufficiently high to overcome the resistance of the sphincter and force some colonic content back into the ileum.

Bibliography

Anderson, I.H., Levine, A.S. and Levitt, M.D. (1981). Incomplete absorption of the carbohydrate in all-purpose wheat flour. *New England Journal of Medicine* **304**, 891–2.

Bolondi, L., Gaiani, S., LiBassi, S., Zironi, G., Casanova, P. and Barbara, L. (1990). Effect of secretin on portal venous flow. *Gut* **31**, 1306–10.

Booth, I.W., Patel, P.B., Sule, D., Brown, G.A., Buick, R. and Beyreiss, K. (1988). Glucose-galactose malabsorption: demonstration of specific jejunal brush border membrane defect. *Gut* **29**, 1661–5.

Brandtzaeg, P., Sollid, L.M., Thrane, P.S., Kvale, D., Bjerke, K., Scott, H., Kett, K. and Rognum, T.O. (1988). Lymphoepithelial interactions in the mucosal immune system. *Gut* **29**, 1116–30.

Bronner, F. (1987). Intestinal calcium absorption: mechanisms and applications. *Journal of Nutrition* **117**, 1347–52.

Brown, N.J., Read, N.W., Richardson, A., Rumsey, R.D.E. and Bogentoft, C. (1990). Characteristics of lipid substrates activating the ileal brake in the rat. *Gut* **31**, 1126–29.

Brunsson, I. (1987). Acute inflammatory diarrhoea in the small intestine. Thesis, University of Göteborg, Sweden.

Burman, J.F., Jenkins, W.J., Walker-Smith, J.A. *et al.* (1985). Absent ileal uptake of IF-bound vitamin B_{12} *in vivo* in the Imerslund–Grasbeck syndrome (familial vitamin B_{12} malabsorption with proteinuria). *Gut* **26**, 311–14.

Carpenter, C.C.J., Greenough, W.B. and Pierce, N.F. (1988). Oral-rehydration therapy – the role of polymeric substrates. *New England Journal of Medicine* **319**, 1346–48.

Carroll, K.M., Wong, T.T., Drabik, D.L. and Chang, E.B. (1988). Differentiation of rat small intestinal epithelial cells by extracellular matrix. *American Journal of Physiology* **254**, G355–G360.

Christensen, H.N. (1990). Role of amino acid transport and countertransport in nutrition and metabolism. *Physiological Reviews* **70**, 43–77.

Code, C.F. and Marlett, J.A. (1975). The interdigestive myo-electric complex of the stomach and small bowel in dogs. *Journal of Physiology* **246**, 289–309.

Conrad, M.E. (1987). Iron absorption. In Physiology of the Gastrointestinal Tract, 2nd edn., pp 1437–53 Ed. by L.R. Johnson. Raven Press, New York.

Crissinger, K.D., Kvietys, P.R. and Granger, D.N. (1988). Autoregulatory escape from norepinephrine infusion: Roles of adenosine and histamine. *American Journal of Physiology* **254**, G560–G565.

Dahms, V., Prosser, C.L. and Suzuki, N. (1987). Two types of 'slow waves' in intestinal smooth muscle of cat. *Journal of Physiology* **392**, 51–69.

Field, M., Rao, M.C. and Chang, E.B. (1989). Intestinal electrolyte transport and diarrheal disease (2 parts). *New England Journal of Medicine* **321**, 800–06, 879–83.

Goodlad, R.A. (1989). Gastrointestinal epithelial cell proliferation. *Digestive Diseases* **7**, 169–7.

Gor, J. and Hoinard, C. (1989). Na^+/H^+ exchange in isolated hamster enterocytes. *Gastroenterology* **97**, 882–7.

Granger, D.N. and Barrowman, J.A. (1983). Microcirculation of the alimentary tract. 1. Physiology of transcapillary fluid and solute exchange. *Gastroenterology* **84**, 846–68.

Granger, D.N. and Kvietys, P.R. (1985). Recent advances in measurement of gastrointestinal blood flow. *Gastroenterology* **88**, 1073–6.

Granger, D.N., Zimmerman, B.J., Sekizuka, E. and Grisham, M.B. (1988). Intestinal microvascular exchange in the rat during luminal perfusion with formyl-methionyl-leucyl-phenylalanine. *Gastroenterology* **94**, 673–81.

Hahn, U., Stallmach, A., Hahn, E.G. and Riecken, E.O. (1990). Basement membrane components are potent promoters of rat intestinal cell differentiation *in vitro*. *Gastroenterology* **98**, 322–35.

Hediger, M.A., Coady, M.J., Ikeda, T.S. and Wright, E.M. (1988). Expression cloning and cDNA sequencing of the Na^+/glucose co-transporter. *Nature* **330**, , 379–80.

Holmes, R. and Lobley, R.W. (1989). Intestinal brush border revisited. *Gut* **30,** , 1667–78.

Holt, P.R. (1985). The small intestine. Chapter 3 in Gastrointestinal disorders in the elderly. *Clinics in Gastroenterology* **14(4)**, 689–723. W.B. Saunders, London.

Hopfer, U. (1987). Membrane transport mechanisms for hexoses and amino acids in the small intestine. In *Physiology of the Gastrointestinal Tract*, 2nd edn., pp 1499–1526. Ed. by L.R. Johnson. Raven Press, New York.

Ikeda, T.S., Hwang, E.-S., Coady, M.J., Hirayama, H.A., Hediger, M.A. and Wright, E.M. (1989). Characterization of a Na^+/glucose cotransporter cloned from rabbit small intestine. *Journal of Membrane Biology* **110**, 87–95.

Israel, E.J. and Walker, W.A. (1988). Host defense development in gut. *Pediatric Clinics of North America* **35**, 1–15.

Jodal, M. and Lundgren, O. (1986). Countercurrent mechanisms in the mammalian gastrointestinal tract. *Gastroenterology*, **91**, 225–41.

Jodal, M., Eklund, S. and Sjovall, H. (1988). Enteric nerves and function of intestinal mucosa. *Digestive Diseases* **6**, 203–15.

Jones, A.J. (1984). The intestinal immune system: a time for the reaper. *Gastroenterology* **87**, 234-7.

Joyce, N.C., Haire, M.F. and Palade, G.E. (1987). Morphologic and biochemical evidence for a contractile network within rat intestinal mucosa. *Gastroenterology* **92**, 68–81.

Karasov, W.H. and Diamond, J. (1983). Adaptive regulation of sugar and amino acid transport by vertebrate intestine. *American Journal of Physiology* **245**, G443–G462.

Karbach, V. (1989). Mechanism of intestinal calcium transport and clinical aspects of disturbed calcium absorption. *Digestive Diseases* **7**, 1–18.

Kessler, M. and Semenza, G. (1983). The small intestinal Na^+,D-glucose cotransporter: an asymmetric gated channel (or pore) responsive to $\Delta\Psi$. *Journal of Membrane Biology* **76**, 27–56.

Komuro, T. (1985). Fenestrations of the basal lamina of intestinal villi of the rat. Scanning and transmission electron microscopy. *Cell and Tissue Research* **239**, 183–8.

Krejs, G.J. (1986). Physiological role of somatostatin in the digestive tract: gastric acid secretion, intestinal absorption and motility. *Scandanavian Journal of Gastroenterology* **21** (Suppl. 119), 47–53.

Kromer, W. (1990). Endogenous opioids, the enteric nervous system and gut motility. *Digestive Diseases* **8**, 361–373.

Lang, R.E., Unger, T. and Ganten, D. (1987). Atrial natriuretic peptide: a new factor in blood pressure control. *Journal of Hypertension* **5**, 255–71.

Levin, R.J. (1982). Assessing small intestinal function in health and disease *in vivo* and *in vitro*. *Scandinavian Journal of Gastroenterology* **17**, (Suppl. 74), 31–51.

Lönnroth, I. and Lange, S. (1987). Intake of monosaccharides or amino acids induces pituitary gland synthesis of proteins regulating intestinal fluid transport. *Biochimica et Biophysica Acta* **925**, 1 7-23.

McNeil, P.C. and Ito, S. (1989). Gastrointestinal cell plasma membrane wounding and resealing in vivo. *Gastroenterology* **96** 1238–48.

Moore, R., Carlson, S. and Madara, J.L. (1989). Villous contraction and repair of intestinal epithelium after injury. *American Journal of Physiology* **257**, G274–G283.

Murer, H. and Kinne, R. (1980). Membrane vesicles to study epithelial transport processes. *Journal of Membrane Biology* **55**, 81–95.

Neale, G. (1990). B_{12}-binding proteins. *Gut* **31**, 59–63.

Neild, T.O., Shen, K.-Z. and Suprenant, A. (1990). Vasodilatation of arterioles by acetylcholine released from single neurones in the guinea-pig submucosal plexus. *Journal of Physiology* **420**, 247–65.

O'Donnell, L.J.D. and Farthing, M.J.G. (1989). Therapeutic potential of a long lasting somatostatin analogue in gastrointestinal diseases. *Gut* **30**, 1165–72.

Perry, M.A., Kvietys, P.R. and Granger, D.N. (1990). Circulation and vascular disease of the small intestine. *Current Opinion in Gastroenterology* **6**, 264–69.

Phillips, S.F., Quigley, E.M.M., Kumar, D. and Kamath, P.S. (1988). Motility of the ileocolonic junction. *Gut* **29**, 390–406.

Quigley, E.M.M. (1988). Motor activity of the distal ileum and ileocecal sphincter and its relation to the region's function. *Digestive Diseases* **6**, 229–41.

Ramasamy, M., Alpers, D.H., Tiruppathi, C. and Seetharam, B. (1989). Cobalamin release from intrinsic factor and transfer to transcobalamin II within the rat enterocyte. *American Journal of Physiology* **257**, G791–G797.

Read, N.W. (1989). Small intestinal motility: current opinions. *Current Opinion in Gastroenterology* **5**, 226–30.

Roman, C. and Gonella, J. (1987). Extrinsic control of digestive system motility. In *Physiology of the Gastrointestinal Tract*, 2nd edn., pp 507–53 Ed. by L.R. Johnson, Raven Press, New York.

Rose, R.C. (1987). Intestinal absorption of water-soluble vitamins. In *Physiology of the Gastrointestinal Tract*, 2nd edn., pp 1581–96. Ed., by L.R. Johnson, Raven Press, New York.

Roubaty, C. and Portmann, P. (1988). Relation between intestinal alkaline phosphatase activity and brush border membrane transport of inorganic phosphate, D-glucose and D-glucose-6-phosphate. *Pfluger's Archives* **412**, 482–90.

Rumessen, J.J. and Gudmand-Høyer, E. (1986) Absorption capacity of fructose in healthy adults. Comparison with sucrose and its constituent monosaccharides. *Gut* **27**, 1161–68.

Sarna, S.K. (1985). Cyclic motor activity; migrating motor complex: 1985. *Gastroenterology* **89**, 894–913.

Schjønsby, H. (1989), Vitamin B_{12} absorption and malabsorption *Gut* **30**, 1686–91.

Shepherd, A.P. and Riedel, G.L. (1982). Continuous measurement of intestinal mucosal blood flow by laser Doppler velocimetry. *American Journal of Physiology* **242**, G668–G672.

Sjövall, H. (1984). Sympathetic control of jejunal fluid and electrolyte transport. *Acta Physiologica Scandinavica* Suppl. **535**, 1–63.

Sjövall, H., Abrahamsson, H., Westlander, G. *et al.* Intestinal fluid and electrolyte transport in man reducing circulating blood volume. *Gut* **27**, 913–18.

Spiller, R.C., Trotman, I.F., Adrian, T.E., Bloom, S.R., Misiewicz, J.J. and Silk, D.B.A. (1988). Further characterisation of the 'ileal brake' reflex in man – effect of ileal perfusion of partial digests of fat, protein and starch on duodenal motility and release of neurotensin, enteroglucagon and peptide YY. *Gut*, **29**, 1042–51.

Stewart, C.P. and Turnberg, L.A. (1989). A microelectrode study of responses to secretagogues by epithelial cells on villus and crypt of rat small intestine. *American Journal of Physiology* **257**, G334–G343.

Stremmel, W. (1988). Uptake of fatty acids by jejunal mucosal cells is mediated by a fatty acid binding membrane protein. *Journal of Clinical Investigation* **82**, 2001–10.

Taylor, R.H., Barker, H.M., Bowey, E.A. and Canfield, J.E. (1986). Regulation of the absorption of dietary carbohydrate in man by two new glycosidase inhibitors. *Gut* **27**, 1471–8.

Terasaka, D., Bortoff, A. and Sillin, L.F. (1989). Postprandial changes in intestinal slow wave propagation reflect a decrease in cell coupling. *American Journal of Physiology* **257**, G463–G469.

Tso, P. (1985) Gastrointestinal digestion and absorption of lipid. *Advances of Lipid Research* **21**, 143–86.

Ugolev, A.M. (1974). Membrane (contact) digestion. In *Biomembranes*, Vol. 4A, pp 285–362. Ed. by D.H. Smyth. Plenum Press, London.

Valori, R.M., Kumar, D. and Wingate, D.L. (1986). Effects of different types of stress and of 'prokinetic' drugs on the control of the fasting motor complexes in humans. *Gastroenterology* **90**, 1890–1900.

Vidon, N., Chaussade, S., Merite, F., Huchet, B., Franchisseur, C. and Bernier, J.-J. (1989). Inhibitory effect of high caloric load of carbohydrates or lipids on human pancreatic secretions: a jejunal brake. *American Journal of Clinical Nutrition* **50**, 231–36.

Volkheimer, G., Schulz, F.H., Aurich, I., Stauch, S., Beuthin, K. and Wendlandt, H. (1968). Persorption of particles. *Digestion* **1**, 78–80.

Watson, A.J.M., Lear, P.A., Montgomery, A., *et al.* (1988). Water, electrolyte, glucose and glycine absorption in rat small intestinal transplants. *Gastroenterology* **94**, 863–9.

Weinman, H.D., Allan, C.H., Trier, J.S. and Hagen, S.J. (1989). Repair of microvilli in the rat small intestine after damage with lectins contained in the red kidney bean. *Gastroenterology* **97**, 1193–1204.

Weisbrodt, N.W. (1987). Motility of the small intestine. In *Physiology of the Gastrointestinal Tract*, 2nd edn., pp 631–63. Ed. by L.R. Johnson, Raven Press, New York.

Wilson, T.H. and Wiseman, G. (1954). The use of sacs of everted small intestine for the study of the transference of substances from the mucosal to the serosal surface. *Journal of Physiology* **123**, 116–25.

Womack, W.A., Tygart, P.K., Mailman, D., Kvietys, P.R. and Granger, D.N. (1988). Villous motility: relationship of lymph flow and bloodflow in the dog jejunum. *Gastroenterology* **94**, 977–83.

Wood, J.D. (1987). Physiology of the enteric nervous system. In *Physiology of the Gastrointestinal Tract*, 2nd edn., pp67–109. Ed. by L.R. Johnson, Raven Press, New York.

Wood, S.M., Kraenzlin, M.E., Adrian, T.E. and Bloom, S.R. (1985). Treatment of patients with pancreatic endocrine tumours using a new long-acting somatostatin analogue. Symptomatic and peptide responses. *Gut* **26**, 438–44.

6

The large intestine

In many courses of physiology, the large intestine receives less attention than any other region of the gastrointestinal tract. This is perhaps the result of the large bowel being 'at the end of the road' and hurried lecturers devoting less time to a consideration of its functions. The large intestine is also less accessible to be studied and our understanding has not progressed at the same rate as, for example, the small intestine.

In this chapter absorption, secretion and motility are discussed. In addition, sections are devoted to dietary fibre and to the bacteria of the gastrointestinal tract. The gases in different regions are also described.

Structure of the large intestine

The large intestine includes the caecum and appendix, the colon, rectum and anal canal. It is about 1.5 metres long. The caecum is a large cul-de-sac continuous with the proximal colon. Projecting from the caecum some 2 cm or so below the level of the ileum is the vermiform appendix.

The colon can be divided into four regions, the ascending (15 cm), transverse (50 cm), descending (25 cm) and sigmoid (40 cm) (Fig. 6.1). Continuous with the sigmoid colon is the rectum, which passes towards the anal canal. The rectum is about 12 cm long and differs from the sigmoid colon in having no mesentery or sacculations (see below). In the empty rectum a number of longitudinal folds of mucous membrane can be seen. Two types of transverse or horizontal folds (semilunar) are also recognized. One of these involve the mucous membrane, circular and longitudinal muscle, the other has no longitudinal muscle component. The number of the latter folds present is variable, although commonly three can be detected. The anal canal, about 4 cm long in man, begins where the rectum suddenly narrows (Fig. 6.2). The upper half of the anal canal presents 6–10 vertical folds or columns. The lower ends of the columns are joined together by folds of mucous membrane, the anal valves. Above each of these lies a small recess or anal sinus, which may retain faeces and become infected to produce anal abscesses, or be torn and develop anal fissures. The subsequent part of the anal canal is known as the transitional zone, or pecten, which has a stratified epithelium but contains no

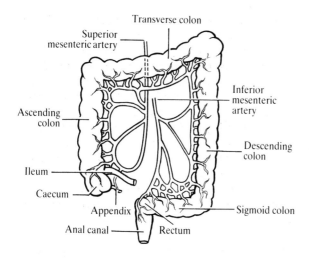

Fig. 6.1 The regions of the large intestine and their blood supply

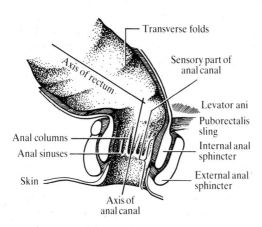

Fig. 6.2 A longitudinal section of the rectum and anus showing the angle between the axes of the rectum and anal canal (After Duthie, H.L. (1975). *Clinics in Gastroenterology* **4**, 467–77.)

no sweat glands. It ends in a region lined by true skin containing sweat and sebaceous glands.

Anal glands are to be found in the region of the anal sinuses. Many of these are mucus secreting. These glands are important clinically as they can also become infected and result in abscess or fistula formation. Muscular sphincters surround the anal canal. At the anorectal junction the circular muscle coat of the rectum becomes thickened to form the internal anal sphincter and surrounds the upper three-quarters of the anal canal. An external anal sphincter surrounds the whole anal canal. This is composed of striated muscle. The tone of both internal and external anal sphincters normally maintains the anal canal closed.

The layers of the large intestine are the same as in the small intestine. The longitudinal muscle forms a continuous layer. However, it is thickened to form conspicuous longitudinal bands, the taeniae coli. In the caecum and colon three taeniae coli are present. These bands are said to be shorter than the other coats of the intestine and contribute to the characteristic sacculations and haustrations. In the rectum the longitudinal muscle fibres spread out to form a layer which is thicker on the anterior and posterior surfaces so that two broad bands can be recognized. Circular muscle fibres form a thin layer over both the colon and caecum. The mucous membrane is smooth and devoid of villi and raised into folds corresponding to the interhaustral regions. In the caecum, colon and upper rectum, columnar absorptive cells with striated borders and mucus-secreting goblet cells are observed on the surface and lining the walls of the glands. Thus a large surface area is available for the absorption of electrolytes and water, and lubrication of the faeces can assist their passage to the exterior.

Both branches of the autonomic nervous system are represented in the large intestine. Up to the distal third of the transverse colon the parasympathetic supply is via the vagus and the sympathetic nerves are derived from the coeliac and superior mesenteric ganglia. Subsequently, until the lower half of the anal canal is reached, the nervi erigentes provide the parasympathetic fibres. The sympathetic nerves from the lumbar spinal cord and the superior hypogastric plexus follow a pathway via plexuses on the branches of the inferior mesenteric artery. The external anal sphincter is supplied by branches of nerves arising from the sacral cord (2, 3 and 4).

Electrolyte transport by the large intestine

When the contents excreted through the anus are analysed and compared with those entering the colon from the ileum each day, it is found that the faeces contain less water (1350 ml), sodium (200 mmol), chloride (150 mmol) and bicarbonate (60 mmol). One has to remember that these differences do not represent the total absorption by the colon as they do not account for any movements of water and electrolytes from the gut wall into the lumen.

The mechanisms involved in electrolyte absorption are incompletely understood. The picture is complicated by the existence of species differences and the fact that transport processes are not uniformly distributed along the large intestine. As regards Na^+ absorption, active transport mechanisms are necessary. These may transfer Na^+ from fluids containing very low concentrations (15 mmol/l) against potential differences of 40 mV (lumen negative with respect to the serosal surface). Two different systems have been proposed (Fig. 6.3). One involves an electrogenic mechanism and has been studied extensively in the distal colon of rabbits. In it Na^+ is transferred from the lumen by amiloride*-sensitive channels down electrical and chemical gradients.

---

*Amiloride is a drug used clinically to block Na^+ reabsorption in renal distal tubules (and secondarily inhibiting K^+ secretion).

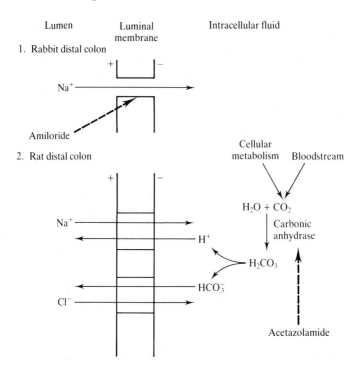

Fig. 6.3 Models for Na+ uptake. 1. In rabbit distal colon an electrogenic mechanism has been proposed. 2. In rat distal colon an electrically neutral process is available coupled to Cl^- : HCO_3^- exchange. Dotted arrows (- - →) represent inhibition

A different mechanism is dominant in rat distal colon where $Na^+:H^+$ exchange occurs at the luminal membrane. This process, inhibited by the carbonic anhydrase inhibitor, acetazolamide, is coupled to intracellular pH. Na^+ removal from the epithelial cells against an electrochemical gradient can be achieved via the energy-requiring Na^+,K^+-pump.

Cl^- absorption is not simply the passive movement of anions following Na^+ to maintain electrical neutrality. There is strong evidence that Cl^- can exchange with HCO_3^- at the luminal membrane. For example:

1. If Cl^- and Na^+ are present in the luminal contents in equal concentrations, then more Cl^- may be absorbed than Na^+.
2. When the pH of the luminal contents is low the absorption of Cl^- is increased. This has been explained in terms of an increased acidity of the contents stimulating HCO_3^- secretion so as to increase pH.
3. If the colon is perfused with Cl^--containing salines the luminal fluid $[Cl^-]$ decreases while the $[HCO_3^-]$ rises markedly. The $[HCO_3^-]$ achieved may be greater than those recorded in the plasma. In contrast, $[Cl^-]$ may fall below plasma levels.

The $Na^+{:}H^+$ and $Cl^-{:}HCO_3^-$ exchange systems appear to be coupled although a Na^+-independent $Cl^-{:}HCO_3^-$ exchange has been proposed (as has passive Cl^- movement down its electrochemical gradient). The absence of Cl^- from the lumen can markedly reduce the absorption of Na^+ and vice versa.

The question remains as to which Na^+ transport mechanisms are present in different regions of the large intestine. Human studies indicate that the electrogenic process is the principal mechanism in the distal colon (as in the rabbit). In the proximal colon (ascending) electroneutral events dominate. One should not forget that the caecum makes a contribution, although this region, in many mammals, may not have the enormous Na^+ absorptive capacity reported in the rabbit.

Na^+ transport in the adult colon, unlike the situation encountered in the small intestine, is not coupled to sugars and amino acids. In the fetus and newborn rat, however, villi line the colon and both glucose and amino acids are absorbed. The mechanisms involved are similar to those found in the small intestine. Glucose stimulates net Na^+ absorption. Such processes disappear rapidly following birth.

Transport of K^+ by the colon involves both secretory and absorptive processes (Fig. 6.4). In a model of secretion K^+ can be seen entering the cell

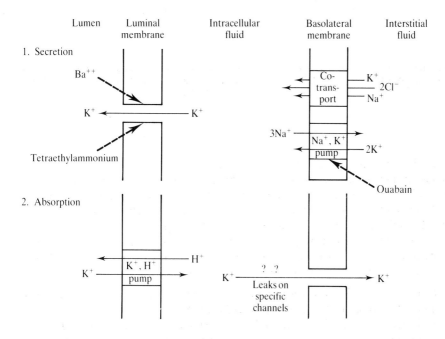

Fig. 6.4 Handling of K^+ by the colon. Both absorptive and secretory mechanisms have been demonstrated. During absorption K^+ is thought to 'leak out' of the cells into the interstitial fluid. Might a more specific channel, similar to that providing a 'safety valve' for epithelial cells of the small intestine, limit intracellular K^+ accumulation (see page 164). Dotted arrows (- - →) represent inhibition. Thus the luminal membrane K^+ channel is sensitive to barium and tetraethylammonium while the Na^+,K^+-pump can be inhibited by the cardiac glycoside ouabain

via the Na^+,K^+-pump or an electrically neutral process transferring Na^+, K^+ and Cl^- in the ratio of 1:1:2 (see page 164). Subsequently it is released to the lumen through barium- and tetraethylammonium-sensitive channels. For K^+ to be absorbed a K^+,H^+-pump provides a means for cation uptake. Was such a mechanism not described in the parietal cell? Leaks down electrochemical gradients account for K^+ reaching the interstitial fluid. The net result of these two processes, absorption and secretion, depends on the state of the animal. It has been suggested that the colon contributes significantly to K^+ homeostasis. Thus dietary K^+ depletion enhances active K^+ absorption. On the other hand, dietary K^+ loading and Na^+ depletion, with resulting secondary hyperaldosteronism, leads to the induction of active K^+ secretion. It appears that the whole of the colon can secrete K^+. Only the distal colon, however, effectively absorbs the cation. Whether both mechanisms exist in the same cells and/or whether one process influences the other is still being debated.

Although the net result of the various processes in the colon is that Na^+, Cl^- and water are absorbed while K^+ and HCO_3^- are secreted, it must be remembered that Cl^- secretion is an important function of the large, as well as the small, intestine. A similar mechanism exists in both epithelia (see page 164). The primary event by which Cl^- secretion can be altered is by changing the permeability of the Cl^- channel in the luminal membrane. However, the presence of K^+ channels in the luminal membrane results in a K^+-rich secretion in the colon. The secretion of Cl^- is usually regarded as a function of the crypt, rather than the surface, epithelial cells. This does not mean that surface cells are incapable of secreting. Indeed, using a patch clamp* technique, Cl^- channels have been recognized within the luminal membrane of the surface cells suggesting that the distinction between secretory and absorptive cells is not as clear cut as we tend to think.

Factors modifying electrolyte transport

Absorption

Several hormones influence water and electrolyte movement across the colon. These include both mineralo- and glucocorticoids. Thus, aldosterone stimulates Na^+/H_2O absorption, and patients with primary aldosteronism have decreased $Na^+:K^+$ ratios in their stools. Aldosterone increases the Na^+,K^+-pump activity and the surface area of the basolateral membrane as well as inducing Na^+ channels in the apical membrane. Some have recently suggested that the effects on the basolateral membrane may be, at least partially, attributed to the greater apical membrane Na^+ permeability resulting in increased intracellular $[Na^+]$. Aldosterone also induces the separate and distinct K^+ channel in the apical membrane.

Glucocorticoids have effects which are generally similar to the mineralocor-

---

*The patch clamp technique is one in which a 'patch' or area of membrane is isolated from the rest of the cell by forming a high-resistance electrical seal within the isolated membrane.

ticoids. However, quantitative and qualitative differences in the responses of the colon to these steroids have been reported. One view is that specific receptors exist for glucocorticoids. These are distinct from those accepting mineralocorticoids. When they are activated the result is the stimulation of electroneutral but not electrogenic Na^+ transport. Two other hormones modifying transport are angiotensin II and antidiuretic hormone. The former stimulates while the latter decreases Na^+ absorption, effects which might have been anticipated of substances which contribute to the maintenance of the volume and tonicity of the extracellular fluid, respectively. Their mechanisms of action in the colon are not known. However, it has been suggested that angiotensin II may produce its effects indirectly by facilitating the release of noradrenaline from sympathetic nerve endings and by stimulating the release of adrenal catecholamines. Noradrenaline stimulates net Na^+ absorption at least in the small intestine.

Undoubtedly the nervous system has a role to play in the regulation of electrolyte transport. The colonic mucosa is extensively innervated although the dense network of nerve fibres appears to be spontaneously inactive. The epithelium is set for near to maximum absorption. When cholinergic enteric nerves are activated Na^+ and Cl^- absorption are inhibited. One can only speculate as to the functional significance of this effect. An interesting possibility is that because the proximal colon extracts a large fraction of the electrolytes and water from the ileal effluent, the neural inhibitory effect might be important for maintaining some fluidity of the luminal contents. An inhibition of absorption may also be a factor in the pathophysiology of diarroheal disease.

Secretion

Many factors increase colonic secretion. The list includes bacterial toxins, e.g. Shigella toxin, hormones, neurotransmitters, local metabolites and laxatives. One should remember that a particular agent may produce its effects by modifying more than one cellular process. Furthermore, by causing damage to the mucosa metabolites are released which may also stimulate secretion.

Among the secretagogues recognized are bradykinin, 5HT, VIP, adenosine, several prostaglandins and cholinergic agents, e.g. bethanechol. Some bile acids also increase fluid movement to the lumen. For example, the primary conjugated bile acid taurochenodeoxycholate inhibits Na^+ absorption and stimulates Cl^- secretion. The latter effect is achieved when the bile acid enhances the activity of adenylate cyclase in the basolateral membrane. (NB. Taurochenodeoxycholic acid stimulates secretion via a cyclic AMP-dependent mechanism. In contrast cholinergic agents and 5HT appear to induce Ca^{++}-dependent effects.) Taurochenodeoxycholate also causes a general increase in the passive permeability of the epithelial barrier. By altering the integrity of the tight junctions between epithelial cells, water can be more readily attracted osmotically from the interstitial fluid.

Greater secretions can also be recorded in the colon during immune responses to antigens. Sensitization of the guineapig colon to trichinella induces changes reflecting increased Cl^- secretion. At least some of the effects could be accounted for by histamine and prostaglandin E_2. Such agents are released from cells involved in inflammatory responses, e.g. mast cells. Thus the contribution of the numerous cells in the gastrointestinal immune system to the regulation of electrolyte transport may be greater than previously thought and an exciting area for future research.

Finally, one has to consider K^+ secretion. K^+ is the major cation in faecal fluid. Its concentration in the distal colon is normally 10 times greater than in the extracellular fluid. Had passive diffusion down electrochemical gradients been the only mechanism by which K^+ appeared in the lumen such concentrations would not have been achieved. Active K^+ secretion by the colonic epithelium has now been established. Its possible importance in K^+ homeostasis has not been overlooked. It is recognized that the body may have to tolerate acute K^+ loads when (a) K^+-rich diets are ingested, (b) large amounts of K^+ are released from muscles etc. during severe exercise or trauma, and (c) there is renal insufficiency. Aldosterone is one of the important factors increasing K^+ secretion in response to acute-K^+ loading. Another may be the interstitial fluid $[K^+]$. The K^+ secretory pathway appears to be more sensitive to the mineralocorticoid than the mechanisms concerned with Na^+ absorption. The Na^+ and K^+ transport systems can be dissociated.

The large intestine may also have a greater role to play than expected in Na^+ conservation. This applies particularly in the preterm neonate (Table 6.1). Although high circulating levels of aldosterone can be measured in such individuals urinary salt wasting occurs because of immature renal tubular functions. However, even before birth the large intestine has well developed salt-conserving mechanisms. These have been detected early in the last trimester of gestation. Such processes would appear to be valuable to the very young at a time when adequate nutrition and the conservation of fluid and electrolytes are vital for optimal growth. The importance of mineralocorticoids in the regulation of colonic electrolyte transport can also be seen in the data obtained from studies of children with various forms of disordered aldosterone metabolism, e.g. pseudohypoaldosteronism (end-organ unresponsiveness), congenital adrenal hyperplasia (aldosterone deficiency) or the secondary hyperaldosteronism associated with congenital chloride-losing diarrhoea (Table 6.1).

Mucus secretion by the colon

Both the crypts and the surface epithelium have a high density of goblet cells. These cells contribute to a colonic secretion which is alkaline and rich in mucus. The mucus provides a juxtamucosal layer in which a stable and neutral pH can be maintained even when the pH of the luminal contents is altered between 6 and 9. Interestingly, the $[K^+]$ of the colonic microclimate is also buffered. Studies with guinea pigs have revealed that changing the luminal $[K^+]$ from 0 to 70 mmol/l increases the surface $[K^+]$ but only from 6.3 to 21.3 mmol/l. These findings may help to explain why the colonic epithelium continues to function in spite of fluctuations of pH and $[K^+]$. The luminal $[K^+]$ may approach 140 mmol/l.

Table 6.1 Rectal Na$^+$ absorption, K$^+$ secretion and plasma aldosterone concentrations in children of different age groups, and children with various forms of disordered aldosterone metabolism. The data presented are average values except when only two or three subjects were studied. In these instances individual measurements are given. Electrolyte transport was measured by a non-equilibrium dialysis method using dialysis bags of 3 or 4 cm in length depending on the size of the child. The initial electrolyte concentrations introduced were isotonic and contained Na$^+$ 140 mol/l, K$^+$ 20 mmol/l, Cl$^-$ 130 mmol/l and HCO$_3^-$ 30 mmol/l (From Jenkins, H.R., Fenton, T.R., McIntosh, N., Dillon, M. J. and Milla, P. J. (1990. *Gut* **31**, 194–7.

Description	Age	Number of subjects	Absorption of Na$^+$ (nmol/min/cm^2)	Secretion of K$^+$ (nmol/min/cm^2)	Plasma [aldosterone] (pmol/l)
Preterm neonates	30–33 weeks	15	315	38	5464
Preterm neonates	34–37 weeks	14	302	37	3085
Term neonates	38–44 weeks	5	243	47	1248
Children	1–12 months	17	203	27	780
Children	1–8 years	19	149	33	240
Children with pseudohypoaldosteronism	6–12 months	2	71, 105	0.5	3900, 10500
Children with congenital chloride-losing diarrhoea	10–24 months	2	368, 312	107, 50	9750, 1240
Children with congenital adrenal hyperplasia: (a) 48 hours without mineralocorticoid supplements	6–18 months	3	55, 68, 46	0, 2, 6	0, 0, 0
(b) receiving corticosteroids			148, 153, 130	31, 37, 15	Not estimated

The alkaline mucous secretion also helps to neutralize the products of fermentation in the faeces. Thus the surface of a faece may be neutral while its centre has a pH under 5.0. Surface irritants (e.g. mustard oil) stimulate a secretion, as does mechanical irritation caused by the contact of the colon with the faecal mass. These secretions can be independent of extrinsic nerves. Nevertheless, a central nervous system component has been identified mediated by the nervi erigentes. Certainly, extreme emotional disturbances can lead to large mucous secretions and excursions to the toilet every half hour.

The mucus released by the colon is not identical with that produced in more proximal regions of the gut. Its sialic acid content and degree of sulphation are greater making it more resistant to bacterial enzymes. Nevertheless, some bacteria, e.g. *Bifidobacterium bifidium*, can secrete glycosidases enabling them to break down and utilize mucus as their only source of energy. Should the numbers of such bacteria increase the protection offered by mucus to the colonic epithelium against toxins might be seriously compromised.

Short chain fatty acids (SCFAs) in the colon

Some glucose can be taken up by the colonic mucosa but its movement has little influence on blood sugar concentrations. Any sugars not absorbed are likely to be metabolized to form SCFAs. These make the major anion component of human faeces. The fatty acids produced have never been completely described although volatile SCFAs account for about 47% of them – e.g. acetate, propionate and butyrate. In herbivores these acids provide a major source of the animals energy needs. Up to 22% of its basal requirements can be satisfied. In man, however, the contribution is much smaller. Nevertheless, it can be increased considerably if the intake of dietary fibre is high. For example, the ingestion of 10 g dietary fibre when eating wholemeal bread can provide 100 mmol acetate.

Volatile SCFAs are avidly absorbed by the colon. At the same time they stimulate Na^+ and water absorption. This finding was unexpected, particularly as it was thought that SCFAs provided a potent osmotic force contributing to the diarrhoea associated with carbohydrate malabsorption. How might volatile SCFAs increase Na^+ absorption? They can provide energy for the absorbing epithelial cells. Another possibility has recently been proposed. In the rat distal colon, where electroneutral NaCl absorption can result from $Na^+:H^+$ and $Cl^-:HCO_3^-$ exchange, it has been found that butyrate is as effective as HCO_3^- in promoting the electroneutral process. To explain this it has been suggested that SCFAs diffuse into the epithelial cells (because of their lipid solubility) and are subsequently recycled by a $Cl^-:SCFA$ exchange process.

Decreased SCFA production, resulting from a reduction of bacterial metabolism, may be of particular significance for patients receiving antibiotic therapy and fed liquid diets via enteral tubes, e.g. nasoduodenally. Such patients show an increased incidence of diarrhoea. This may be the result of the unavailability of SCFAs to enhance Na^+ absorption. Some SCFAs are products of carbohydrates, poorly utilized by man, being intentionally introduced into the diet. An example is lactitol or 4-O-β-D-galactopyranosyl-D-glucitol, a disaccharide alcohol produced by the hydrogenation of lactose. It has acceptable taste and is not digested or absorbed by the small intestine. Because of these properties it has been recognized as a possible substitute for sucrose and glucose, providing a low-calorie sweetener for foodstuffs. In man only about 55% of the potential energy of the sugar derivative is utilized. Lactitol can, therefore, be regarded as a reduced calorie substitute, undoubtedly good for the teeth and the pancreas. However, the warning has been given that its widespread incorporation into the diet could lead to intakes approaching its laxative threshold and, therefore produce, unacceptable bowel habits.

SCFAs have effects other than providing an energy source and promoting NaCl absorption. Some can stimulate either colonic secretion, motility or epithelial cell division. An increase in Cl$^-$ secretion is produced by propionate although not by acetate. The response to propionate is not direct. A mechanism similar to that by which secretagogues act in the small intestine may account for the effects of propionate (Fig. 6.5). It has been proposed that the SCFA activates endocrine-like cells which release peptides and/or amines into the interstitial fluid. As a result nearby nerve fibres are excited and a secretion elicited which releases acetylcholine close to the muscarinic cholinergic receptors on the basolateral membranes of secreting cells. Volatile SCFAs stimulate colonic mucosal growth. Butyrate is more potent than either acetate or propionate. They may exert direct trophic effects on the colonic epithelium. However, SCFAs probably increase mucosal proliferation in several other ways.

Their release lowers the luminal pH. Increased luminal acidity stimulates mucosal growth. Furthermore, SCFAs increase intestinal blood flow, providing

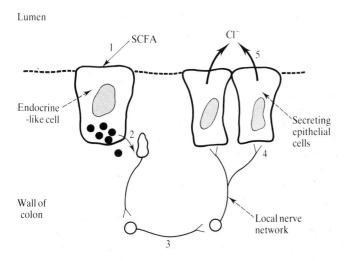

Fig. 6.5 An incomplete, but useful model illustrating the effects of SCFAs on colonic secretion. (1) SCFAs act on endocrine-like cells releasing peptides and/or amines which (2) activate a local nerve reflex (3). The release of acetylcholine (4), which binds to muscarinic receptors on colonic epithelial cells, results in increased Cl$^-$ (and fluid) secretion

conditions which facilitate growth. One other possibility has also been recognized and that is that SCFAs may release growth promoting factors from the intestinal mucosa. Crypt cell production rates in the proximal colon are not greatly increased by poorly fermentable dietary fibre providing inert bulk. In contrast, feeding a readily fermentable fibre (purified wheat bran) which releases SCFAs, causes a large proliferative response. What might SCFAs release? One candidate is the hormone enteroglucagon which is elaborated by cells located predominantly in the colon and terminal ileum. It is thought likely to be implicated in promoting intestinal cell renewal.

The handling of urea in the colon

Urea might appear to be an unnecessary substance to consider. However, the daily urea synthesis exceeds the urinary output by some 20% and it has been calculated that the remaining 6–9 g urea are secreted into the colon, metabolised by bacteria and their products absorbed. The metabolizm takes place at some juxtamucosal site, as intravenously administered urea is more rapidly metabolized than urea perfused through the lumen. Approximately 200–300 mmol ammonia and 100–150 mmol HCO_3^- are formed each day. At the pH of the colonic contents, ammonia occurs mainly in the form of NH_4^+ and it has been suggested that NH_4^+ and HCO_3^- are converted to NH_3 and CO_2, which are able to diffuse freely across the mucosal barrier and reach the circulation. The ammonia is taken to the liver where it can be available for amino acid synthesis.

Dietary fibre

Until recently dietary fibre was not given the important recognition it deserved. This was because of the persistent belief in its inertness and non-nutritive character in man. Dietary fibre has been described as the remnants of plant cells resistant to hydrolysis by the gastrointestinal enzymes. It is extremely difficult to classify partly because the major fraction is composed of hundreds of polysaccharides. These contain more than 100 sugars and sugar derivatives. Lignin provides a further complication. This fibre, which contributes to the structural rigidity of cell walls, is not a polysaccharide. Indeed, it is a phenylpropane polymer, molecular weight 1000–4500.

One way of describing dietary fibre is to divide it into three groups:-

1. Structural fibres, making up the plant cell wall. These include cellulose, lignin, hemicelluloses and pectins.
2. Gums and mucilages involved in the repair of injured areas.
3. Storage polysaccharides. Guar gum provides an example of this group, which is distinct from the digestible polysaccharides such as starch.

A number of other substances, such as phytic acid, silica, cell wall protein, aromatic constituents and non-metabolizable sugars (e.g. raffinose), are regarded as dietary fibre-associated substances. These and the dietary fibres themselves are referred to as the dietary fibre complex.

So what is the value of dietary fibre? A pointer perhaps is given when one compares the diseases of Western populations with those of rural Black populations in Africa or other developing countries. The Western diets are often of low fibre, low starch, high sucrose and high fat content with 10–14% protein, many vegetables and fruit and 5–10 g salt each day. In contrast, the diet of the African Black is almost the opposite, having a high fibre and starch content. Among the Western-risk diseases are constipation, diverticular disease, haemorrhoids, polyps and cancer of the large bowel, irritable colon and ulcerative colitis. Adding fibre in the form of bran regularly to a Western-type diet remedies constipation, eases haemorrhoids and relieves the symptoms of diverticular disease.

This suggests, therefore, that dietary fibre is of considerable value to man. How can it modify the functions of the gastrointestinal tract? A number of effects are attributable to dietary fibre. These include the following:

1. Altered transit time.
2. Water holding.
3. Cation binding.
4. Gel formation.
5. Provision of substrates for bacterial metabolism.
6. Altered digestion and absorption.

Altered transit time

In general, adequate quantities of cellulose-rich food (e.g. wheat bran) decrease transit time and increase faecal bulk. Intestinal propulsive movements are likely to be stimulated by greater volumes of luminal contents.

However, the view that high fibre diets will increase the rate of transit is an oversimplification. Pectins may delay gastric emptying and slow intestinal transit because of their gel formation.

Water holding

Dietary fibre has considerable water holding capacity, the water being either adsorbed to the surface or trapped within the fibre matrix. It has been found that most polysaccharides swell in the presence of water to form gels. Pectins, gums, storage polysaccharides and mucilages have high affinities. Even structural polysaccharides bind water, at least to a limited extent. Those fibres with a lower affinity for water, e.g. bean, are thought to be relatively inert in the gut and less available for bacterial enzyme fermentation.

Cation binding

This is related to the presence of acidic sugars, e.g. those with uronic acid groups. Binding may modify the ability of the fibre to form gels. Over the short term at least, calcium, iron, magnesium and zinc excretion may increase. Whether over the long term the faecal content of these cations remains high has still to be investigated. However, whole wheat products have been implicated in the development of osteomalacia in Bedouins and rickets in chappati-eating immigrants in Britain.

Gel formation

A variety of fibres form gels in the small intestine and a gel filtration system similar to that used in column chromatography may be established. This could remove molecules (or bacteria) because of their size or charge and thus interfere with digestion and absorption.

Provision of substrates for bacterial metabolism

Dietary fibre is partially digested via the colon. This process depends on the bacteria present within the lumen. For many bacteria dietary fibre is a major nutrient and energy source. Most of the enzymes breaking down plant polysaccharides, e.g. cellulases, hemicellulases and pectin esterases appear to be bound to bacterial cell walls. Some, however, are released extracellularly. Many are inducible. In general, pectin is completely digested in man while cellulose and hemicelluloses are only partially broken down. One should ask why cellulose is less well utilized. Part of the answer lies in the relative insolubility of cellulose and the limited surface area to which bacterial polysaccharidases have access. When bran is finely ground its surface area is greater than that offered by coarse bran with the result that cellulose breakdown is increased.

Because cellulose digestion is a relatively slow process the time available for cellulytic enzymes to act is obviously an important factor. If colonic transit is slow cellulose digestion will be more complete. Clearly preparations containing senna or codeine sulphate, which increase and decrease colonic propulsive activity respectively, will alter the proportion of dietary cellulose hydrolysed. The presence of lignin within cell walls also reduces fibre degradation. This polymer appears to be completely resistant to colonic fermentation. Some cellular structure is, therefore, maintained and bacterial activity is obstructed.

The products of fibre metabolism are volatile SCFAs and gases, e.g. CO_2, CH_4 and H_2. The SCFAs that are not absorbed provide a valuable source of energy for colonic micro-organisms. Indeed, it has been suggested that a major function of dietary fibre is to be the substrate for bacterial metabolism, and so provide for their growth and maintenance.

Altered digestion and absorption

A number of substances present in the diet or in the gastrointestinal secretions are handled differently in the presence and absence of dietary fibre. For example, bile acids entering the colon can be deconjugated and further metabolized to secondary bile acids. These are more lipid soluble than the conjugated forms and can diffuse through the lipid barrier of the colonic epithelium. Thus the 5–20% of the bile acid pool that enters the colon each day can be absorbed. However, bile acids can be strongly bound to dietary fibre. Some may also be dissolved in the water of hydrated fibre. These bile acids may be excreted in the faeces.

Dihydroxy-bile acids, e.g. chenic acid, appear to bind to a greater extent than the trihydroxy-forms, e.g. glycocholic acid. This can be demonstrated using small amounts of kidney beans, string beans and potato. Bile acid binding could be of clinical significance in patients with ileal resection. To illustrate this problem patients with 28–60 cm of terminal ileum resected were fed either a solid diet containing vegetables, fruit, meat and eggs and including non-digestible fibre (about 5 g per day) or an isocaloric non-residue mixture of corn oil, dextrose, egg white and flavouring. Both cholic and chenic acids were absorbed more efficiently in patients on the liquid diet while chenic acid was preferentially found bound to the stools of patients on fibre-containing diets.

In the normal subject, the handling of both fat and protein is modified by dietary fibre. When whole-wheat products such as bran are fed faecal fat rises, although not pathologically. The question arises as to whether this represents an alteration of fat digestion and absorption directly or an association between fibre and fat (and its products) in such a way as to make it unavailable for absorption. At least part of the answer is that fatty acids and fibre combine so that there is malabsorption of the former.

Faecal nitrogen excretion rises also when whole-wheat products are fed. Possible explanations are:

(a) an increased endogenous nitrogen excretion;
(b) the presence of unavailable protein complexes formed as a result of cooking or other pretreatment of food;
(c) an interference of normal pathways of protein digestion.

Plant fibres have been shown to inhibit *in vitro* activity of both trypsin and chymotrypsin.

Carbohydrate absorption is also modified by dietary fibre. In fact, it has been suggested that a fibre-deficient diet may be related to the development of diabetes mellitus. Certainly, this condition is rare in communities consuming high-fibre diets. Furthermore, the addition of certain dietary fibre to a breakfast of bread and butter, marmalade and tea flattened blood glucose responses and significantly lowered serum insulin levels in healthy voluntees (Kg 6.6). The inference for the diabetic patient is obvious. When eight non-insulin requiring patients were offered the breakfast with or without dietary fibre their glucose levels were better controlled after the fibre-containing meal. Indeed, some who tested positive for urinary glucose one or two hours after the control meal excreted a glucose-free urine after ingesting the meal with added fibre.

The question remains as to how dietary fibre might alter carbohydrate absorption. Increasing the viscosity of the gut contents is probably the most important effect it produces, causing glucose absorption to take place over a longer period of time. Greater viscosity may slow the rate of absorption by :

1. Reducing gastric emptying. The stomach empties its contents more slowly when viscous fibre such as pectin and guar gum is added.
2. Thickening the unstirred water layer and decreasing the accessibility of the absorptive surface to nutrients.

3. Decreasing pancreatic enzyme activity. Enzyme–substrate interactions may be reduced because of the increased viscosity and more acidic nature of the luminal contents.

Earlier in this chapter is was pointed out that haemorrhoids could be eased with a fibre-containing diet. How? Defaecation should be almost effortless. Soft bulky stools should be expelled in response to contractions of the gut and not by muscles of the abdominal wall. If too little residue is present, the gut cannot act effectively, and voluntary straining is necessary. Straining in the presence of relaxed anal sphincters is regarded as the cause of haemorrhoids. Thus haemorrhoids should be largely preventable by providing dietary fibre.

Dietary alterations, e.g. a change from white to wholemeal bread are considered to be useful measures. Not only are these measures proposed as a preventive policy, but surgeons are now finding that some patients with less advanced haemorrhoids, awaiting admission to hospital and provided with fibre, do not subsequently require inpatient treatment. Burkitt and Graham-Stewart (in 1975) made the observation that Napoleon at Waterloo was troubled by piles.

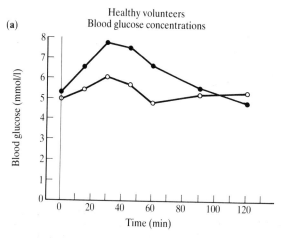

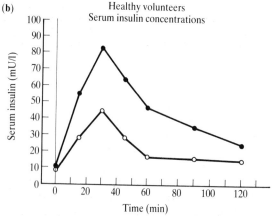

(c)

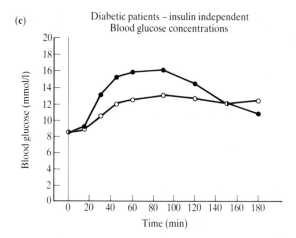

Diabetic patients – insulin independent
Blood glucose concentrations

(d)

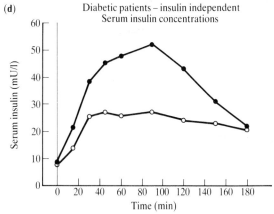

Diabetic patients – insulin independent
Serum insulin concentrations

Fig. 6.6 Blood glucose (**a** and **c**) and serum insulin concentrations (**b** and **d**) after a breakfast consisting of bread and butter, marmalade and tea. It was taken by normal healthy volunteers (**a** and **b**), and by eight non-insulin requiring patients with diabetes mellitus who were managed either by diet or diet and hypoglycaemic drugs (**c** and **d**). The control experiments (●–●) were those in which the breakfast alone was taken. A second study was conducted in which 10 g pectin was added to the marmalade and 16 g guar flour to the bread (o–o). (Data redrawn from Jenkins, D.G.A., Leeds, A.R., Gassull, M.A., Cochet, B. and Alberti, K.G.M.M. (1977). *Annals of Internal Medicine* **86**, 20–23; and Jenkins, D.G.A., Leeds, A.R., Gassull, M.A. *et al.* (1977). *Lancet* **ii**, 172–4.)

They posed the question as to whether or not a pound of bran incorporated into the French commander's larder might have altered the course of history.

It has been recognized that colonic cancer is more prevalent among Western communities than in those of rural Africa. A major cause of this is thought to be the fibre-depleted diets of the former group. This possibility gains support when one considers the different groups within particular countries. For example, the Seventh-Day Adventists in the USA, who are predominantly vegetarians, have a lower incidence of colonic cancer than many of the omnivores around them.

Fibre-rich diets may give protection by diluting the colonic contents because of the increased residue from fibre and by reducing the transit time. In this way, the concentrations of any carcinogens and the time available for their syntheses would be limited. Some dietary fibre may also provide protection against chemically induced tumours by absorbing potentially harmful agents. This is one means by which wheat bran reduces the incidence of colonic carcinoma in rats exposed to 1,2-dimethylhydrazine (DMH).

Finally, another area in which dietary fibre has excited many workers has been obesity. Obesity is uncommon among populations where calories are consumed as vegetables undepleted of their fibre content. The ways in which dietary fibre might contribute to the prevention of excessive energy intake are that fibres:

1. Reduce the calorie density of the diet.
2. Slow the rate at which ingestion of calories can occur.
3. Interfere with the efficiency of absorption of energy-containing compounds.
4. May promote satiety by adding volume to the postprandial gastrointestinal contents. As regards the latter, it is known that dietary fibre sequesters water and swells. If it fills the stomach sufficiently, it may suppress meal size and prolong the length of intervals between meals.

Intestinal microflora

The normal human organism is composed of more than 10^{14} cells. Of these, only about 10% are animal cells. The majority are microbial, colonizing the various body surfaces and the gastrointestinal tract. Thus man has evolved an intimate association with micro-organisms. In 1885 Pasteur went as far as to say that life without microbes would be impossible. The subsequent rearing of germ-free animals would appear, at first sight, to contradict this view. However, germ-free animals, which must be maintained in isolation, are morphologically, physiologically and immunologically ill equipped to survive normal environments and readily succumb to infection. The development of gastrointestinal flora is considered to be essential for the transition from the germ-free existence of the fetus *in utero* to an independent life.

The stomach, duodenum, jejunum and upper ileum have a sparse microflora consisting of Gram-positive facultative organisms, e.g. streptococci, aerobic lactobacilli and fungi. Their total concentration is generally less than 10^4 per ml luminal content. Many are derived from the mouth. The stomach provides an important barrier to microbial overgrowth. Most ingested species are destroyed by gastric acid, although other factors may be involved. Thus the stomach contents of suckling rabbits are usually devoid of living micro-organisms despite a high pH (5.7–6.0) which would normally favour the development of an abundant alimentary flora. It has been suggested that a substrate in rabbit's milk, together with an enzyme secreted by the stomach results in the production of antimicrobial activity.

The distal ileum in about one-third of normal individuals maintains the same meagre flora. However, in the majority of subjects Gram-negative micro-organisms, e.g. aerobic coliforms, start to appear. Across the ileocaecal region a striking change in numbers and types of micro-organisms can be observed (Table 6.2). In the colon the anaerobic population can outnumber the aerobic and facultative flora by more than $10^3:1$. More than 99% of the total bacteria in human faeces (10^{11} per g) are non-sporing, anaerobic rod-shaped organisms. The major species are *Bacteroides fragilis*, *Bifidobacterium aduloscentis* and *Eubacterium narofaciens*. The remainder are mainly *Escherichia coli*, *Streptococcus viridans*, *Streptococcus salivarius* and *Lactobacilli*. In addition, there is a host of minor components.

A count of these organisms, however, may not reflect the distribution of those growing in close association with the mucosal surface. Some microbes adhere physically to the surface with which they associate. Others may enter and remain in an area because they are mobile and are attracted by chemotaxis. Most indigenous micro-organisms associate with the mucosal surfaces in such a way that the epithelium is not altered architecturally by the interaction. An exception in human colon is where spirochetes change the histological appearance.

The numbers and types of organisms are regulated by many factors, some exerted by the host, others by the microbes themselves. For example, a major defence against overpopulation by bacteria is intestinal peristalsis. Race, climate and sex are not regarded as major influences on the flora although polar bear faeces in the Arctic have been reported sterile. When polar bears were transferred to a more temperate zone a faecal flora was observed.

The sterility of the faeces could have been due to a dietary rather than a climatic factor. For example, Antarctic birds have a sparse enteric flora. This has been attributed to the birds consuming algae containing acrylic acid, an antimicrobial substance. In several instances, diet can be seen to modify the bacterial population. In patients with massive bowel resection large quantities of unabsorbed nutrients may reach the colon. In a patient with less than 30 cm small bowel remaining and fed a high-carbohydrate, low-fat diet, Broitman

Table 6.2 Bacterial flora of the lower intestine in man (From Hill, M. J. and Drasar, B. S. (1975). *Gut* **16**, 318–23.)

Species	Mean $\log_{10}$ viable count per g intestinal material		
	Terminal ileum	Caecum	Faeces
Enterobacteria	3.3	6.2	7.4
Enterococci	2.2	3.6	5.6
Lactobacilli	<2.0	6.4	6.5
Clostridia	<2.0	3.0	5.4
Bacteroides	5.7	7.8	9.8
Gram-positive non-sporing anaerobes (Eubacteria and Bifidobacteria)	5.8	8.4	10.0
No. of samples	6	2	100

and his colleagues (in 1966) measured the microflora during the post-operative recovery period. The totals per gram faeces were:

Anaerobes	10^9
Lactobacilli	10^8
Coliforms	10^5
Yeast (saccharomyces)	10^8

Three months later, by which time carbohydrate and protein absorption had improved, the coliforms had gradually replaced the yeast populations.

Low concentrations of unconjugated bile acids inhibit growth of some microflora. Such bile acids are to be found in the colon as a result of bacterial metabolism and may regulate the composition of the flora in that region.

Microbial populations undoubtedly exert strong forces to maintain their communities. These forces may include the formation of bacteriocins and toxic end products, such as SCFAs, e.g. butyric and propionic acids. Bacteriocins are highly specific protein macromolecules produced by various organisms which are capable of destroying members of their own or closely related species. For example, colicins are elaborated by some *Escherichia coli* and cause death by interfering with metabolism rather than bacteriolysis after their adsorption to specific receptor sites on susceptible cell surfaces. Interestingly colicinogenic *Escherichia coli* persisted in normal individuals over a 6-month period while other non-colicinogenic *Escherichia coli* disappeared. Bacterial metabolism may promote as well as inhibit the growth of other species. For example, facultative bacteria, which can grow either aerobically or anaerobically, utilize oxygen and thus help to provide an environment in which sensitive anaerobic bacteria can survive.

In what ways do the bacteria modify the intestines? Morphologically, the intestines of a germ-free animal are not the same as those of the conventional animal. The lymphoid tissue is poorly developed and inflammatory cells of the lamina propria are virtually absent in the former. This may contribute to the increased susceptibility of the germ-free animal to infection. Furthermore, the villi of the small intestine are taller and show an absence of degenerative changes in the lining epithelia. The walls of the caecum are extremely thick and elastic.

A number of examples of bacterial involvement in physiological functions of the body can be found in other parts of the book. Thus the metabolism of bilirubin to urobilinogens (see page 103), the conversion of primary conjugated bile acids to secondary unconjugated bile acids (see page 99) and gas production (see page 225) will not be considered here. Microflora contribute further by the degradation of endogenous proteins, e.g. digestive enzymes, mucoproteins and cellular debris. Trypsin and invertase are excreted in the faeces of germ-free animals, and it is suggested that the normal flora rather than autodigestion play a major role in the inactivation of some digestive enzymes.

Intestinal bacteria are also able to synthesize vitamins, e.g. K, B_{12}, thiamin and riboflavin. Formation of the first mentioned is particularly important as the amount of the vitamin in foods ingested is normally insufficient. Furthermore, vitamin K is lipid soluble and can be absorbed by the large intestine. With dietary deficiencies, blood clotting is abnormal in the germ-free animal. For example, conventional and germ-free rats have been fed vitamin K-deficient diets. All the germ-free animals had hypoprothrombinaemia, many were found to have haemorrhages at autopsy and several died. None of the conventional animals showed any of these symptoms. On the other hand, disturbances in coagulation of germ-free animals could be alleviated by transferring the animals to a contaminated environment.

While the intestinal microflora play vital roles in the development and survival of the host, they can exert deleterious effects by utilizing the luminal nutrients so that they are unavailable to the host and by causing mild forms of toxaemias. In addition, the question is being asked as to whether the intestinal bacteria are involved in the genesis of colonic and rectal cancers. Such malignancies are among the most common in both males and females, accounting for approximately 20% of deaths caused by malignant disease in the USA. The view has been expressed that the microflora may convert the bile acids to potentially co-carcinogenic compounds. In support of this concept is the finding of a positive correlation between faecal levels of steroid metabolites and the population risk of colonic cancer. Further, in experiments with rats (Table 6.3) intrarectal administration of taurodeoxycholic or lithocholic acids was found to increase the frequency of colonic cancer in the presence of a carcinogen (N-methyl-N[1]-nitro-N-nitrosoguanidine).

Bacteria may also initiate neoplastic changes by metabolizing relatively inactive compounds to more toxic forms. Such procarcinogens may be present in the diet as natural products, food preservatives, dyes, food additives or pollutants. How might the microflora act? Several possibilities should be considered. One of these involves a contribution of either β-glucosidases or β-glucuronidases. Both are widely distributed within the microflora. The former enzyme is thought to contribute to the production of mutagenic agents when human faecal bacteria are incubated with tea or red wine. Bacterial β-glucosidases can also hydrolyse cycasin, the β-glucoside of methylazoxymethanol. This glycoside, found in cycad gymnosperms, is not carcinogenic in germ-free animals.

Table 6.3 The incidence of tumours in the distal colon and rectum of rats in response to N-methyl-N[1]-nitrosoguanidine (MNNG) and the increase in frequency observed when lithocholic acid (LC) or taurodeoxycholic acid (TC) is administered. MNNG was given intrarectally as a single dose (4 mg in suspension). LC and TC (1 mg doses in 0.5 ml peanut oil) were administered five times a week for thirteen months. There were sixteen ♂ and sixteen ♀ rats (6–7 weeks old) in each group initially (From Narisawa, T., Magadia, N. E. Weisburger, J. H. and Wynder, E. L. (1974). *Journal of the National Cancer Institute* **53**, 318–23.)

Treatment group	No. of rats with neoplasms	Total no. of neoplasms
LC	0	0
TC	0	0
MNNG + LC	15	30
MNNG + TC	18	28
MNNG	8	10

However, following hydrolysis the parent aglycone can induce tumours in both conventional and germ-free rats. Glucuronidases remove glucuronic acid from numerous potentially toxic compounds secreted from the liver into bile. Thus the polycyclic hydrocarbon benzo(a)pyrene, found in charcoal-broiled meats, may appear in bile in a conjugated form, but subsequently be hydrolysed to mutagenic products.

Recently, other mutagens produced by faecal bacteria have generated interest. These are fecapentaenes (FPs) and 2-amino-3,6-dihydro-3 methyl-7H-imidazo(4,5-f)quinoline-7-one (7-OH-IQ). FPs are produced mainly by Bacteriodes. These agents induce considerable genetic damage of human cells in culture, e.g. lymphocytes. Information is anxiously awaited as to the effect of FPs on colonic epithelial cells and the identity of the precursors from which they are produced. It is not known whether they are derived from dietary components gastrointestinal secretions or intestinal bacteria. They are not produced in all human faeces. The other bacterial metabolite, 7-OH-IQ, can be detected in the faeces of volunteers ingesting meals rich in fried meat. Its mutagenic properties have been recorded using Salmonella, and its derivatives induce tumours of the large intestine in rats and mice. The activity of 7-OH-IQ, however, on mammalian cells remains to be tested.

Gastrointestinal gas

Carbon dioxide, hydrogen, oxygen, methane and nitrogen make up more than 99 per cent of the gastrointestinal gases. The proportion of these gases can vary widely, as can be seen by examining Table 6.4. The data presented were obtained from an analysis of the intestinal luminal contents using an argon washout technique.

Note the low oxygen content. All the gases above are without smell, so that traces of other gases must be present to provide the mixture issuing from the anus with its frequently unpleasant odour. Thus ammonia, hydrogen sulphide, indole, skatole (the 3-methyl derivative of indole) SCFAs, and volatile amines

Table 6.4   The major constituents of intestinal gas in man. Eleven healthy male subjects were intubated with mercury-weighted polyvinyl tubes. The tube was allowed to pass 105 cm from the teeth, a distance usually just beyond the ligament of Treitz in the proximal jejunum. The stomach was constantly aspirated through a second tube to prevent swallowed air from entering the intestines. Argon bubbled through water was then infused through the intestinal tube at a rate of 45 ml/min. Gas appearing in the rectum was collected and anaylsed (From Levitt, M. D. (1971). *New England Journal of Medicine* **284**, 1394–8.)

Gas	Percentage
N_2	26–88
CO_2	5.5–27
CH_4	0–20
H_2	0.2–49
O_2	0.1–1.8

can be detected. In a fasting man, the mean intestinal volume is about 100 ml (range 30–200 ml) while in normal subjects 500 ml per day (range 300–2000 ml per day) can be collected via a rectal tube. There are three sources of intestinal gas:

(a) swallowed air;
(b) production in the lumen as a result of either neutralization of acid or bacterial metabolism;
(c) diffusion into the lumen from the blood (only a small contribution).

In the stomach, the gas mixture closely resembles expired air in composition (N_2 = 79 per cent, O_2 = 17 per cent and CO_2 = 4 per cent). Each time one swallows, approximately 2–3 ml air enters the stomach. A greater volume may be swallowed while eating and drinking. In addition, some air is found in food either as a result of processing, e.g. bread, or in its structure, e.g. 20 per cent of the volume of an apple is gas.

Little gas is normally present in the small intestine. This does not mean, however, that the gas volumes passing through the small intestine are insignificant. For example, in 1973 Fordtran and Walsh suggested that the normal stomach produces approximately 30 mmol acid per hour after a meal. If this acid were to be neutralised completely by the bicarbonate secretions from the liver and pancreas, a considerable volume of CO_2 would be liberated.

$$HCl + HCO_3^- \rightarrow CO_2 + H_2O + Cl^-$$

1 mol acid is associated with 22.4 litres CO_2
∴ 30 mmol acid is associated with $22.4 \times 30/1000$ = 0.672 litres

An additional source of acid is dietary fat. Suppose 20 g fat are ingested in a meal. If one assumes the molecular weight of a triglyceride to be about 900 and its hydrolysis within the intestinal lumen to be two-thirds complete, then the neutralization of the fatty acid with bicarbonate will be associated with the release of nearly 1.5 litres of carbon dioxide. Fortunately, this gas can be readily absorbed by the small intestine and excessive distension does not take place.

Bacterial fermentation processes are regarded as major sources of colonic gas. Hydrogen is not excreted by either the germ-free rat or new born infants. For this gas to be produced, a supply of protein or carbohydrate is required. Thus in the fasting human subject hydrogen production is low. A number of non-absorbable substances which can be utilized by colonic bacteria are present in a variety of foodstuffs, e.g. beans contain stachyose, a tetrasaccharide (-D-galactosyl (1→6)--D-galactosyl (1→6)--D-glucosyl (1→2)--D-fructoside) which is not hydrolysed by intestinal enzymes. Other dietary components regularly causing excessive gas production because they contain carbohydrates resistant to man's digestive enzymes include onions, cabbage, brussel sprouts, prunes and nuts. Subjects eating them may complain of cramping abdominal pain and borborygmi (the crushing and explosive sounds produced by gases in the gastrointestinal tract). Methane is excreted by only one-third of the population. Some believe that dietary factors are unimportant for its production and that there is a familial tendency to harbour methane-producing organisms.

Although uncommon, malabsorption is an important cause of excessive production, e.g. flatulence may accompany malabsorption of lactose. In this case, disaccharidase deficiency results in the availability of lactose to colonic bacteria. In fact a convenient means of establishing lactose intolerance is to measure the output of hydrogen in the breath after lactose ingestion.

Both hydrogen and methane are combustible and in the presence of oxygen provide a potentially explosive mixture. A spark from an electrosurgical device could lead to extensive colonic perforation. Indeed, explosions, one fatal, have been reported. These have led surgeons to question the practice of asking their patients to drink 10 per cent mannitol as a means of bowel preparation. Mannitol, a sugar alcohol, is poorly absorbed by man. However, it can be metabolized by bacteria and may lead to the production of dangerous amounts of hydrogen. Certainly the gas content of the colon, as estimated by the measurement of colonic gas shadows, is greater in patients drinking mannitol solutions than in those drinking saline or treated with castor oil. At least the problem has been recognized. Several measures have been taken to minimize the risks. These include:

1. Fasting the patients prior to endoscopy. This is a normal procedure whereby faecal bulk is reduced. At the same time less hydrogen is produced.
2. Giving enemas and cathartics which remove hydrogen- and methane-forming bacteria and helps to lower the concentrations of these gases towards safe levels.
3. Perfusing the lumen with inert gases. The routine insufflation of CO_2 has been recommended for polypectomy.

Furthermore it has been proposed that a knife rather than diathermy should be used to incise the bowel even when it appears to be completely clean. The risk of an explosion is not limited to the large intestine. A recent diathermy-elicited accident during gastrotomy has been reported in a patient with ileal obstruction resulting from ischaemia. The explosion was attributed to bacterial proliferation and the production of combustible gases not normally found in the stomach and small intestine.

Motor function of the colon

The motor function of the colon is to continue the mixing of the luminal contents arriving from the distal ileum and to propel them eventually towards the anus. NB. The contents entering the human colon are liquid and not semi-solid as many research workers, who have observed the consistency of the material in rat ileum, might have expected. While in the colon, most of the water arriving there is absorbed and the residual matter becomes solid, although not hard. The contents reaching the large intestine remain in this region for longer periods of time than in other parts of the alimentary tract. Passage through the stomach and small intestine seldom takes longer than twelve hours. However, it can take many hours more before the residue is finally excreted as faeces. This has been investigated by administering tiny, coloured glass beads in gelatine capsules to volunteers and subsequently recovering them from the stools. It was concluded that residues from a meal can be retained in the colon for a week or more, although normally 80 per cent have been extruded by the end of the fourth day. The time taken for the first appearance of ingested material in the faeces varies remarkably.

In a study of 150 young adult males given carmine in capsules, this time varied between 6.5 and 98 hours. These extremes might be interpreted as data from subjects with diarrhoea on the one hand and constipation on the other. However, the subjects could not be categorized thus.

The question remains as to the types of movement that can be recorded in the large intestine. As in the small bowel, a number of terms have been introduced to describe the processes by which residues are mixed and propelled. These include haustral shuttling, segmental propulsion, multihaustral propulsion and peristalsis. The former is the most frequently observed in the fasting subject and results from apparently random contractions of circular muscle. As a result of these contractions, the mucosa is folded into sacs which form and reform at different sites and the luminal contents are shuttled in either direction. Such movements are not propulsive, but the contents are slowly kneaded or mixed.

Segmental propulsion occurs when the haustral contents are displaced towards the anus through several haustra without being returned. Movements in the reverse direction have frequently been described as well. Multihaustral propulsion occurs when several segments contract virtually simultaneously and propel their contents distally. The region receiving these contents may contract in a similar manner or, as less frequently occurs, reform their haustra.

Peristaltic movement has already been described in the oesophagus, stomach and small intestine. In the colon, a progressive wave of contraction behind the contents pushes them slowly caudad (1–2 cm/min). As might be anticipated, the muscle preceding the contractile wave is relaxed.

Propulsive movements can result in the colonic contents passing caudad at approximately 8 cm/h. However, events propelling the contents in the reverse direction result in a net forward movement of about 5 cm/h.

Several types of muscular activity have been described above. Are these found throughout the large intestine or are different regions characterized by particular movements? In man, retrograde peristalsis, ring contractions moving cephalad, is the dominant activity of the proximal colon. Segmentation, either stationary or progressive over short distances in either direction, is the common event in the transverse and descending colon. Infrequently, a powerful ring contraction moving caudad occurs in the transverse and descending colon also. One should ask how and when these different patterns of contraction are induced, and what controls them. A possible approach in an attempt to answer these questions would be to measure the electrical changes that occur in colonic smooth muscle. Such measurements in the stomach and small intestine have contributed appreciably to our understanding of the motor functions of these tissues. Electrical signals (BER or slow waves - see pages 66 and 178) were found to be responsible for the timing of contractions. Slow waves can be recorded in the colon but they are different from those recorded in more proximal regions:

1. Their frequencies are faster than those generated in the stomach but slower than in the small intestine. Approximately 4.5 and 6 cycles per minute have been recorded *in vitro* from cat proximal and distal colon respectively.

Similarly, human distal colon, *in situ*, produces about 6 cycles per minute.

2. Slow waves are generated in the submucosal border of the colon's circular muscle layer and not in the longitudinal layer, or cells lining its boundary, as occurs in other regions (see page 187). Slow waves spread quickly around the circumference and slowly along the length of the colon.

3. Slow waves in the small intestine migrate caudad. This contrasts with what has been reported in the colon. In the proximal colon slow waves originating in the ascending colon close to the hepatic flexure migrate cephalad. One might have anticipated such an event as retrograde peristalsis is the major contractile feature of this region. Slow waves and antiperistaltic contractions must, presumably, be reversed at times for the proximal colon to be emptied towards the rectum. Occasionally the reversal of slow waves *in vitro* can be observed. What initiates this is not known. Beyond the hepatic flexure slow waves tend to migrate caudad although movements in both directions are recorded.

4. Unlike the small intestine, the circular and longitudenal muscle layers of the colon have different electrical activities. Slow waves can be monitored in the circular muscle. However, the cable characteristics of circular muscle provides a barrier against the migration of slow waves to the longitudinal muscle. As a result electrical changes not associated with slow waves can be observed. These are described as periods of membrane high frequency potential oscillations (about 41 cycles per minute), lasting for about 12 seconds, which lead to action potentials and muscle contractions. These changes are dependent on stimuli such as stretch. The involvement of intrinsic cholinergic nerves is indicated by the finding that spontaneous activity of longitudenal muscle *in vitro* is inhibited by TTX and atropine.

5. The slow waves in the circular muscle layers appear to be capable of generating contractions themselves. Small rhythmic contractions are commonly recorded accompanying slow waves without the occurrence of bursts of action potentials (spike bursts) that usually correlate with muscle contractions. Furthermore, contractions can take place over several slow wave cycles. The duration of slow waves is not constant (Fig. 6.7) and is increased by cholinergic agents, substance P, pentagastrin and CCK octapeptide. Slow waves developing spontaneously or evoked by acetylcholine are associated with action potential-independent strong contractions. It has been suggested that the slow waves as well as serving their classical role of timing contractions, can also provide sufficient depolarization to induce excitation:contraction coupling. NB. The finding that atropine decreases the duration of the slow wave, and that TTX subsequently causes a further shortening implies that slow waves are modified by the spontaneous activity of both cholinergic and non-cholinergic intrinsic excitatory fibres.

Control of colonic movements

Colonic contractile activity is influenced by at least four factors. These are the intrinsic smooth muscle properties, intrinsic nerves and circulating or locally

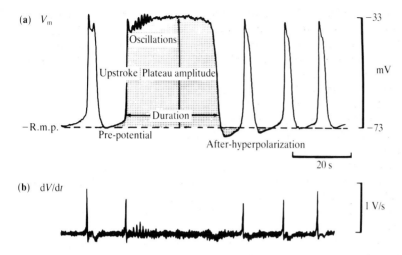

Fig. 6.7 Characteristics of variable slow waves in the circular muscle of canine proximal colon. (*a*) Changes in membrane potential (V_m) associated with a series of spontaneous slow waves. (*b*) The rate of change (dV/dt) of membrane potentials recorded in (*a*). It should be noted that many cells exhibit a slow depolarization (prepotential) between slow waves as distinct from a constant resting membrane potential (Rmp). The plateau phases of slow waves are of variable duration (2–40 secs) and some show oscillations. The two slow waves following the slow wave of longer duration are associated with after-hyperpolarization. Furthermore, their uptake velocities are reduced when compared with the first spontaneous slow wave on the trace (From Sanders, K.M. and Smith, T.K. (1986). *Journal of Physiology* **377**, 297–313.)

released chemicals. The electrical signals generated in smooth muscle have already been referred to. These coordinate and indeed can induce colonic contractions. Muscle of the large intestine exhibits automaticity and responds to stretch by contracting. If muscle shortening is not possible an increase in tension can be recorded. A study with strips of human colonic muscle has recently been published (Fig. 6.8). The results show that the active tension curves of both circular and longitudinal muscle in the ascending and transverse colon are less affected by length changes than those of the descending and sigmoid colon. The contractile frequencies of strips of circular muscle from the right colon (6.25 per min) were almost twice that of strips from the left colon (3.35 per min). These data are consistent with the view that the right colon is more distensible than the descending and sigmoid colon and that it functions as a reservoir in which temporary storage, mixing and absorption of the luminal contents and bacterial fermentation can take place.

Despite the automaticity of colonic smooth muscle the intrinsic nervous system is essential for its normal functioning. This is illustrated by Hirschsprung's and Chagas' diseases. In the former, intramural ganglion cells are missing from a narrowed distal part of colon. The result is that, if sufficient colon is affected, the coordinated propulsive activity of the normal bowel is unable to propel the contents through the aganglionic segment. This leads to severe constipation and, if untreated, many deaths from perforation of the colon or enterocolitis. Chagas' disease, prevalent in South America, is caused by infection with *Trypanosoma cruzi*. The trypanosomes live in the wall of the viscera and apparently produce an agent that destroys intramural ganglion cells. The clinical picture resembles Hirschsprung's disease and treatment depends on the resection of the aganglionic segment. However, the whole colon is likely to be infected and, in contrast to Hirschsprung's disease, a recurrence is not unexpected.

It has been appreciated that the intrinsic or enteric nervous system is not

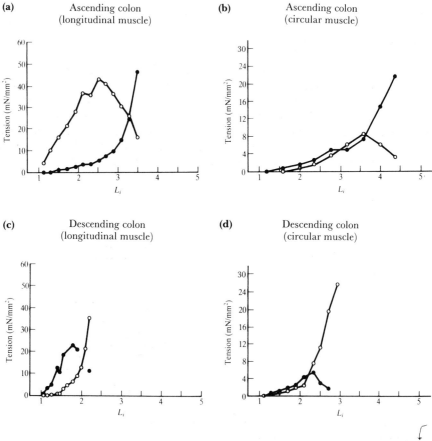

Fig. 6.8 Spontaneous contractile activity and response to stretch, *in vitro*, of human colonic muscle. Strips of muscle were allowed to equilibrate in a Krebs–Ringer solution for 30 minutes. The length of each strip was then measured. The longitudinally and circularly oriented strips used were 10–15 mm and 8–10 mm respectively. After equilibration the strips were stretched by 1 mm every 15 minutes. As the muscle was stretched a length was reached at which baseline tension increased. (This tension then decreased over a 5 minute period to a constant value as the strip, at least partially, accommodated to its new length.) The length of the muscle strip at which baseline tension first increased was taken as the initial length Li. In these experiments changes in active (○) and passive (●) tension are expressed in mN/mm^2 and related to *Li*. Active tension was calculated as the difference between the maximum and minimum force during a cycle of contractions (Redrawn from Gill, R.C., Cote, K.R., Bowes, K.L. and Kingma, Y.J. (1986). *Gut* **27**, 1006–13.)

simply a relay station for signals from extrinsic sympathetic and parasympathetic nerves. Certainly it can perform that function. However, it is also an independent, integrative system possessing the circuitry to process information from sensory receptors (and the CNS) and generate precise patterns of neural output to effector organs (Fig. 6.9). It eliminates the requirement for long neural pathways between the gastointestinal tract and the CNS and allows corrections of gut functions to be made continuously and discretely. J.D. Wood has recommended that the enteric nervous system should regarded as an 'intelligent terminal' in a computer based system, providing a microprocessor in close proximity to the gut, programming its behaviour and automatically making adjustments. The main computer (or CNS) also monitors sensory information and issues commands to the gut which are appropriate for the overall state of the individual.

A number of colonic reflexes can be accounted for by the enteric nervous system. The neural mechanisms for both segmenting contractions and peristalsis are thought to exist within the gut wall. Thus, for example, when the mucosal surface is mechanically stimulated, an increased force of contraction can be measured proximal to the point of stimulation. This can also be recorded in the colon of a dog following the removal of its extrinsic nerve supply. In contrast, there is inhibition of muscular activity at sites distal to the stimulus.

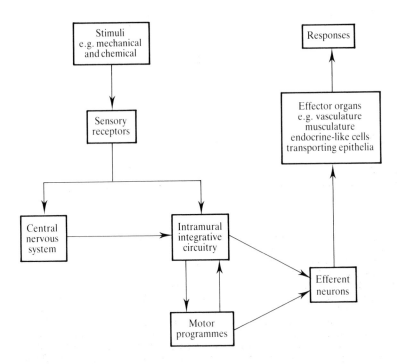

Fig. 6.9 The concept of the enteric nervous system

Extrinsic nerves undoubtedly modify the movements of the large intestine. Thus sectioning the extrinsic nerves abolishes the inhibition of motility resulting from distending or handling the intestine. This reflex response, the colo-colonic inhibitory reflex, is similar to that described by Bayliss and Starling (1899) in the small intestine and subsequently called the intestino-intestinal inhibitory reflex. A demonstration that extrinsic nerves are important for a reflex reaction does not necessarily mean that the CNS makes a contribution. This point is illustrated by the finding that a colo-colonic inhibitory reflex can be elicited *in vitro* provided that prevertebral ganglia (coeliac, superior and inferior mesenteric) and their nerve connections are intact. The inhibitory response can be observed in proximal segments when those more distally located are stimulated and vice versa. It has been concluded that neural circuitry exists for extrinsic reflexes which are independent of the CNS. Thus prevertebral ganglia, as well as ganglia in the wall of the gut, are not simply relay stations for impulses from the spinal cord to effector organs (Fig. 6.10).

Both sympathetic and parasympathetic nerves can influence motility. Their effects, however, have been difficult to assess particularly as excitatory and inhibitory neurons are found in both these branches of the autonomic nervous system. The excitatory effects of the parasympathetic nervous system can be seen when pelvic nerves are sectioned and the distal stump then stimulated.

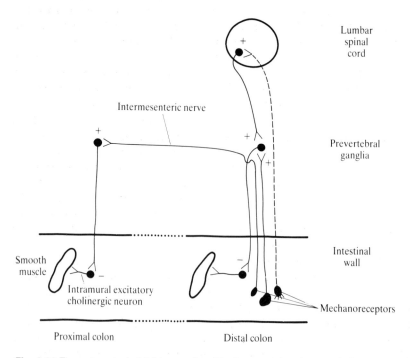

Fig. 6.10 The colo-colonic inhibitory reflex. The intramural excitatory cholinergic neurons are a part of the intrinsic network and stimulate the contraction of smooth muscle. By inhibiting their activity the motility of the colon is depressed. The symbols + and − represent stimulation and inhibition respectively

A role for the sympathetic fibres has been acknowledged for over half a century. In 1933, Garry noted that an interruption of the lumbar pathways to the colon enhanced its motility. This observation indicates a tonic inhibitory influence of sympathetic nerves. The origin of the sympathetic outflow, however, is undecided. One possibility is that it is generated by endogenous oscillator circuits in the lumbar spinal cord. Certainly supraspinal mechanisms are not essential as an inhibitory outflow remains after transection of the thoracic spinal cord (T10–T13). The efferent firing of the lumbar colonic nerves is enhanced by stretching the proximal colon. This effect is blocked by sectioning the lumbar dorsal roots. However, the spontaneous firing of the lumbar colonic nerves is independent of traditional reflex pathways because it is not influenced by destruction of lumbar dorsal roots. This has led to the view that either an endogenous oscillator exists or ventral root afferent pathways are involved. The question remains as to whether higher centres modify lumbar sympathetic activity. It appears that they do. Patients with high cord transection have reduced colonic motility. This has been interpreted as suggesting supraspinal facilitation of the spinal inhibitory centre. However, little is known of the mechanisms involved.

A clear picture of the role of extrinsic nerves and the CNS has yet to emerge. Several studies appear to be contradictory and the responses observed very variable. Nevertheless, the involvement of the CNS can be appreciated by the finding that in some subjects, emotion brings about motility changes. For example, Grace, Wolf and Wolff (1951) made observations of four patients with colostomies. In each case the colon had prolapsed through the original wound. They found that discussion evoking anger, resentment and hostility increased the activity of the prolapsed segment. One of the patients was easily depressed and on such occasions a pronounced inhibition of colonic motility was recorded. Cheering him up by talking about his hobbies increased the motor activity.

Not all people experience marked changes in colonic motility when faced with stressful, emotional situations. Nevertheless, many of my colleagues and I can be observed regularly making a visit to the toilet several minutes before delivering a lecture. Perhaps we belong to the group that has been described as the 'physiological overreactors'. The variable reactions recorded in the colon to a given stimulus are reminiscent of those encountered when one measures the responses of the cardiovascular system to stress. Those who have measured the changes in diastolic blood pressure when the human forearm is plunged into ice-cold water will readily agree.

Increased colonic motility has also been recorded after ingested food reaches then stomach. In man, at least, distension of the stomach alone is an ineffective stimulus. If, however, the energy content of a meal is increased, e.g. from 350 to 1000 Calories (from 1.5 to 4.2 MJ), colonic responses are magnified. The changes observed, i.e. increased frequency and amplitude of contractions of both proximal and distal colon, have been regarded as the result of a *gastrocolic reflex*. Leaders in the field of motility would like to see the term gastrocolic reflex abandoned. It represents an oversimplification of what actually takes place. Neural mechanisms do provide a major contribution, and patients with degenerative lesions of the nervous system no longer exhibit colonic responses to eating. However, hormones such as gastrin and CCK may also have excitatory roles to play. Colonic motility is significantly increased when gastrin is infused into normal human subjects at rates which maintain serum gastrin levels similar to those established after a meal. Increases are also observed when the octapeptide of CCK is continuously infused at rates submaximal for increasing gall-bladder contractions. Thus the response to eating may not be simply a nerve reflex. Furthermore, not only the stomach takes part. Patients with gastrectomies have increased colonic motor activity when fatty acids and amino acids are introduced into the duodenum.

There remains the question of luminal and circulating factors influencing large intestinal contractions. Numerous agents have been proposed to alter motility. However, their effects on the large intestine as a whole and their physiological significance are difficult to establish. In the ever increasing list of putative factors are fatty acids, SCFAs and secondary (but not primary) bile acids.

When lipids are infused into the proximal colon of human volunteers the oleic acid liberated can induce abnormal motility and accelerate colonic transit. Early defaecation is observed. These changes may well mirror what occurs in patients with steatorrhoea. Intraluminal SCFAs also stimulate contractions of the large bowel. They exert their effects at physiological concentrations on the distal colon. More proximal regions do not respond. The stimulatory effect is probably mediated by a local enteric reflex with sensory receptors close to the epithelial cell layer. It is abolished by scraping off the mucosa. A final example is provided by the secondary bile acids, e.g. deoxycholic acid. These, like SCFAs, are products of bacterial metabolism and also stimulate motor activity of the colon. The capacity of bile acids and SCFAs to increase both motility and secretion (see pages 102 and 212) suggests how larger and/or abnormal bacterial populations could result in diarrhoea. The increased propulsive activity caused by deoxycholic acid is blocked by the local anaesthetic procaine and by TTX, atropine and phentolamine but not by hexamethonium. Such observations suggest a complex neural pathway requiring intact muscarinic cholinergic and α-adrenergic neurons but not involving nicotinic synapses.

Defaecation

A simple picture

Usually the rectum is virtually empty. When propulsive movements cause the faeces to enter this region of the large intestine, the desire to defaecate is experienced. This desire can be induced experimentally by distending the rectum with a balloon. Sensory receptors are not restricted to the wall of the rectum. The near normal sensations of patients who have had the rectum removed with its place being taken by descending colon imply that nerve endings in the muscles of the pelvic floor can be stimulated and give rise to a call to stool. Distension initiates signals that spread over the myenteric plexus to cause peristaltic waves in the descending colon, sigmoid and rectum. Thus the faeces are forced towards the anus. As the peristaltic wave nears the anus, the internal anal sphincter relaxes. Normally this smooth muscle is tonically constricted. If the voluntarily controlled external anal sphincter is also relaxed, defaecation occurs. Defaecation is also assisted by relaxation of the puborectalis sling. Normally this muscle, attached to the symphysis pubis, pulls the junction of the rectum and the anal canal forwards. By doing so it creates the rectal angle which provides a resistance for the movement of luminal contents and is important for maintaining continence.

The defaecation reflex is regarded as the event occurring in the absence of CNS modification. That such a reflex can occur was established by the finding that men with various neurological lesions effectively separating the bowel from the CNS were capable of producing a normal response. However, this reflex is very weak and is fortified by a further reflex which includes the sacral spinal cord. When receptors in the rectum are stimulated, the signal is transmitted to the spinal cord and then back to the descending colon, sigmoid and rectum via parasympathetic fibres in the nervi erigentes. The result is that the waves of contraction are made more powerful. Other responses also occur when afferent impulses are transmitted from the rectum to the spinal cord and brain. These include straining movements in which, after a deep inspiration, the diaphragm is fixed and the abdominal and chest wall muscles are contracted while the glottis is closed (Valsalva manoeuvre). The result is a considerable rise in intra-abdominal (and intrathoracic) pressure. Pressures of up to 200 mm Hg act on the large intestine and assist in the expulsion of the faecal mass. At the same time, the pelvic floor is pulled outwards and upwards on the anus to evaginate the faeces downwards.

Accommodation and sampling responses

The defaecation responses referred to above are activated when relatively large amounts of material are present in the rectum. When smaller amounts enter, accommodation and sampling responses take place. This view is supported by the finding that at routine examination of the rectum there are often considerable amounts of faecal matter present even though the subject is not aware of it.

To study the effects of entry of material into the rectum, balloon techniques have been used (Fig. 6.11). Although sensory nerve endings in the anal canal are unavoidably stimulated by the presence of the tubing necessary for the inflation of the balloon and recording systems, this method has contributed significantly to our understanding. Only a small volume of gas (approximately 10 ml.) has to be introduced into a rectal balloon to produce a response. Initially, an increase in pressure within the rectal ampulla occurs, which is maintained for about a minute and then followed by a pressure decrease to preinflation levels. This adjustment is thought to consist of receptive relaxation of the rectal ampulla to accommodate the faecal mass. When greater volumes of air are introduced into the rectal balloon, the intrarectal pressure does not return to pre-inflation pressures and at a variable pressure the urge to defaecate is experienced, although this passes off within seconds as the rectum accommodates.

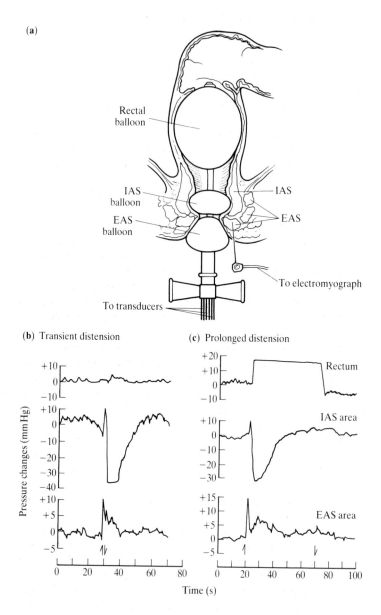

Fig. 6.11 (a) A technique for the simultaneous recording of pressures in the internal (IAS) and external anal sphincter (EAS) areas during distension of a rectal balloon. The activity of the external anal sphincter can also be measured electromyographically using a concentric needle electrode. (b) and (c) Responses of anal sphincter areas to transient (b) and prolonged (c) rectal distension. The arrows indicate the times when the rectal balloon was inflated (↑) and deflated (↓). Note the increase in pressure in the external anal sphincter area reflecting muscle contraction. In contrast, the internal anal sphincter relaxes. However, these responses are not maintained and with a prolonged distension tone returns to baseline levels before the stimulus has been released (From Schuster, M.M., Hookman, P., Hendrix, T.R. and Mendeloff, A.I. (1965). *Bulletin of the Johns Hopkins Hospital* **116**, 70–88.)

To appreciate the sampling of rectal contents one has to recognize the importance of:

(a) the mechanisms controlling the anal sphincters,
(b) the effect of reducing the degree of contraction of the internal anal sphincter, and
(c) the sensory receptors in the upper part of the anal canal.

At least part of the resting tone of the internal anal sphincter is myogenic. However, sympathetic nerves also have a role to play. Spinal anaesthesia (T6–T11) is accompanied by a decrease in the anal canal pressure. It appears that in man parasympathetic nerves do not have a direct effect on resting tone nor do supraspinal structures. The pressures recorded in control subjects and in patients with transection between C6 and L1 are identical.

The external anal sphincter depends on neural control via the pudendal nerve. This striated muscle is unique in that it is continually active and not electrically silent. Tonic contractions can be detected even during sleep. Furthermore, except on one occasion, tone increases when any activity raises the intra-abdominal pressure, e.g. coughing, laughing and lifting weights. The one situation when sphincter tone does not increase is during an attempt to defaecate. The external anal sphincter can also be voluntarily controlled, at least for a limited period of time.

When the rectum is distended transient responses can be induced in man (Fig. 6.11). These responses provide time for sampling and accommodation, and for decisions to be made whereby, if necessary, the subject can reach a socially acceptable site before the urge to defaecate becomes overwhelming. Even in normal, healthy subjects an urgent call to stool occasionally threatens continence. In diarrhoeal states the threat is more frequently experienced. It is important to remember that the contractions of the external anal sphincter are not maintained. Even if 'the alarm is raised' and subjects consciously constrict this voluntary muscle, the squeeze produced by the contraction can be held only for some 40–60 seconds.

Relaxation of the internal anal sphincter accompanied by contraction of the external anal sphincter allows the rectal contents to come into contact with the sensory epithelium of the canal to a level 1.5 cm cranial to the anal valves. Nerve endings associated with touch, temperature and pain have been located in this region. When the urge to defaecate is experienced, conscious sampling of the contents can be achieved by slightly increasing the abdominal pressure and increasing the activity of the external anal sphincter. If the hips are extended so that the angle between the rectum and the anal canal is maintained, then solids can be retained while gas is expelled and the intrarectal pressure is relieved. If fluid is present, conscious activity ensures the closure of the external anal sphincter until rectal accommodation develops. Thus continence is maintained.

Two mechanisms have been proposed to account for the relaxation internal anal sphincter in response to rectal distension. One involves a tion of sympathetic tone (Fig. 6.12), the other a non-cholinergic, non-a mechanism acting more directly on the sphincter. The relaxati

(a)

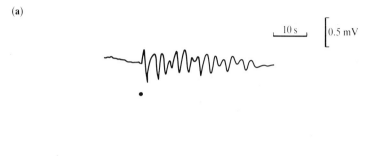

(b)

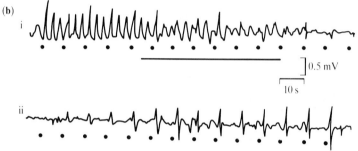

Fig. 6.12 Rectal distension inhibits the electrical activity of cat internal anal sphincter induced by sympathetic nerves *in vivo*. (**a**) An electromyogram (emg) of sphincter muscle when a single stimulus (1 ms; 10 V), indicated by the dot (●), is given to the hypogastric nerve. (**b**) The effect of rectal distension (black bar) on the emg of sphincter muscle during hypogastric nerve stimulation (single shocks: 1 ms; 15 V given at times indicated by the dots (●). (i) and (ii) represent a continuous record). Note the marked reduction of electrical activity during rectal distension which persists after the stimulus has been removed (From Bouvier, M. and Gonnella, J. (1981). *Journal of Physiology* **310**, 457–69.)

independent of peristalsis. It can be induced by a weak distension stimulus that is ineffective in causing rectal contractions. The inhibition of sympathetic tone can be removed by sectioning sacral spinal roots and suppressed by atropine. These observations point to the involvement of an extrinsic reflex needing parasympathetic cholinergic nerves. It is thought that acetylcholine, delivered from parasympathetic fibres, binds to muscarinic receptors on sympathetic varicosities and prevents the release of noradrenaline, i.e. presynaptic inhibition (Fig. 6.13).

Rectal distension also relaxes the internal anal sphincter in the presence of atropine and the α- and β-receptor antagonists phentolamine and propranolol. To explain these findings non-cholinergic, non-adrenergic mechanisms have been proposed possibly involving both intrinsic and extrinsic nerve pathways. What might the neurotransmitter be? Evidence supporting a role for VIP has been gathered. For example, experiments have been conducted with strips of rabbit internal anal sphincter muscle. This *in vitro* preparation exhibited resting tone and relaxed with electrical stimulation. Electrically induced relaxation

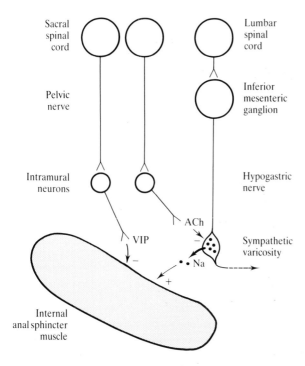

Fig. 6.13 A model for the neural control of the internal anal sphincter

was (a) blocked by TTX, indicating a neural effect, and (b) reduced by VIP antiserum in concentrations that inhibited the relaxation produced by VIP.

Thus yet another process may well be controlled by VIP. Twelve years ago, I considered setting the following examination question: 'Is there a region of the gastrointestinal tract not affected by VIP?' Perhaps the advice, that I should not do so on the grounds that a student would be entitled to answer simply 'no', was sound!

Controlled defaecation

In the simple picture presented, the presence of faeces in the rectum leads to defaecation. However, in man, the time at which defaecation occurs is dependent on environmental factors and on a complex cortical inhibition of reflexes from the rectum and anus. Except in the very young, the conscious mind controls the external anal sphincter and either allows or prevents the expulsion of faeces. If contraction of this sphincter is maintained, the defaecation reflex dies out after several minutes and does not return until more material enters the rectum. This may not take place for several hours.

In most people, defaecation is a matter of habit. Some defaecate before, some after breakfast. Others defaecate in the evening following a meal or hot drink.

Some defaecate numerous times each day while others, considered normal, accede to the urge only once in several days. The 'normal' range in the UK is usually stated to be between 3 per day and 3 per week. Man's environment has a considerable effect on his habits. Many feel ill at ease in homes not their own and refrain from defaecating. How many people in the Middle East, accustomed to squatting on the floor refuse to use the facilities in the United Kingdom?

Having decided to defaecate, a position is taken whereby the subject squats or sits so as to straighten out the angle between the rectum and the anal canal. A Valsalva manoeuvre increasing the rectal pressure, an increase in large intestinal motility (defaecation reflex) and relative inhibition of the external anal sphincter permit the passage of the faeces to the outside. Stimulation of the anal canal by the faeces maintains the inhibition of the external anal sphincter. When the rectum is empty, the external anal sphincter regains its resting activity, and the anal canal is closed.

Continence

The distal large bowel is maintained in an empty and collapsed state. Several factors contribute to this. The angulation, from which the sigmoid colon derives its name, and spiral folds (valves of Houston) exert resistance against movement of material in the distal colon. These areas provide resistance because of their narrowings. The weight of solid faeces accentuates their barrier effect.

Increases in intra-abdominal pressure while lifting weights further accentuate the angulations producing a 'flap valve' effect at the sharp bends and a 'flutter valve' (Fig. 6.14) at the collapsed slit-like anorectal region. The 'flutter valve' is, perhaps, a concept which needs some explanation. In 1965, Phillips and Edwards described it as follows:

> 'If a soft compressible tube passes through a slit in a diaphragm so that the tube walls are in gentle apposition without being squeezed, a gentle pressure within the lumen will meet with little resistance to flow. If, however, pressure is applied outside the tube (intra-abdominal as distinct from intrarectal) the pressure will tend to push the walls of the tube together into the slit, so closing the tube. The greater the pressure the firmer the closure. The walls of the slit do not compress the tube. The full force of the difference in pressure across the slit is sustained by the stiffness of the diaphragm forming the walls of the slit. In the abdomen this is synonymous with the tone of the muscle of the diaphragm and of the pelvic floor.'

Physiological mechanisms also contribute to maintain the rectum empty. Motor activity is more frequent and contractile waves are of greater amplitude in the rectum than in the sigmoid colon. The reverse gradient may provide a barrier to resist the progress of faeces from sigmoid to rectum. It may also account for the cephalad movement of material when barium-impregnated retention enemas or suppositories are introduced into the rectum.

Finally one might ask the question as to which of the anal sphincters, the internal or the external, is the most important for maintaining continency. This has been a controversial issue. The two sphincters work together. Many have pointed to the value of the internal anal sphincter which contributes the most in the resting state. In contrast, the external anal sphincter contracts only 'as much as necessary' but can constrict further when stimulated, e.g. by

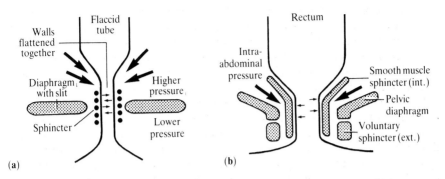

Fig. 6.14 The flutter valve. (a) The principle of the flutter valve at a slit opening. (b) The application of the flutter valve principle to the anal canal (From Phillips, S.F. and Edwards, A.W. (1965). *Gut* **6**, 396–406.)

rectal distension. The importance of the external anal sphincter is illustrated by studies with patients having gross faecal incontinence as a result of:-

1. Neurological impairment, following partial transection of the spinal cord because of tumours,
2. Myopathy, or
3. Anal sphincter injuries secondary to surgical trauma, e.g. haemorrhoidectomy.

These patients had normal internal anal sphincter reflexes but the responses of the external anal sphincter were absent. Is any question easily answered in physiology?

Bibliography

Alva, J., Mendeloff, A.I. and Schuster, M.M. (1967). Reflex and electromyographic abnormalities associated with fecal incontinence. *Gastroenterology* **53**, 101–6.

Bergman, E.N. (1990). Energy contributions of volatile fatty acids from the gastrointestinal tract in various species. *Physiological Reviews* **70**, 567–90.

Biancani, P., Walsh, J. and Behar, J. (1985). Vasoactive intestinal peptide: a neurotransmitter for relaxation of the rabbit internal anal sphincter. *Gastroenterology* **89**, 867–74.

Bouvier, M. and Gonella, J. (1985). Nervous control of the internal anal sphincter of the cat. *Journal of Physiology* **310**, 457–69.

Bridges, R.J., Rack, M., Rummel, W. and Schreiner, J. (1986). Mucosal plexus and electrolyte transport across the rat colonic mucosa. *Journal of Physiology* **376**, 531–42.

Broitman, S.A. and Glannella, R.A. (1971). Gut microbial ecology and its relationship to gastrointestinal disease. In *Absorption Phenomena*, pp265-321. Edited by J.L. Rabinowitz and RM Myerson, Topics in Medicinal Chemistry Volume 4, Wiley Interscience, New York.

Burkitt, D.P. and Graham – Stewart, C.W. (1975). Haemorrhoids – postulated pathogenesis and proposed prevention, *Postgraduate Medical Journal* 51 (559), 631-36.

Christensen, J. (1987). Motility of the colon. In *Physiology of the Gastrointestinal Tract*, 2nd edn, pp 665–93. Ed. by L.R. Johnson. Raven Press, New York.

Clauss, W., Hoffmann, B., Schäfer, H. and Hörnicke, H. (1989). Ion transport and electrophysiology in the rabbit cecum. *American Journal of Physiology* **256**, G1090–G1099.

Diener, M., Rummel, W., Mestres, P. and Lindemann, B. (1989). Single chloride channels in colon mucosa and isolated colonic enterocytes of the rat. *Journal of Membrane Biology* **108**, 21–30.

Duthie, H.L. (1982). Defaecation and the anal sphincters. *Clinics in Gastroenterology* **11**, 621–31.

Edmonds, C.J. and Willis, C.L. (1988). Potassium secretion by rat distal colon during acute potassium loading; effect of sodium, potassium intake and aldosterone. *Journal of Physiology* **401**, 39–51.

Engelhardt, W.V., Kuck, U. and Krause, M. (1986). Potassium microclimate at the mucosal surface of the proximal and the distal colon of guinea pig. *Pflgers Archiv European Journal of Physiology* **407**, 625–31.

Gill, R.C., Cote, K.R., Bowes, K.L. and Kingma, Y.J. (1986). Human colonic smooth muscle: spontaneous stretch contractile activity and response to stretch. *Gut* **27**, 1006–13.

Gonella, J., Bouvier, M. and Blanquet, F. (1987). Extrinsic nervous control of motility of small and large intestines and related sphincters. *Physiological Reviews* **67**, 902–61.

Grace, W.J., Wolf, S. and Wolff, H.G. (1951). *The human colon: in an experimental study based on direct observation of four fistulous objects.* Paul Hoeber, New York.

Grimble, G. (1989). Fibre, fermentation, flora and flatus. *Gut*, **30**, 6–13.

Grimble, G.K., Patil, D.H. and Silk, D.B.A. (1988). Assimilation of lactitol, an 'unabsorbed' disaccharide in the normal human colon. *Gut* **29**, 1666–71.

Jenkins, D.J.A., Jenkins, A.L., Wolever, T.M.S., Rao, A.V. and Thompson, L.U. (1986). Fiber and starchy foods: gut function and implications in disease. *American Journal of Gastroenterology* **81**, 920–30.

Jenkins, H.R., Fenton, T.R., McIntosh, N., Dillon, M.J. and Milla, P.J. (1990). Development of colonic sodium transport in early childhood and its regulation by aldosterone. *Gut* **31**, 194–7.

Joyce, F.S. and Rasmussen, T.N. (1989). Gas explosion during diathermy gastrotomy. *Gastroenterology* **96**, 530–531.

Kreulen, D.L. and Szurszewski, J.H. (1979). Reflex pathways in the abdominal prevertebral ganglia: evidence for a colo-colonic inhibitory reflex. *Journal of Physiology* **295**, 21–32.

Kuwahara, A. and Radowicz-Cooke, H.J. (1988). Epithelial transport in guinea-pig proximal colon: influence of enteric neurons. *Journal of Physiology* **395**, 271–84.

Mallett, A.K. and Rowland, I.R. (1990). Bacterial enzymes: their role in the formation of mutagens and carcinogens in the intestine. *Digestive Diseases* **8**, 71–9.

Read, N.W. (1988). Motility and related disorders. *Current Opinion in Gastroenterology* **4**, 43–51.

Rhodes, J.M. (1989). Colonic mucus and mucosal glycoproteins: the key to colitis and cancer. *Gut* **30**, 1660–6.

Roman, C. and Gonella, J. (1989). Extrinsic control of gastrointestinal motility. In *Physiology of the Gastrointestinal Tract*, 2nd edn, pp 507–30 Ed. by L.R. Johnson., Raven Press, New York.

Russell, D.A. and Castro, G.A. (1989). Immunological regulation of colonic ion transport. *American Journal of Physiology* **256**, G396–G403.

Sanders, K.M. and Smith, T.K. (1986). Extrinsic neural regulation of slow waves in circular muscle of the canine proximal colon. *Journal of Physiology* **377**, 297–313.

Silk, D.B.A. (1989). Fibre and enteral nutrition. *Gut* **30**, 246–64.

Simon, G.L. and Gorbach, S.L. (1987). Intestinal flora and gastrointestinal function. In *Physiology of the Gastrointestinal Tract*, 2nd edn. Roman, C and Gonella, J. (1989) Ed. by L.R. Johnson. Raven Press, New York. pp 1623–48.

Vahouny, G.V. (1987). Effects of dietary fiber on digestion and absorption. *In Physiology of the Gastrointestinal Tract*, 2nd edn, Roman, C. and Gonella, J. (1989) Ed. by L.R. Johnson., Raven Press, New York. pp 1623–48.

Wood, J.D. (1987). Physiology of the enteric nervous system. In *Physiology of the Gastrointestinal Tract*, 2nd edn, Roman, C. and Gonella, J. Ed. by L.R. Johnson., Raven Press, New York. pp 67–109.

Yajima, T. (1988). Luminal propionate-induced secretory response in the rat distal colon *in vitro*. *Journal of Physiology* **403**, 559–75.

Index